"Parents and professionals are often encouraged to support the development of the whole child but are rarely taught how to do it—until now. Dr. Scott Shannon's new book offers us a big-picture view of integration and wellness together with a treasure trove of practical tools that we can use every day to support the health and well-being of children and their families."
—Susan Kaiser Greenland, co-founder, Inner Kids;
author of *The Mindful Child*

"Dr. Scott Shannon is a physician living the truth of balance and wellness in a time when aging models of disease and disorder so often fail to truly serve our children. This book draws on his clinical experience and vast knowledge base to provide excellent advice on what works, while expressing an immense kindness for children and their families."
—Howard Glasser, creator, Nurtured Heart Approach; chairman of the board and founder, Children's Success Foundation

"This book offers just what the title promises—a brilliant guide to health and wholeness for children. Dr. Scott Shannon has long been a pioneer in bringing genuine holism back to psychiatry. In *Mental Health for the Whole Child*, he distills years of study, clinical experience, and hard-fought wisdom to provide a practical, positive, and effective tool for families and clinicians who care, as he does, about our beautiful, hurting, incredibly resilient children."
—Henry Emmons, MD, creator, Resilience Training Program;
author of *The Chemistry of Joy* and *The Chemistry of Calm*

"A handy and insightful resource for all trainees, practitioners, parents, educators, and advocates, this book presents a valuable model of comprehensive mental healthcare. Describing a whole, integrative method of practice, Dr. Shannon reminds us of the many aspects of healing. Reading it has changed the way I practice."
—Robert L. Hendren, DO, professor and director, Child and Adolescent Psychiatry at the University of California, San Francisco; past-president, American Academy of Child and Adolescent Psychiatry

"An accessible guide to the 'whole child' approach from a 'whole therapist' who is not only knowledgeable about a broad spectrum of treatments, but also skilled in remaining centered, attentive, and clear. Dr. Shannon's 30 years of clinical experience give him a unique perspective on both the relevance and the limitations of scientific research, and a sensible, systematic approach to diagnosis and treatment that extends the benefits of integrative mental health into the realm of pediatric psychiatry. He eloquently builds a solid foundation for an emerging field: integrative pediatric mental health care."
—Patricia L. Gerbarg, MD, co-author of *Non-Drug Treatments for ADHD, How to Use Herbs, Nutrients, & Yoga in Mental Health*, and *The Healing Power of the Breath*

"Dr. Shannon's fine book is a valuable contribution to the emerging field of integrative mental health care. Pediatricians, psychiatrists, and psychologists will find valuable insights into mental health, along with an up-to-date review of holistic approaches to preventing and treating mental health problems in children and adolescents."
—James Lake, MD, author of *Textbook of Integrative Mental Health Care* and *Integrative Mental Health Care: A Therapist's Handbook*

"With pharmaceutical prescriptions at an all-time high for our children, this refreshing resource provides a guide to self-healing mechanisms that can reduce the role of chemicals in treating them. I have tremendous respect for Dr. Shannon's expertise in this area and his ability to combine science with common sense to promote healthy outcomes. I highly recommend this book for clinicians and parents wishing to stack the deck in favor of a child's whole health."
—David Rakel, MD, director, University of Wisconsin Integrative Medicine program; associate professor of Family Medicine, University of Wisconsin School of Medicine and Public Health

MENTAL HEALTH
for the
WHOLE CHILD

Moving Young Clients
from Disease & Disorder
to Balance & Wellness

SCOTT M. SHANNON, MD
with
NOAH GALLAGHER SHANNON

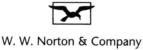

W. W. Norton & Company
New York • London

For information about permission to reproduce selections from this book,
write to Permissions, W. W. Norton & Company, Inc., 500 Fifth Avenue,
New York, NY 10110

For information about special discounts for bulk purchases,
please contact W. W. Norton
Special Sales at specialsales@wwnorton.com or 800-233-4830

Manufacturing by Courier-Westford
Book design by Bytheway Publishing Services
Production manager: Leeann Graham

Library of Congress Cataloging-in-Publication Data

Shannon, Scott M.
  Mental health for the whole child : moving young clients from disease &
disorder to balance & wellness / Scott M. Shannon, M.D. with Noah Gallagher
Shannon. — First edition.
      pages cm.
  "A Norton Professional Book"—
  Includes bibliographical references and index.
  ISBN 978-0-393-70797-7 (hardcover)
  1. Problem youth—Counseling of.   2. Adolescent psychotherapy.
  3. Youth—Mental health.   4. Mental illness—Alternative medicine.
  I. Shannon, Noah Gallagher. II. Title.
  RJ506.P63S49 2013
  616.89'140835—dc23
                              2013006168

ISBN: 978-0-393-70797-7

W. W. Norton & Company, Inc., 500 Fifth Avenue, New York, N.Y. 10110
www.wwnorton.com
W. W. Norton & Company Ltd., Castle House, 75/76 Wells Street,
London W1T 3QT

1 2 3 4 5 6 7 8 9 0

For Suze and Sarah, of course

CONTENTS

ACKNOWLEDGMENTS

This book grows from the web of support and community that sustains me and makes my work possible.

My deep appreciation goes to the staff and professionals at the Wholeness Center in Fort Collins, Colorado, who share my passionate vision for creating a loving and practical model of what integrative mental health can be. Thank you for your dedication, your wisdom, and your endless support.

All of the ideas contained in this work flow seamlessly from my mentors and teachers. Thanks especially to Andrew Weil, MD, who took me under his wing when I was a rough-hewn twenty-something brimming with passion and ideas. My other teachers are too numerous to enumerate, but Harvey Gurian, Gladys McGarey, Bob Anderson, and C. G. Jung stand out.

I would like to thank Andrea Dawson and her team for their belief in my work and her enlightened efforts to make this book better. Gail Ross of Ross Yoon has been my superstar agent for over a decade and has been a profound catalyst for sharing my ideas with the world at large.

Integrative mental health has been a small world for many years. Although it is now rapidly expanding, the early years felt very isolated and intimate. I would like to thank all of my peers who have inspired and encouraged me over the years. The Colorado group in particular—Larry Cormier, Janet Settle, Mic Braud, and Will Van DerVeer—has been a source of strength and support for over a decade. My national colleagues have also been crucial to my development: James Lake, Kathi Kemper, Larry Rosen, Tim Culbert, Sandy Newmark, and many others are beacons of wisdom as we try to give voice to a new vision.

I would like to share my appreciation for all of my colleagues at the American Academy of Child and Adolescent Psychiatry. Old friends like

Steve Adelsheim, Bob Hendren, and Charles Popper have joined with new friends like Wayne Batzer and Jenna Saul to create change in our profession. I would also like to reach out and thank the countless professionals who are following their hearts, looking for new ways to help and be of service. I would also like to thank Marianne Wamboldt and all of the folks at the University of Colorado who believed in me and asked me to teach their residents.

The American Board of Integrative Holistic Medicine is my tribe, my professional family. Their bottomless love and connection have made my last decade of work so much more vibrant. Healers like Lee Lipsenthal, Rob Ivker, Nan Sudak, Patrick Hanaway, Mimi Guarneri, Dave Rakel, Wendy Warner, and the rest of the board have given so much to me in terms of love and instruction. They inspire me to make myself a more complete healer. I am forever in their debt.

But, as you know, it all comes down to family. As the very core of who I am and who I can be, my family fills me every day. My parents, Howard and Pat, gave me the best foundation possible and they remain inspirations for what health and vitality can be well into their eighties. My daughter, Sarah, carries my heart forward in the health care profession as a wise, sensitive, and compassionate young woman. My wife of thirty-some years, Suze, taught me how to love and teaches me every day how to be more open and loving.

This book owes its greatest debt, however, to my son, Noah. He co-wrote it, edited it, shared my vision, and helped me give voice to my experience. Luckily, he is much smarter than I am and has a profound gift for both language and organization. He challenged me to make this a better book every step of the way. He tolerated my extensive elaborations on the profound, which often came at the dire expense of the relevant. If this book reaches you on a deep level it is because of him. I dedicate this effort to my son. Thank you, Noah.

INTRODUCTION
TWO TALES

Although my life at times has been driven forward by ideas, more often it has pivoted on unexpected personal encounters. My experience with Henry is one of those defining events.

In 1989, behind the wheel of a large U-Haul truck, I drove across the country from New York to Albuquerque, New Mexico. I was fresh from a psychiatric residency at a Columbia University–affiliated hospital in New York, a landscape formal, traditional, and conservative in almost every respect. Standing in stark relief, the child psychiatry program at the University of New Mexico, where I had just accepted a fellowship offer, enchanted me with the lure of multicultural orientation. It promised an approach to medicine and psychiatric care that drew from the traditional healing models of neighboring First Nation peoples, respected the consent of various belief systems, and even offered exposure to Jungian analysis.

Albuquerque, wide-open, bright, and dry with the omnipresent waft of roasted chili, offered wild separation from the looming forest, hazy days, and meandering streams of upstate New York. My family's new home, made of thick, rammed adobe, was lined with a threadbare ocotillo fence and sat near the wide bed of the Rio Grande River. At the hospital, many of my attending physicians sported Navajo bolo ties—a rare, if not outrageous, sight in the East. And to put me at a further remove, frenzied notes of Spanish and other native tongues buzzed through the perimeters of the building as I moved between assignments. My patients were mostly First Nation or Hispanic (or both), populations and cultures I was little exposed to in my training, and almost all of the families were poor and chronically unemployed.

As a child psychiatry fellow I was assigned to the Children's Psychiatric Hospital (CPH), where I would work for the next 8 months. The CPH campus was located on spacious grounds north of the main campus and was divided into eight separate "cottages" housing the kids. These cottages were named after outlying New Mexico counties and broken down by age group. CPH functioned as the state's de facto mental health crisis intervention center; kids with the most severe cases of psychiatric and behavioral issues usually ended up at CPH for in-depth assessment and treatment. They came from every corner of the state and were fully funded in their stay. New Mexico has always been desperately poor and very rural, but over the last few decades the state has quietly become a leader in mental health programming for the underserved.

Children between the ages of 6 and 8 ended up at Cibola Cottage, and so did I. My attending physician, Dan Kerlinsky, a recent graduate and open-minded iconoclast, had one principal message for me as he walked me in the door for my first day: Give kids time, a sense of safety, and consistent affection. The vast majority of the kids at CPH ended up there because of a history of unspeakable abuse and neglect. Most suffered from trauma and posttraumatic stress similar to the worst of Vietnam War veterans—but unlike those sufferers, these kids' developing brains had no real understanding of the war to which they had been ruthlessly subjected.

Soon after this curt introduction, as one of the first-year fellows, I was assigned to Henry. Like most of the kids at CPH, Henry's early life was painful and marred by difficulty and tension. His First Nation mother, herself a victim of years of sexual abuse, lived life on the streets of Albuquerque as a prostitute and a severe alcoholic with a penchant for violence. In Henry's first 18 months of life, there were numerous visits from social services and reports of neglect and abuse, but no concrete action taken against the mother. The camel's back finally gave out one day when she passed out drunk at a local bar and the owner called social services once more. After this, the agency collected Henry and, as procedure mandated, placed him with one of his mom's distant relatives. But there was no reprieve for young Henry. Over the next 5 years, Henry continued to experience abuse and neglect, and this time the abuse turned sexual at the hands of his new family. Nearing the end of his stay with them, Henry became increasingly violent and aggressive.

After a series of violent incidents, social services took custody once more and this time moved Henry into state foster care for the next 2 years. His behavior continued to deteriorate with manic outbursts and unmanageable behavior. He became wild, explosive, and brutally violent. He blew out of one foster home after another. Countless hours of therapy with psychiatrists and counselors as well as a laundry list of neuroleptics and other powerful medications could not temper his rage. Henry found his way to Cibola Cottage unimproved and unmanageable.

Prior to his arrival, Henry, like most of the kids at CPH, had accumulated a litany of psychiatric labels—pediatric bipolar disorder, posttraumatic stress disorder, reactive attachment disorder, attention-deficit/hyperactivity disorder, oppositional defiant disorder, and disruptive disorder. Luckily for both Henry and me, this was a different era of psychiatric care, in a state with progressive mental health policy. I was not expected to medicate his symptoms aggressively and discharge him within a week or 10 days. In fact, at CPH the average length of stay was measured in months, not days. The administration was committed to providing kids the intimate care and attention their growing brains deserved, without much of a thought to per-diem cost and length of stay. So Henry and I had time to get to know one another, to build a relationship. And in light of this, the plan was simple: discontinue his medications and assess his baseline.

Thin, sullen, and dark skinned, Henry avoided all eye contact. He had been nonverbal at the hospital for weeks, with both the other kids and the warm staff. I was nervous. What would our sessions be like together? How would I manage his aggressiveness, which had already grown legendary in the cottage? Would he accept or reject me? The freedom, creativity, and magic of working with children had drawn me in as an adult resident, where the work felt too structured and formal—and not always responsive. Yet at this moment the lack of structure felt intimidating. Would I have the ability to move from the insightful and wise to the warm and accepting, like my mentors in New York so deftly could? Could I set the firmest of limits without provoking anger and resentment? This was a massive first step on my path to becoming a child psychiatrist, and not only did I feel insecure, but there was also a vague premonition of something out of reach, something beyond comprehension.

Henry came willingly into my small nondescript office on our first day and sat in the chair near the door. He did not look at me. I told him this session was his time and we could cover or do whatever he would like. He gave no response, his body motionless in the small chair. I asked him about what he liked to do for fun. No response. I tried every angle I thought might reach him—nothing. His intensity was palpable, with the coiled potential of a cornered animal. I felt uncomfortable. I could not reach him. I finished the session after a clockless hour of desolate conversation. Completely exhausted, I went home defeated. As I reflected on the session, I couldn't shake his isolation. There was no eye contact, no facial expressions—no real acknowledgment of my presence at all. He was remote, secluded in his suffering.

The next four sessions went the same way. At that point I began to think I had failed as a child psychiatrist. I started to doubt my career choice and skills—Henry felt not only remote but unreachable. I was powerless to affect him. Perhaps he was so damaged and traumatized that nothing would work. Maybe we should heavily medicate his aggression and recommend him to one of the long-term care facilities for a life of institutionalized care. Maybe he needed a smarter or more caring doctor.

The cottage staff was starting to ask questions about his treatment. Henry was almost 1 month into his stay at CPH but remained extremely violent and had not spoken a word to anyone. The team's support of my treatment was beginning to flag. My supervisor, Dr. Kerlinsky, however, remained supportive and encouraging: "Just create a safe and accepting holding environment for him, Scott. And don't doubt yourself." But I did. Restless before his next session, I sat up in bed through the night trying to make sense of my training and my experiences thus far with Henry. His mind and past were locked away. And nothing in my education gave me the hint of a key.

One day, I led Henry into my small office, now getting warm by the bright New Mexico afternoon sun. We sat together in silence for a moment, Henry looking away with his affectless stare. At the end of my rope, I needed to try something completely different. I knew initiating speech would be the first and most important step in working through his trauma and unlocking his pain, but direct verbal contact had little effect on him. It seemed, for Henry, language no longer held any purpose. After what he had been through, it was like language no longer could accomplish what he needed. So instead of attempting direct verbal contact, I wanted to see if he cared to communicate in another, more indirect way.

I laid a brush, a palate of watercolors, and a canvas in front of both of us. Wordlessly, I began to paint. I painted without looking over at Henry, trying to make him feel comfortable and unencumbered. After some time, he picked up a brush and began to paint. This simple act started one of the most pivotal experiences of my professional life. Over the next hour Henry painted nonstop, never looking over at me.

Stark, bold, and outlined with dexterous precision, a black and tan horse took shape on the paper. The pure, fluid beauty of this image floored me. Henry painted with intensity—but very slowly. Fully absorbed in the moment, he paid fastidious care to each shape and texture, often tilting his head to get a sense of different perspectives. At the end of our session, he laid his brush down and scanned the paper with furrowed brow and without a word turned and walked out. Even if no words were spoken, I had made contact. Art, it seemed, offered him dimensions of expression language could not. I couldn't wait for our next session.

The next time, Henry stepped into my office as though nothing had changed. We sat down together in front of the watercolors and Henry jumped right in—still completely silent. With the same slow rigor, he began to paint a herd of running horses. Still staring straight ahead, fixed on the paper, he suddenly announced, "This is the story of Runner, the horse." It was my turn for silence. After so many hours with Henry, his small, delicate words seemed strange and out of place. But over the next hour, I grew to know his voice. He told the story of Runner, while I transcribed word for word and carefully watched his thought process and turns of expression. It was as if he was slowly coming out of a long, stiff sleep—his language and gestures at first muted and rigid but over time softening and evolving in complexity.

After that session Henry began to use a few words in the cottage. The aggression also toned down over the next few weeks. After 10 more weeks Henry was fully verbal, cooperating with staff and other kids. His aggressive outbursts continued to fade over time. He was never prescribed any medications during his stay.

Over the course of our time together Henry told the story of Runner the horse in a series of 17 spirited watercolors dominated by warm tones of gold, brown, and red. Initially separated from his herd, Runner endured a series of challenges that included desert storms, lightning, an erupting volcano, and even an airplane crash. Somehow Runner survived all of these travails and in time regained his herd. Each of Henry's successive narrative installments came in more forceful laconic language. For someone who had studied Jungian psychology for years, I was captivated, almost intoxicated, by the vivid narrative material gushing from Henry's unconscious. Runner's story unfolded as a classic hero's quest— a timeless tale of trial and redemption: life, death, and renewal.

After 4 months in the hospital, Henry's behavior had transformed from violent and speechless to cooperative and verbal. Henry could still be irritable or oppositional at times, but my team felt that he could be managed outside the hospital. His story was transcribed; his images preserved. And in the end, he left the hospital with a book that made his imaginary journey concrete, real—an expression of his own transformation.

For Henry, the fairy tale ending was not to be. There would be no perfect family waiting to adopt him and love him. He was discharged on no medications into a group home. I followed him as his psychiatrist over the next year and a half. After I left New Mexico I maintained an avuncular relationship with him, trading cards, letters, and occasional visits, even teaching him how to drive a car on one of his visits with my family in Colorado.

Given his deep history of horrific abuse, vulnerable genetics, frank neglect, and attachment trauma, Henry should be a shell of a man. Yet somehow he continues to rise above all of that to find joy and success in life. Now some 20 years later, he is a celebrated artist working in silver. Happily married with two lovely daughters, Henry lives a solid middle-class American life. He keeps a passionate interest in playing basketball, working on his art, and, most of all, his family. He has no substance abuse, depression, or sequelae of his brutal introduction to this world.

Henry left me with more questions than I could answer. I couldn't fit him into any of the psychiatric models I was learning at the time. He challenged the very essence of what I was learning in psychopharmacology, psychodynamics, and attachment theory. Beyond that, his recovery occurred by a process without a clear mechanism. Was it simply my caring attention to him over time that helped him to heal? What role did his artwork play? What does his archetypal journey, as described by Jung and elaborated by Joseph Campbell, mean? And how can I apply these lessons to other kids? Did the narration of his imaginative story alter his neurochemistry or did he just "grow out of it"?

Even now I struggle with these questions. The conventional framework of psychiatric assessment and treatment doesn't provide a means through which to understand Henry's recovery or apply its lessons. The best advice from psychiatry might be to celebrate Henry's return to health and happiness, write his recovery off as an anomaly—and move on. This kind of limited perspective, unfortunately, was consistent with what I expected.

I entered psychiatry as a bit of a skeptic, willing to be convinced but weary of the conventional wisdom. Much of the reason for this is that prior to entering medical school my first interface with medicine came through the study of holistic health care models and alternative medicine. As part of my undergraduate honors thesis on theories of consciousness at the University of Arizona, the department of psychology sent me to meet with a possible advisor, an "odd doctor" who lived far out in the desert near the saguaro-lined rim of the Catalina Mountains.

On our first visit, Dr. Andrew Weil implored me to do away with many of my preconceptions about the brain and instead embrace new, bold thinking and a skeptical attitude. His mentorship turned into a backroom tutelage. Over the next few months, we sat together in his adobe portico each Monday until the desert sun receded over the mountains. In that time we shared ideas and research about health, consciousness, and human happiness. He helped me to think about the mind and brain on a broader scale, understanding and incorporating many seemingly divergent disciplines in order to unravel one central problem: how health and illness are expressed in the brain.

Dr. Weil became a close friend who over the course of my medical and psychiatric training continually reminded me to challenge the accepted paradigms and trust my physician's intuition. And so I learned as I went, always asking questions and testing alternative hypotheses. My encounter with Henry, many years later, further enforced my intuition that psychiatry needed a more broad and hopeful paradigm to understand the human psyche and its health. It needed a model to understand kids like Henry—and kids like Caley.

Caley, unlike Henry, was born to a functional nuclear family. Her early development was typical and without exception. Caley was an eager learner who did well in school and played with friends in her quiet suburban neighborhood outside of Denver, Colorado. Jeremy, her father, traveled for work and was gone a few weeks a month but doted on Caley and her older sister when he was around. Courtney, her mother, had previously been diagnosed with bipolar disorder but had been stable on the same two medications for many years.

All was good in Caley's home until just after her seventh birthday when she began to rage and scream, seemingly without provocation. She would throw tantrums that lasted for hours. The appearance of visual and auditory hallucinations finally drove her parents to seek help. Caley spent 16 days in a local psychiatric hospital and left on two psychiatric medications. One year later, she had been tried on five other medications with no sign of benefit. The psychiatric symptoms grew more consistent and severe as time dragged on, debilitating her school performance and social connections. In response, she began to dialogue mainly with an imaginary friend and became extremely fearful of any contact outside her family.

By the time she got to the University of Colorado psychiatric clinic at Children's Hospital, Denver, where I was assistant clinical professor of psychiatry, things had continued to break down for young Caley. She lived in a fearful, chaotic world of hallucinations and social ostracism. In-depth psychological testing identified core psychotic processes characterized by disorganized rage, delusions, and stark immaturity. She had lost significant ground in every sphere of her development. She looked much younger than her 9 years. Eight different psychiatric medications in aggressive dosage failed her, and her parents were desperate. On our first visit, her mom handed me a disc containing her complete medical records including the battery of psychological tests. Even in the digital age, this was a rare gift. I pored through her records right away. I knew this story needed elaboration and careful scrutiny.

When we met, Caley had to be dragged into my office. A brief glimpse of a round cherubic face and a short, cropped haircut was all I caught before she crawled under my desk and hid herself. For the rest of the session she kept out of sight behind furniture and the basket of stuffed animals I kept in the corner. Her folks told me that she was often cheerful, but only if she could stay in her own world undisturbed by others. After Caley had relaxed a bit I asked her about her world and what she did and saw. She told me about seeing corpses and strange animals. The more she told me, the more she appeared to become alarmed and frightened by her own words. She quickly went silent and retreated back behind the desk.

Joining us with the family was a child psychiatry fellow, Mike, whom I was mentoring in the clinic. CPH was unique in that we provided integrative child psychiatry, offering options that included nutritional and natural supplement-based treatments. Mike chose this fellowship elective because he was curious and eager to learn about more progressive tools. And, like me so many years before, he was growing tired of conventional psychiatry's failings. The parents, however, had no vested interest in my approach or me. I just happened to be a child psychiatrist with an open appointment.

After the first visit, Mike and I reviewed Caley's records together, paying close attention to the medication trials and testing. The current diagnosis was pediatric bipolar disorder with psychotic features. The medication trials of Abilify, Seroquel, Risperdal, Geodon, lithium, Depakote, and Tegretol were aggressive, extended, and well documented. The response had been negligible. Mike and I agreed the first step was to taper her off her current medication in order to document her baseline. We did—and nothing changed over the next 6 weeks. The conventional treatments not only had failed her but seemed to have no marked effect on her whatsoever—beyond significant weight gain. Her psychotic features remained intact, and she was as fearful as ever. Since she showed no benefit from medications, Mike and I considered alternative options.

On Caley's next visit, we told her parents that we would like to initiate treatment with a vitamin- and mineral-based supplement called EMPowerplus (see glossary and Chapter 13). They looked at us as if we were mad. Their little girl was very sick; clearly she needed powerful medicine, not a vitamin. Caley's grandmother, who also attended this visit because she had provided some respite care in the last few years, finally spoke up. "All of those medications failed Caley," she said. "Let's try this. It might work." The parents were hesitant, but agreed to give informed consent. I reviewed the studies for the supplement and let the parents know what the remaining conventional options were (a few off-label medications). The parents were concerned about potential side effects from the supplement. They had lived through too much already. For the family, new medicine always meant new unpredictable, strange side effects, and a little less of their old Caley. I told them that we occasionally see mild upset stomach or loose stools at first but that generally as treatment goes on those things go away. After years of sedation, motor abnormalities, insomnia, lethargy, headaches, weight gain, and nonresponse, hearing about these relatively innocuous side effects turned the corner for Caley's folks. "Okay. Let's try it," her father said as her mother nodded slowly in agreement.

Frankly, I wasn't expecting much. I had used the supplement to good effect in kids with bipolar disorder before, but Caley seemed different, more severe—almost unreachable. Caley walked into our next visit under her own power, standing tall, and with a bright smile blurted, "I don't see things anymore. My voices are gone." Her father quickly corroborated: "She is clearly better. This is the first treatment that has helped. Caley has not been aggressive with us—at all."

Three weeks later, the improvements not only continued, they grew. Her mother told us that she could pay attention in school again and, better yet, she was making friends again. Over the next 3 months she lost 20 pounds, made more friends, and stopped talking to her imaginary friend. For the first time in years she slept through the night in her own bed. During our next few visits, Mike and I could have a genuine discussion with her, talking about her favorite subjects in school and her new friends. Caley remained somewhat immature and silly, however (a reasonable outcome given the years "lost" to her illness). But she also seemed to no longer fear adults or new, more mature situations. To Mike and me she was a different girl altogether. To her family she was simply back. The crowning moment came when her dad beamed and said, "Caley has been named the most improved student at her school this month."

Once skeptical, her parents were now convinced that the natural supplement had worked a miracle. This was further confirmed by the fact that if she missed two or three doses the old Caley would briefly return, but only until dosage began again. Because we were in a teaching clinic within a university department, Mike and I decided to more completely document this case for review and consideration. At 6 months, we had a psychologist completely redo her battery of tests. The results were again startling: significant improvement in all areas of functioning, resolution of psychotic features, and a substantial improvement (5 to 20 points) in IQ testing—unheard of in the literature. Our department chair decided we should present this case at a national psychiatry meeting. The proposal, unfortunately, was routinely turned down as "anecdotal" or "anomalous."

Difficult Questions

There are important lessons to learn from Caley, Henry, and other "anomalies." Yes, one might with good cause deem them anecdotal. They are, after all, somewhat unexpected, unexplained success stories. But labeling their cases as such does nothing to help us parse, understand, and learn from their healing process. The very soul of science is to ask seemingly impertinent questions about oddities, peculiarities, and inconsistencies so that we may arrive at a new earned perspective. So perhaps the more respectful and wise choice would be to shrug off labels and instead ask, How can we understand and learn from such unexpected cases of success? And what can we apply from such cases to failed or failing ones? Henry and Caley are not easily accounted for by the literature or by our standard models of assessment and care. But we must begin with trying cases and tough questions to learn anything.

However dubious the results of cases such as Henry and Caley first appear, they are not random events. It's not totally accurate to label these cases as anomalies, because it implies that the conventional treatments are, on average, safe and consistently efficacious, which the mounting evidence base roundly disproves. Conversely, at the time of Caley's treatment seven studies of this natural supplement, EMPowerplus, in the psychiatric literature strongly supported its efficacy (there are now 20). Charles Popper, MD, professor of child psychiatry at Harvard's McLean Hospital and founding editor of the *Journal of Child and Adolescent Psychopharmacology*, reported similar results over a decade ago (Popper, 2001).

But it's also true that these data are a lot to digest, perhaps too much yet for the profession. They go against much of the conventional wisdom of the chemical imbalance hypothesis and the societal belief that psychopharmacological interventions mark the psychiatric revolution. If nothing else, when you witness such a complete and total transformation in a young girl with a very serious, chronic, and well-documented psychiatric illness after several failed years of aggressive medication management, it certainly gives you pause.

We must begin to grapple with and examine these seemingly anomalous cases—and we all have them—for what they are: lessons about mental illness's individuality, adaptability, and mercurial nature. So as I reflect on Henry and Caley, and if I'm to learn anything, I have to begin by asking some basic questions. Did Henry cure himself or did I play some role? Was Caley ill or just deficient in some necessary enzyme co-factor for her brain, such as magnesium?

If I dilate these questions even further, and try to apply them to psychiatry as a whole, a few more poignant questions come up. Are we medicating too many kids like Henry, instead of meeting their intimate emotional needs? And are we simply missing the metabolic needs of many kids like Caley?

The more difficult questions, however, arise after some thought about our current model of assessment and care. Does the profession of psychiatry have a theoretical model that can account for both of these cases? Is there any formal consideration for the healing power of the mind? Can the neurotransmitter model of modern psychiatry account for nutritional and environmental issues? If children can be so transformed as Henry and Caley were, are we doing some harm by continuing to aggressively medicate them? Might these drugs actually impair the innate power of the psyche to heal in certain kids? Clearly, psychiatric medications do help people. The testing, however, is too limited in children. And we don't have a reasonable model that can separate those who benefit from those who don't—it's still hopelessly, and dangerously, trial and error. That being said, should we save medications for those cases that do not respond to other treatments instead of using them as the first line of defense as we do now?

My Path

Over the last 20-some years, questions like these have rattled around in my head as I worked with kids like Henry and Caley, and kids very unlike Henry and Caley. My first job as a psychiatrist involved setting up an adolescent inpatient psychiatry and day treatment program at a rural hospital. After a few years, I became medical director of both the hospital and the substance abuse program. I spent the morning doing crisis intervention and inpatient work, and the afternoons seeing children in my private practice. After 7 years working in this setting, I felt the urge to move to a practice less crisis driven and more fully integrative in care.

My opportunity came when the CEO at a neighboring hospital heard of my work, took a personal interest in holistic medicine, and invited me to start a hospital-based care center for holistic medicine. At this new center, I began to focus all my practice in integrative psychiatry, researching and utilizing safe, effective treatments. At the same time, I also helped organize integrative services for the hospital and its cancer center. As the setup process calmed, my work at the center eventually moved to half time. I wanted to direct more attention to my new job as medical director for three residential treatment centers for children, teens, and young adults spread across Colorado's Front Range. At these centers I incorporated and improved on many of the lessons I had learned about integrative medicine and medication management at the first few hospitals. We got kids healthier faster and discharged them into more stable family environments by employing tools such as diet, supplements, yoga, movement, acupuncture, and excessive hugging. And in the last two years I've had the opportunity to lead the development of an integrative mental health clinic in Fort Collins, Colorado. The Wholeness Center is now the largest and most comprehensive integrative mental health clinic in the United States.

My work is driven by questions like those asked above. In certain settings with certain kids, I've been able to answer many of them. And it is rewarding, fulfilling progress toward a better psychiatry. But in certain settings with certain kids, I've also been humbled and have had to go back to the drawing board. During my career, I have struggled to develop a philosophy consistent with the findings of modern science; a model that reasonably accounts for variability of response; and a standard of care consistent with the lessons of adaptability and individuality learned from cases like Caley and Henry.

This book represents my philosophical and practical findings. My vision does not invalidate modern psychiatry; rather, it makes room for it as one part of a more broad and comprehensive perspective for assessing and treating mental illness in kids. This philosophy is mental health for the whole child.

Wholeness: A New Perspective for Mental Health

Health is a comprehensive phenomenon, a celebration of all parts of the intact person working together. Since our bodies directly react and interface with the environment, this series of external interactions is also a crucial part of the working definition of health.

If we take this working definition of wholeness and apply it to children's mental health, we begin to understand that all parts of children's bodies, as well as the myriad interactions they have with their environment, influence their mental health. All these factors coalesce as a kind of web of interactions and influences, every strand playing a part in the consolidation or loss of mental health.

This is not a new idea. In fact, the more we study the complexity of the child—and health and mental health in general—the more we come to realize that these are systemic problems. They cannot be understood in isolation or as distinct from each other. Psychiatry needs to widen its view of illness in order to understand and treat complex, little-understood maladies. The problem psychiatry has run into so far is that if you underrepresent the complexity of a problem, inevitably, you will arrive at an unrepresentative solution.

So as we begin to take a wider, more whole look at mental health, factors like school, nutritional health, and home life all influence and form critical links in the child's web of health and mental health. Their mutual harmony and balance, in turn, build the child's foundation for health and happiness. For example, stabilizing Henry's rage was only possible once he became more expressive. These two problems—rage and not talking—had to be considered as connected before they both could be resolved. Thus proper appreciation of this web of factors and its dynamic interactions paves the way for a new understanding of mental health care.

A good model for understanding whole-child mental health already exists in science: ecology. Ecological science studies and describes the connections linking and influencing all organisms. According to ecology, the various interconnected and interdependent interactions of nature and its constituents lie at the heart of the "web of life." Ecology is derived from the Greek *oikos*, meaning "household," reinforcing the connection between the stability of life, its many relationships, and the environment in which it lives. Ecology, in this way, is contextual thinking. In ecology, what we might think of as distinct—an individual child, tree, or cell—is really just a pattern at one level of a larger system of interaction. Every being and thing, in this sense, is a dynamic part of an open system of interplay—continually influencing and being influenced.

Thus, by applying ecology to mental health as a metaphor, we dilate the perspective of psychiatry to include the myriad interactions of the child at the cellular level of the brain and metabolic system as well as at the environmental level of school, home, and society. Really, this metaphor honors what we observe in children's mental health—the symbiotic roles of relationship, environment, nutrition, and other external factors.

Consequently, through the metaphor of ecology, the solitary influence of biochemistry is de-emphasized and instead the power of relationship between the various parts of the body, the mind, and its environment is re-emphasized. This idea also builds on the many insights of neural plasticity and epigenetics, sciences that demonstrate the many ways in which the human brain and heredity continually react and respond to the environment. Similar in character, ecological science downplays the internal features of any discrete creature and instead tries to identify and highlight the crucial strands in the creature's web of external influences morphing and affecting its life.

Obviously, in looking at a child's mental health we have to acknowledge the importance of some internal factors such as basic temperament, genetic predisposition, and specific gifts. But the ecological framework allows us to probe these factors a little more and see the role of external factors in their expression. Thus, in this view, the internal features of the child are a rough scaffolding given form and texture by external interplay.

If we apply this understanding to the case of Henry, one explanation for his troubles is that he simply carried a unique inner quality that took advantage of a cathartic artistic expression in order to help him heal. And maybe Caley just possessed a specific metabolic inefficiency that, when corrected, freed her to health and happiness. Effectively, these kids reflect the powerful reactions possible between internal and external factors, and how, if properly catalyzed by the physician, they can create change and healing. They also demonstrate how balance between the many factors contributes to health and happiness.

Once we embrace this understanding of external and internal factors, it's possible to move on and examine each strand of influence and look at how imbalance in any of these strands can potentially contribute to illness and disorder. Caley's story, for example, shows how metabolic distress can be manifested as mania and how, when that imbalance is corrected, the whole system can be effectively returned to balance and happiness. In this sense, true prevention is possible by promoting balance in all the spheres of the child's life. Assuredly, this is a complex task, as the child's brain and environment is a complex web of interactions and interdependence—but they deserve the effort.

From here, a pithy but workable definition of whole-child mental health care becomes possible: the ecologically sound care of the whole child. By giving due value to the vast ecosystem that each child is immersed in, this new model is able to embrace the influences of factors such as media exposure, parenting style, attachment, genetics, nutrition, toxins, and relationships. For this reason, it is also prepared to draw from the lessons of neural plasticity and epigenetics and truly honor the adaptability of the child. Each kid has a proven ability to change his or her own brain and to sidestep or express various genetic predeterminations. Acknowledging and working within this model, then, also improves preventative care. If each kid is a responsive, adaptive being within a web of influences, promoting balance and wellness in the web will ensure healthy development and growth.

A number of implications grow from this new perspective.

First, one can understand the child's mental health only through the appreciation of the whole child and his or her diverse web. Thus, an extremely comprehensive assessment becomes essential. A superficial workup of current symptoms paints an unrealistically narrow and an unnecessarily pessimistic view.

Second, the acknowledgment of these outside influences creates a model of prevention through the appreciation of triggers and cofactors. Debilitating factors such as inactivity, obesity, isolation, poor diet, and the like can all trigger a cascade of effects, one of those perhaps critically detrimental to mental or emotional health. As ecology teaches us, it is also clear that none of these factors operates or exists in isolation— one cofactor may have to be remedied to cure another ailing one. Supporting factors such as exercise, good sleep, and social support, then, offer some hope for prevention and the maintenance of health and happiness for our kids.

Third, our palette of available treatments expands massively with this understanding. Supplements, diet change, social skills, and cognitive exercises all get a seat at the table, as they can dramatically influence any of the web's strands. Diet and nutrition thus move out of the shadow of allopathic medicine and onto center stage as powerful tools to influence change in the body.

Fourth, a system built on health and wholeness transforms the pessimism of pathology-based psychiatry into a model based on an optimistic psychology of health. This potential is not generally appreciated today, either by medicine or its patients. That's because medicine and psychiatry today are predominantly allopathic. This widely used term, which in the original Greek means "other than the disease," was first coined by Samuel Hahneman, founder of homeopathy, to describe the tendency to treat only the superficial symptoms of disease. But it's no secret that our medical paradigm is disease centered rather than health centered. In fact, the task of our profession has largely become waging war on disease. We see examples of this everywhere we look in our health care system.

In the same way, psychiatric practice now relies almost solely on identifying pathology and prescribing a corresponding pharmaceutical treatment. And most often, this process occurs without any consideration of what health really means to the patient or what other treatment tools could potentially be used in that pursuit. In point of fact, doctors rarely look beyond the prescription pad. And as the psychologist Abraham Maslow once said, "When all you have is a hammer, everything looks like a nail." It seems, then, that every patient in a psychiatric office is on a pathway to some psychiatric illness. This drive to pathologize will only amplify further with the dimensional alterations of *DSM-V* when it is introduced in 2013 (Frances, 2011; Frances 2012b). Health care has lost sight of the fundamental nature of human health, especially as it relates to mental health.

This is an important point for medicine and particularly psychiatry, because the dominant scientific paradigm informs our values, our treatments, and, most crucially, how we think about ourselves. Thus our health care, in its unswerving quest to label the disease as the enemy and wage war on its symptoms, undermines the preventative values of healthy living, the empowering freedom of choice, and the enormous potential of the individual to change and heal. In error and in frank opposition to the current developments in hard science, this sclerotic disease-centered mentality gives us a pessimistic vision of a human brain that's static, isolated, and hardwired for failure.

With the shift to a whole-child perspective, however, we open our understanding of children to include their expansive web of life and their vast potentiality for health. In this model, the narrow pessimism of conventional care transforms into an expansive landscape of options, choice, empowerment, and potential. Unbridled optimism and potential are the birthright of every child.

Mental Health for the Whole Child

PART ONE

Philosophy & Practice

CHAPTER ONE

The Nature of Health and Healing

A whole-child approach to mental health promises to palliate and prevent much of the suffering facing our younger generation. But in order to broaden our scope to the whole child, we must first pivot and answer an important, albeit it perplexing, question: What exactly does mental health look like?

Let's first review what psychiatry teaches us about it. Interestingly, the majority of psychiatric training involves just two topics: specific illnesses encountered and techniques employed to treat them. On one level, this makes perfect sense. Clinicians need to be prepared for what they will face in everyday practice. Consequently, during training practitioners come to understand mental health simply as a lack of mental illness. This hardly seems like an appropriate answer to our question, though. It doesn't seem nearly precise, elaborate, or positive enough to describe mental health.

It might seem odd that psychiatry offers little wisdom on a topic as central to its ethos as mental health, but it's a direct consequence of the profession's restrictive philosophy. The training and instruction reflect this perspective. By narrowly focusing instruction and training to the degree it has (illness identification and treatment), psychiatrists have limited exposure to topics (e.g., general health, nutrition, or the psyche) potentially germane to a description of mental health. For example, less than 1% of educational time and material is spent on something as seemingly critical to mental health as prevention. Certainly no one learns anything about nutrition in their psychiatric training. Moreover, and strangely enough, most psychiatric institutions do not cover anything on the human psyche in health and wellness.

Our field has become so narrowly focused on specific illnesses and treatment techniques that mental health is rarely, if ever, discussed. It was not covered in my two years of fellowship training. In Mel Lewis's well-annotated *Textbook of Child and Adolescent Psychiatry*, for instance, there are three minor entries for mental health over 23 index pages of small print with three columns and thousands of entries (Martin & Volkmar, 2007). Two other significant textbooks of child and adolescent psychiatry had no mention of this topic at all in the index or table of contents. (Some professions may cover this topic better than others— e.g., counseling or psychology—but generally these professions deliver much less impact to the policy and practice of mental health care than psychiatry does.) In some sense, psychiatry doesn't really need a definition of mental health because it operates in an allopathic medical model, which is inherently focused on illness.

Because of psychiatry's focus on illness, the majority of the funding for experimental research and treatment in mental health care goes toward pharmacological interventions. Without question, advancements have been made in the discovery of helpful treatments for various illnesses. However, in spite of a narrow focus on neurochemical models and pathways, psychiatric science still has not established the pathophysiology for a single psychiatric illness.

Unfortunately, because of psychiatry's solitary focus on the disease model, the preventative value of lifestyle (exercise, diet, sleep) receives lip service but no real engagement or serious application. Similarly, mind-body skills (meditation, yoga, mindfulness, biofeedback) garner little attention and funding. Moreover, despite mounting evidence for its efficacy in the treatment of a myriad of mental illnesses, omega-3 fatty acid supplementation gets to the patient infrequently. Diet is ignored. The placebo effect, which can carry 60% to 90% of the benefit of most medications without any of the risks, is rarely utilized (at least on purpose). The list goes on. Suffice it to say, the typical mental health patient rarely comes into contact with these treatments.

Unfortunately, as you can see, the current psychiatric paradigm offers little clarity on the question of mental health. It's necessary, then, to look for answers elsewhere. And since mental health so far proves elusive, defining health in general might help us sharpen our definitional edges. Let's start, then, by unpacking one of the most basic elements of health: entelechy or "self-completion."

Entelechy and the Science of Self-Completion

Aristotle described the principle of entelechy over 2,300 years ago. Self-completion, according to Aristotle, is the realization of innate potential through development and functioning. Acorns become oaks and tad-poles become frogs. A human embryo matures into an adult. For Aristo-tle, this drive to self-completion carries such power that only a few things short of death or severe trauma can derail it. Truly, it's nothing short of miraculous that in spite of the forces of entropy and disorder and the many disrupting variables facing development and functioning, life continues to develop and find completion.

Self-completion occurs through the mechanisms of "self-correction" and "self-organization." Self-correction, in this sense, describes the ways in which life heals, balances, and reaches homeostasis (a wound heals; blood balances its pH). Self-organization describes the ways in which life adapts, evolves, and finds order (the organization of ontogeny; the adap-tation of gene expression). These two basic functions of life guide a be-ing's development and functioning, ensuring its eventual completion.

Interestingly enough, many years later, in his novel studies of the psyche, C. J. Jung expounded on a principle similar to that of Aristotle. He called it the process of individualization. He saw individualization as the innate drive of biological organisms to reach completion on all levels of being—mental, physical, and spiritual. This completion, according to Jung, occurs through self-correcting and self-organizing mechanisms in-herent to life, such as healing and maturation. In fact, dreams, for Jung, are the subconscious mechanism by which the mind heals, matures, re-stores order, and, eventually, reaches completion.

In similar fashion, Abraham Maslow understood development as the process by which the latent potential of the mental, emotional, and spir-itual spheres becomes a reality (1993). This final reality, then, was a mental, emotional, and spiritual wholeness resembling Jung's individual-ization and Aristotle's completeness. According to Maslow, the real work of the clinician is "to help [patients] to be more perfectly what they al-ready are, to be more full, more actualizing, more realizing, in fact what they are in potentiality" (1993, p. 41). Potential, for Maslow, is essential to the very fabric of the human. And, for that reason, one of the human's most basic drives is to reach its potential.

Whether they call it self-completion, individualization, or the actual-ization of potential, all of these great thinkers, in their own way, de-scribed the process by which humans become complete, healthy, whole people. Perhaps the most incredible aspect of this process is recovery from injury or illness—the ability of the human to turn chaos and disas-ter into order and wholeness.

In my work with young children with severe developmental disabilities or a history of physical or sexual abuse, I continually notice one common element in their presentation. In spite of all that they do not possess, all that was damaged or lost, these youngsters marvelously adapt, find balance, and move toward wholeness. Obviously, these kids have grave limitations, but their drive for completeness, for understanding, for balance, for adaptation never ceases.

Oliver Sacks, the great neurologist and prolific author of such works as *Awakenings* and *The Man Who Mistook His Wife for a Hat*, remarked at length about this phenomenon in his work with people suffering from the gravest of neurological injuries and illnesses:

> This sense of the brain's remarkable plasticity, its capacity for the most striking adaptations, not least in the special (and often desperate) circumstances of neural or sensory mishap, has come to dominate my own perception of my patients and their lives. So much so, indeed, that I am sometimes moved to wonder whether it may not be necessary to redefine the very concepts of "health" and "disease," to see these in terms of the ability of the organism to create a new organization and order, one that fits its special disposition and needs, rather than in terms of a rigidly defined "norm." (Sacks, 1995, p. xvii)

Most of the profound neuroscientists of the past century, including A. R. Luria, L. S. Vygotsky, and even Piaget, the developmental psychologist, came to the same conclusion. In their work and writing, they all emphasized the essential intactness of those with neurological injury; how the brain self-corrects and self-organizes and tries to return to order.

In fact, Sacks sees the ability to recover from injury and illness as essential to the definition of health. For Sacks, "The ability of the organism to create a new organization and order" is synonymous with health. With this in mind, he and others have developed a view of the human brain not as programmed and static but as

> dynamic and active, a supremely efficient-adaptive system geared for evolution and change, ceaselessly adapting to the needs of the organisms, its need above all to construct a coherent self and world, whatever effects of disorders of brain function befell it. . . . The miracle is how they (the minutely differentiated areas of neurological function) all cooperate, are integrated together, in the creation of self. (1995, p. xvii)

For these scientists and thinkers, the brain is more than a pro-grammed organ; it's an intelligent, integrated, adaptive system respon-sible for the creation of the self, continually striving for evolution, adaptation, and change. Andrew Weil, a close friend and mentor, seemed to have Sacks's comments in mind when he dilated this sense of the brain as an "efficient-adaptive system" to include the whole of being:

> The achievement of balance adds an extra quality to a whole. It makes the perfect whole greater than the sum of its parts, makes it beautiful and holy, and so connects it to a higher reality. Health is wholeness— wholeness in its most profound sense, with nothing left out and every-thing in just the right order to manifest the mystery of balance. Far from being simply the absence of disease, health is a dynamic and har-monious equilibrium of all the elements and forces making up and sur-rounding a human being. (Weil, 1983, p. 51)

To Weil's thinking, the brain's self-correcting and self-organizing process-es are simply part of a larger body-wide phenomenon, the brain just one part of the "dynamic and harmonious equilibrium" of the body, where in spite of injury or illness, the body finds balance, health, and wholeness.

Not only does the body return to balance after injury and illness, but the healing process often leaves the body stronger and better adapted than it was before. (Think of bone growth in response to intensive use or injury.) By thinking about the body in this way, the common dictum "whatever doesn't kill you makes you stronger," often attributed to Nietzsche, acquires a new biological import.

This is truly the intelligence of life—the making of order out of chaos.

Interestingly, self-correcting and self-organizing principles are also prevalent in a diverse collection of sciences beside medicine, including chemistry, nonlinear mathematics, and ecology, to name a few. Each of these unique disciplines explains how complex systems self-correct and self-organize to reach a new equilibrium. The Gaia hypothesis, for in-stance, describes all life on the planet as one vast self-regulating organ-ism. Like Gaia, the wholeness model of mental health provides benefits both as a scientific theory and as a metaphor advancing a deeper under-standing and appreciation of complex systems and how they function.

Obviously, as we extend this idea to human health, it forces us to think in a new, very different way. We have to think about human health almost as a massive feedback loop, correcting and organizing as both internal and external forces stimulate the body, as well as the mind and spirit. Thinking about health in this way means that we can no longer arbitrarily isolate physical health from mental and spiritual health.

The Arbitrary Divisions of Health

The Cartesian dualism of mind and body endures in the training and practice of nearly all health professions. Social work, counseling, psychology, marriage and family therapy, and school professionals all selectively target the relational, cognitive, and emotional facets of mental health. In effect, these practitioners work exclusively with the software of the human psyche, whereas physicians, psychiatrists, and primary care physicians (PCPs) handle the hardware of the body.

Psychiatry prides itself on being brain based, firmly on the body side of the Cartesian divide. But in practice, psychiatrists sequester the brain from the rest of the body. They see the brain and its biochemistry as effectively cut off from the rest of the body, operating as the exclusive and independent hub of mental health and illness. You can see proof of this in the fact that epigenetics, gut health, exercise, inflammation, toxic burden, sleep quality, pain, and nutrition are all but ignored in psychiatry as influences on brain health. (As if the molecules we consume in our food don't also make up the structure of our brain.) In general, PCPs are left to sort out these "physical" issues in their examination of bodily health.

Unfortunately, because of this compartmentalization, our understanding of health is confined to arbitrary professional divisions—psychiatry to brain biochemistry, psychotherapists to the psyche, PCP to physical maladies, and so on. Each profession has a focal point of research and intervention and, because of this, we just have snapshots of each professional focal point. We have no sense of a larger context, no cross-disciplinary collaboration. All the professions suffer as a result.

It seems, in trying to get their arms around health, the health professions are like the old parable of six blind men examining an elephant. Each blind man gropes around one isolated part of the animal trying to figure out what lies before him. One calls out that it's a snake as he touches the trunk and another shouts that it's a tree as he grasps a leg. In some sense, there is a bit of accuracy to each of their tactile judgments. But without a sense of the larger context or good communication between the investigating men, they are all blind to the creature's nature.

In the same way, something as multifaceted and complex as health can't be understood compartmentally. It is not an isolated phenomenon, and it cannot be understood according to just the mind or just brain or just body or other specific parts of the body. The mind, body, and spirit, as we have seen, operate in the same way, are driven by the same forces of self-correction and self-organization, and are interconnected and interdependent in their function. And because of this, they drive health together.

This is perhaps most evident in the way mental health informs general health, and vice versa. A wealth of current data shows that mental health drives long-term health outcomes for just about every chronic illness. For example, it's well known that after a heart attack, cardiac patients who have major depression have dramatically reduced survival. Likewise, we have good evidence that health risk factors such as obesity, poor nutrition, and inflammation deteriorate the mental health of the affected population. This all goes to show that mental health and health are inextricably connected. The same forces driving health also drive mental health.

It is time for the health professions to embrace a fairly simple fact: Mental health is merely one specific expression of health.

Just as mental health is but one form of health, mental illness is but one expression of illness. Some mental health issues may be localized to brain function and biochemistry. However, the current trend in the scientific research points us toward a more systemic, body-wide view of mental illness. Increasingly, mental health issues appear to reflect physiological abnormalities throughout the entire body. Autism, for instance, appears to be a pervading health issue affecting all components of body-mind-spirit (see Chapter 15). In this way, it's very difficult, and perhaps impossible, to pinpoint the localization of mental illness and mental health issues. When you do try, you just end up chasing a long chain of interconnected and interdependent reactions. Take depression, for example. It has long been suspected and now is increasingly accepted that major depression is an inflammatory disorder (see Chapter 10), which by its nature therefore involves the endocrine system, which by extension involves the autonomic nervous system, which therefore also involves the hippocampus and so on and so forth, in a long chain of interdependent and interconnected interplay. You could ask where this chain has its origins, but that would be misleading. It's better to recognize the multiple interconnections and interdependencies so that you can help correct imbalances at any level of the chain.

Our compartmentalized view of health and illness limits our ability to heal our children. Stories of recovery like those of Henry and Caley demonstrate the ways in which our current vision of biochemistry and brain-based mental illness restricts not only our understanding of mental illness but also the healing process. If we are to completely understand mental health, and help those afflicted kids, our system of care must expand to include the broadest view of health possible. So instead of reducing the definition of health to something as negative as the "absence of disease," we must begin to view and respect health for what it is: order and balance on all levels of life.

Primum Non Nocere

As healers, we serve life itself. Health care, as a natural extension, must be built on the basis of preserving life. Any time health care in any form diverges from this understanding and becomes too reductionistic, it risks effacing the basic principles of life, and therefore the health and safety of those left in its care.

Primum non nocere in Latin means "first, do no harm." The oft-cited dictum of medicine first appeared as a central premise of the Hippocratic oath over 2,500 years ago. At the center of this ethic is the primacy of life, and it is consistent with the gut reaction most practitioners have to potentially dangerous treatments. This core premise permeates spiritual and political practice as well. From Buddha to Jesus Christ, Martin Luther King Jr. to Thoreau, the avoidance of harm above and beyond other concerns resonates in human thinking. Quite simply, the primacy of life is sacred, and we must do all that we can to not harm it.

Many mental health practitioners now fear that too many of our treatments unnecessarily harm too many patients. In essence, they sense that the conventional paradigm for treatment is in conflict with the basic respect at the heart of medicine's ethic. (Much of the impetus for writing this book, for example, lies in a deep and abiding respect for life and the need to have our mental health treatments better honor it.)

Practitioners experiencing these kinds of misgivings with medicine know intuitively that health is the rule, not the exception. They understand that health can be accomplished by methods not inconsistent with the principles of life and medicine. In short, they know that untested, invasive, or silver-bullet cures are sometimes inconsistent with the goal of getting someone healthy, and that there exist many potential options for getting people healthy again.

Health is not a one in a billion chance; rather, it is the norm, if only a few essential ingredients are in place and well maintained. Caley, the little girl featured so prominently in the Introduction, is a prime example of a case of severe mental illness self-correcting and self-balancing once an essential factor of her diet and metabolism was assisted. As practitioners, then, we best assist our patients' health—and protect the primacy of life—when we work with their core factors of health rather than with their symptoms of a presumed illness.

The Dangers of Risky and Untested Interventions

Sadly, safety is rarely, if ever, the prevailing concern during the introduction of treatment. In fact, side effects—even potentially life-threatening ones—are almost always regarded as subsidiary to efficacy. Psychiatry, in particular, fails to fully comprehend the potential damage that hasty interventions and medications can have, and in this way founders on its own Hippocratic oath.

Instead, each year deep piles of data build up on only a few preferred treatments, with little clarity on long-term effectiveness or safety derived therefrom. It is still contentious, for instance, whether antipsychotic medication helps or hinders long-term outcomes in children. And yet, the use of these agents continues, and spreads. There are many reasons for this paradigmatic loyalty, the least of which is the buttressing of the prevailing model by powerful commercial interests. Surprisingly, despite the rise of psychiatric disability rates in the last 20 years, most mental health professionals feel confident that we walk upon a firm foundation of science, with the data and support needed to validate our current treatments.

While we employ a few treatments that seem to work in the short run, a vast range of possible tools and triggers lie undiscovered. Given that our knowledge of the real underlying causes of any mental illness is shaky, the range of unexplored possible treatments remains incomprehensibly broad. It's possible that 60 years from now we will be embarrassed by the inadequate and inappropriate use of our current tools and our incomplete ideas about mental health.

Such is the history of the treatment of brain-related maladies. Just over 60 years ago, in fact, lobotomy—that most invasive and at the time "effective" of mental health treatments—was broadly accepted in mental health and society at large, even garnering its inventor, Egas Moniz, the Nobel Prize in medicine in 1949. Like lobotomy, insulin-shock therapy, bloodletting, cold-water immersion, teeth pulling, and a variety of other brutal techniques all had their day in the sun and then passed out of practice as another "wonder" treatment was discovered. At the time, each of these treatments was "carefully" studied and robustly supported by clinicians and the literature. But as Sir William Osler, MD, the father of modern medicine, reflected, "the philosophies of one age become the absurdities of the next" (1902, p. 132). Interestingly, over the course of psychiatry's ebb and flow of treatments, the only therapy that has withstood the test of time is lithium carbonate, a salt readily found in nature.

As practitioners, we would do well to keep the ebb and flow of psychiatric history in mind as we treat patients, stopping to ask, is this treatment really safe? Since it is the practitioner's primary responsibility to protect life and health, all other considerations must remain secondary to this. If there is any potential cause for concern, the introduction of risky or untested treatments must be taken off the table. This is especially important in considering medication management, because we do not yet know the manner and degree to which pharmaceutical agents affect the body, mind, and spirit (particularly in the long term).

Health, as we have learned, is a balancing act involving many interconnected and interdependent systems. In the human, as in an ecosystem, the introduction of one affecting variable can have cascading, and sometimes devastating, effects. We have no idea how far the ill effects of powerful medications might reverberate down through the human system. Safety and caution are paramount.

Life Is Interconnected and Interdependent

The science of ecology teaches us that all facets of life are interconnected and interdependent. Consequently, we can well expect a powerful antipsychotic agent, for example, to have effects on many spheres of being, particularly for children, considering the supple nature of their brain and biology. Therefore, it is important, as a practitioner, to respect the interconnectivity and interdependence of each patient's life and resist using interventions that could potentially disrupt it.

In a professional setting, respecting this interconnectivity and interdependence means getting to know a child and the many spheres of that child's life. It means understanding how various spheres overlap: how home life might be affecting school performance, for instance, or how daily gut pain is affecting the child's ability to spend time with friends. Kids lead complicated lives, so take the proper time to learn about them and the potential issues that might be affecting their health.

Most often, as you get to know a kid better you will notice the presence of many issues: pent-up anger at a friend, frustration over chronic insomnia, fear of an upcoming move, or sadness over the recent loss of a pet. Unfortunately, these emotions are often experienced all at the same time—piling up in a big mess of worry and suffering.

All of these emotions, as we know, have an effect on each other. They are interconnected and interdependent. We can easily see that physical issues of the body—pain, fatigue, nutrition—affect the mental and emotional spheres (as we saw with Caley, for example). In turn, we can also see that mental, emotional, and spiritual issues can manifest in the body and upset the physiological sphere (this might be one reason for Henry's mutism). Each kid exists in an ecosystem fluctuating and swaying according to the kid's interactions. So never assume that it is just one isolated issue affecting a kid's health. Try to untangle the whole mess of conflicting and afflicting issues and correct as many of them as you can.

A few general implications for the practitioner flow from this understanding of interconnectivity and interdependence. First, all interventions, regardless of their nature, create a cascading series of effects, many of which are unpredictable. A simple positive interaction with a coach or teacher, for instance, may reverberate in unforeseen and powerful ways. It might decrease cortisol, leading to improved memory or sleep, which then might in turn help abate some symptoms of mental distress. Likewise, a single negative comment or interaction can have devastating, unpredictable effects on a kid. Thus, more powerful interventions like psychiatric medication will be more forceful and wide ranging in effect pattern. For example, the lack of long-term safety data on the neurobiological implications of using psychiatric medication in a plastic, developing brain gives me great pause every time I think about writing a prescription for a kid.

Second, we need to remain humble in our struggle to understand our children. Live in awe and respect of the mystery and complexity contained in every child. Let this mystery and complexity humble you and, in turn, motivate your desire for a better understanding of each kid. Remain open to possibilities, other opinions, and the chance that you are wrong.

Finally, we must remain skeptical of conventional thought and practice, especially if it seems to carry any risk. Kids have enormous potential, not only to heal, but also to overcome hardship and lead an inspired, happy life. As practitioners, then, we cannot afford to put any of this potential at risk.

Appreciate and Protect Potential

Kids are potential manifested. Whether they suffer from horrible illness, a devastating event, or the harshest of challenges, never underestimate the potential that lies within every kid to confront these afflictions and move beyond them. Henry, our little boy from the Introduction, expressed this kind of vast potential. And, simply as a matter of course, potential must be protected, and our philosophy of mental health must embody it.

The effective delivery of relevant psychoeducation or skill building amplifies this potential through a lifetime. It gives children the appropriate skills to awaken their latent potential and the coping mechanisms to keep it alive under duress. Likewise, any tool that increases awareness magnifies personal potential. The concept of physical fitness and all that it implies in terms of training and development should translate to all spheres of our being. Just so, all children should have some reasonable expectation of a clear minimum threshold for emotional, mental, social, and spiritual fitness. A basic competency in these spheres compounds rewards throughout the long arc of human life. If this competency can be trained, why leave it to chance?

On the other side of the coin, any treatment that clouds awareness or decays a child's ability to learn must be held in great suspicion. It is a

Faustian trade to barter immediate symptomatic relief for possible re-strictions on future potential. And that's exactly what we are doing with neuroleptics. While these drugs might be effective in abating aggressive behavior in the short term, as research indicates, they also cloud aware-ness, limit learning, and inhibit frontal lobe development.

Over my many decades in intensive treatment settings for abused children, I have encountered all too many kids heavily sedated on neuro-leptics to control anger and violence. These kids could not learn in the classroom or grow interpersonally while sedated on drugs. Moreover, the medication's ability to control anger would last for only 2 or 3 months. So you have to ask, what is really accomplished by intervening with these agents? Not much.

Kids are complex little people with limitless potential. It is of the high-est importance to appreciate and protect this, so get to know them and try to understand how your treatments might really change, for better or for worse, their character, health, and life trajectory.

Inductive and Deductive Health Care

The ideas of health outlined so far in this chapter serve as a transition between the broad ideas of wholeness as a theory of health and the prac-tical application of assessment and treatment tools. This manner of thinking about mental health and its treatment, then, is deductive rather than inductive, as it is characterized by the inference of particular in-stances of illness from a general understanding of health.

As we discussed at the beginning of this chapter, in its narrow focus on illness and medication, conventional psychiatry is functionally devoid of a working definition of mental health. This is largely because conven-tional psychiatry's paradigm is characterized by the inference of general laws of health as they are informed by specific instances of illness. This inductive reasoning is, of course, less logically sound than its deductive counterpart. It only requires experiential, or else anecdotal, evidence to validate its claims. The early development and promotion of neurolep-tics reflects just this.

In the 1960s, researchers noticed that neuroleptics affected dopami-nergic pathways while at the same time also affecting schizophrenic symptomatology. From there, it was hypothesized that all mental illnesses were diseases of neurotransmitter pathways. Flurries of studies in the following years were dedicated to the demonstration of raised and lowered levels of various neurotransmitters in patients suffering from mental illness. Inductive reasoning had permeated the ranks.

Of course, research has never conclusively reached a consistent estimation of what neurotransmitter, in what amount, is responsible for what illness. There is good clinical research, for instance, documenting that both SSRIs (selective serotonin reuptake inhibitors; increase the level of serotonin) and SSREs (selective serotonin reuptake enhancers; lower the level of serotonin) abate depressive symptoms (Wagstaff, Ormrod, & Spencer, 2001). Moreover, if mental illnesses like schizophrenia and depression were disorders of neurotransmitter function, we would see a documented baseline difference of neurotransmitter function in those affected patients (e.g., a low baseline of serotonin in depressive patients). But research has never shown this. There is no consistent documented abnormality of neurotransmitter metabolites in cerebrospinal fluid of patients suffering from similar illnesses.

Be that as it may, psychiatry remains vehement and guarded in its understanding of mental illness. And this enduring misrepresentation of mental illness does not appear, unfortunately, to be going away anytime soon. Psychiatry is too entrenched in its own inductive logic.

In contrast to psychiatry's thinking, it is easy to see the value of deductive thinking in mental health. Simply put, rather than making general inferences about health from cases of specific illness, it is more logical to make inferences about specific illnesses from general principles of health. In this way, health care becomes health centered.

Conclusion

Health is defined by the intelligence of life—that innate drive in biological organisms to self-correct and self-balance. This is wholeness. As a concept, wholeness is so simple and ubiquitous that everyone simply overlooks it. Yet, in the same way, it is so complex and nuanced that scientists often fail to perceive it. Nevertheless, wholeness guides health by acknowledging the innate intelligence of life. Without wholeness life becomes disorder and disease; with it life can achieve bodily, mental, and spiritual health. When it is lost, anxiety, depression, disease, and chronic pain emerge. When it is found, inner peace, true joy, and physical healing return.

At the beginning of this chapter, I set out to define health and mental health in order to better inform an understanding of what exactly we, as practitioners, are trying to heal and prevent. Parsing definitions of mental illness and mental health and arriving at a more comprehensive estimation of their character aids our understanding not only of the maladies we are charged with fighting but also what winning that fight might look like. In the process, I've demonstrated the ways in which health, in any sense, means achieving balance in mind, body, and spirit. The question, finally, is how to achieve and entrench this living balance in our kids.

CHAPTER TWO

The Seven Building Blocks of Wholeness

Health is not a random event.

In fact, for all living things health is the rule, not the exception. We are healthy by nature; it usually takes the impact of some powerful negative factor to finally make us unhealthy. And more often than not, we get healthy once again. This is because a steady, innate force in biology governs health, a force that keeps our body, mind, and soul working in sync. The synchronization of these healthy elements is wholeness.

To achieve this synchronization, there are a few necessary building blocks. Luckily for all parents, practitioners, and individuals, wholeness does not require a perfect arrangement of building blocks. Since health is the rule and not the exception, a merely good-enough approximation of the needed building blocks will sufficiently support wholeness.

That's not to say that children can remain healthy and whole in a physiological and psychological vacuum. They do need some level of support. They do need our help. But, since the biological drive to wholeness is so strong, it falls to us, as practitioners and parents, to simply foster the factors promoting health, instead of intervening after the fact.

This is why the role of the practitioner in the Wholeness Model is something resembling a construction consultant. He or she advises and explains the building blocks of wholeness, and allows the natural intelligence of health to bring the child back to health and wholeness. It's important that we move away from the idea that we are somehow fixing our patients—because, really, it's almost never true. And this kind of thinking does not empower our little patients. Instill knowledge; educate the kids and parents you see about what keeps them healthy and whole.

This chapter will provide you with the basis to do so. In no particular order, the following pages will detail the seven building blocks of wholeness. The science and logic behind the inclusion of each will be covered so you have a good sense of their role in getting, and keeping, kids healthy and whole. (In Part II I'll show how these building blocks can be used in devising treatment approaches to specific mental health issues.) Where relevant, I've included a case study that crystallizes the matter in question. Hopefully by the end of this chapter you'll have a better sense of the factors that foster health and wholeness, and you'll be better equipped to navigate the many problems you face in practice. Luckily, these building blocks will make sense to most young kids.

1. Proper nutrition (food and gut health)
2. Connection (attachment, goodness of fit, and social competency)
3. Sound sleep
4. Engagement
5. Self-regulation (emotionality, executive functioning, and character)
6. Spirituality (meaning and purpose)
7. Family

Each of the seven building blocks needs to exist in a healthy balance in relation to the others. One cannot be compromised in order to benefit another. It stresses the whole system if even one remains out of balance. For example, if it goes unaddressed, obesity (related to 1 and 4) can compromise the integrity of each of the other building blocks. The child may struggle with identity (6) and self-regulation (5) as a direct result. And the whole system may fall apart. The balance of the whole system is more important than any one block.

Proper Nutrition

The child in front of you went from a one-celled zygote to a machinery of 200 billion neurons in 6 years of intensive growth. This act of neuro-chemical construction requires a vast array of minerals, vitamins, trace elements, fats, and proteins that must be sourced somehow. Needless to say, they come from our diet or, in the early years, our mother's.

Once created, the human brain operates at a level of complexity that's hard to fathom. Hundreds of different chemical reactions occur every second to keep us alive and aware. These reactions typically involve co-factors, enzymes, or catalysts making it all feasible. These cofactors and catalysts are usually vitamins, minerals, or trace elements. For example, we know that folate (folic acid), cobalamin (B_{12}), thiamine (B_1), pyridoxine (B_6), calcium, chromium, magnesium, iron, choline, zinc, vitamin E, and selenium are micronutrients in our diet that alter brain function. Zinc, as a further example, is a cofactor for over 200 different enzymes present in 300 different metalloenzymes functioning in all areas of metabolism. And it plays a key role in the olfactory bulb (smell) and hippocampus (learning and memory) (Milne, 2000).

The integrity of neurons may in fact be dependent on cellular zinc levels. Zinc plays a vital role in synaptic function and is released into the synapse upon firing (Prohaska, 1987). Zinc deficiency may create an overall decrease in neurotransmitter responsiveness, rather than playing a unique role in any specific neurotransmitter pathway. A number of studies have correlated zinc deficiency with ADHD issues (Akhondzadeh, Mohammadi, & Khademi, 2004). Zinc—not just for sunscreen and colds.

Beyond the commonsense role that diet plays in providing these compounds, researchers have demonstrated that simple nutrients such as folate, B_{12}, B_6, B_1, choline, vitamin E, zinc, and selenium have an effect on human brain health (Kaplan, Crawford, Field, & Simpson, 2007).

The work on essential fatty acids (EFAs) alone grows every year. It's well known, for example, that folic acid levels correlate with mood, major depression, and antidepressant response. In fact, an activated form of folic acid, L-methylfolate (Deplin), recently achieved an FDA indication as a prescription treatment for major depression. We find further corroboration of diet's role in mental health if we zoom out from a metabolic level to the 30,000-foot view to look at population studies.

One large cross-sectional study of 5,731 people measured diet quality and mental health. It found that a traditional diet of meat, fruit, nuts, veggies, and whole grains correlated with reduced depression (Jacka, Mykletun, Berk, Bjelland, & Tell, 2011). Another large study of over 1,000 women looked at diet patterns and mood and corrected for age, socioeconomic status, education, and health behaviors. Again, this study found that a traditional diet of fruits, veggies, meats, and whole grains was associated with much lower odds of depression and anxiety (Jacka et al., 2010). In Spain, one researcher prospectively studied over 10,000 healthy college students over 5 years and found that adherence to a Mediterranean diet was inversely correlated with the risk of depression ($p = 0.001$) (Sanchez-Villegas et al., 2009).

In a large prospective study of over 3,000 Australian teenagers followed for over 3 years, researchers found that diet quality was associated with better mental health, and an improving diet with improved mental health, whereas a deteriorating diet was associated with deteriorated mental health (Jacka, Kremer, et al., 2011).

How does diet link so closely to mental health? Kaplan, in her brilliant article "Vitamins, Minerals and Mood," notes four probable metabolic paths between nutrition and mental health (Kaplan et al., 2007):

1. Illness could be an inborn error of metabolism (such as a single-nucleotide polymorphism [SNP] that is inherited. One example of this might be an SNP that reduces the efficiency of EFA. This is a well-documented mutation).
2. Illness could be a deficiency in the methylation process (proper methylation is needed to make neurotransmitters and is affected by folic acid and SAMe, both of which have been demonstrated to effectively treat depression).
3. Illness could be an alteration of gene expression stemming from a nutritional deficiency. This is the epigenetic mechanism Jirtle demonstrated with his agouti mice (Waterland & Jirtle, 2003).
4. Illness could be long-term, latent deficiency of a specific nutrient (studies demonstrate that omega-3 EFA deficiency during pregnancy increases the risk of postpartum depression) (Golding, Steer, Emmett, Davis, & Hibbeln, 2009).

Obviously, there are cross-links between all of these metabolic pathways. And that being the case, it's reasonable to think that for any given individual with mental health issues all (or any combination) of these metabolic pathways might be at fault.

Why did Caley respond so well to a broad-spectrum micronutrient? Was it because one of these metabolic pathways was at fault? It's difficult to say exactly. A single broad-spectrum micronutrient addresses all four pathways of possible illness, so it's difficult to say which one it is correcting. But does Caley really care?

Bruce Ames, the father of modern laboratory medicine, said, "When one input in the metabolic network is inadequate, repercussions are felt on a large number of systems and can lead to disease" (2005, p. S20). Over 50% of Americans do not meet the basic intake requirements for one of these single key nutrients: vitamin E, calcium, magnesium, and vitamin A. These numbers are for mature adults. Just imagine the increased metabolic need and urgency in a growing child with a massive demand for biochemical production.

But how early does nutritional intervention become relevant? During the neonatal period, infancy, preschool? An epidemiologist and physician from England, D. J. P. Barker, has an idea. His work over the last two decades points to the time before delivery as the starting point for nutritional intervention. In his research, he connected low birth weight to death from coronary artery disease later in life (Barker, 1998). Early childhood malnutrition is now understood as a significant risk factor for high blood pressure, stroke, type 2 diabetes, osteoporosis, and certain types of cancer (Lawlor, Ronalds, Clark, Smith, & Leon, 2005). This risk association is known as the Barker hypothesis.

Consistent with the Barker hypothesis, research now links in utero iron deficiency with significant long-term health issues (Black, Quigg, Hurley, & Pepper, 2011). Emerging evidence now also suggests that iron deficiency in early life leads to long-lasting neural and behavioral deficiencies, including risk of schizophrenia (Insel, Schaefer, McKeague, Susser, & Brown, 2008). One study found almost twice the risk of schizophrenia if the mother was diagnosed as anemic during pregnancy (Sorensen, Nielsen, Pedersen, & Mortensen, 2011). A review of inadequate prenatal nutrition found links to schizophrenia, depression, heightened stress response, and impaired cognition (Roseboom, Painter, van Abeelen, Veenendaal, & de Rooij, 2011). Basically, the fetus adapts to inadequate nutrition by compromising certain metabolic pathways ultimately crucial for good health—and survival.

Put simply, early-life nutrition programs the genetics of every child. Clearly, then, dietary intervention makes sense for prevention. That's why sound nutrition is the first building block of wholeness.

The Gut

Every child eats, but every child must also absorb. The nutrients contained in food must be broken down in the gut in order for them to be properly absorbed and contribute toward the building of a body and a brain. This vital step between is often overlooked, however. It depends on a force both internal and external: the flora of the gastrointestinal (GI) tract.

Soon after birth, the colonization of the child's GI tract begins. Quickly, the bacterial cells outnumber human cells 10 to one. In fact, the number of genes that any human embodies is weighted 100 to one in the bacteria's favor. These beneficial microbes are responsible for breaking down our food, predigesting much of it and producing critical nutrients like vitamin K and B vitamins. This vast ecology makes increasing scientific sense as a source of human health (Floch, 2011). In the last 5 years, in fact, research on this topic has exploded, much of it validating the crucial role of the microbiome in health and disease.

A landmark article published in the prestigious *Proceedings of the National Academy of Science* showed that gut flora plays a significant role in brain development and subsequent adult behavior (Heijtz et al., 2011). The researchers found significant differences in behavior between a germ-free (sterile) and normally colonized gut. And these fundamental gut differences altered behavior well into adulthood. They also found that some of these differences affected alterations in critical neurotransmitter levels related to planning and attention and were nonreversible after a critical period in early development had passed. In all, the researchers noted that gut flora levels alter 40 different behavior-affecting genes in the brain.

In fact, new studies suggest that crucial genes—including brain-derived neurotrophic factor (BDNF)—are downregulated in germ-free populations (Bercik et al., 2011). The summary of one of these studies, published in the mainstream journal *Gastroenterology*, says it all: "The intestinal microbiota influences brain chemistry and behavior independently of autonomic nervous system, gasto-intestinal specific neurotransmitters, or inflammation. Intestinal dysbiosis might contribute to psychiatric disorders" (Bercik et al., 2011, p. 599).

Intestinal dysbiosis is a genetic term for a pathological imbalance of gut microbiota. Some of our most severe childhood psychiatric illnesses, in fact, appear to be linked to microbiota pathology. Children with autism spectrum disorder (ASD), for example, have altered GI flora with more pathogenic species, and the severity of pathology in ASD has been linked to severity of gut microbiota pathology (Parracho, Bingham, Gibson, & McCartney, 2005). And we have known for many years that kids with ASD have high rates of severe gut pathology (9–54%) (Wasilewska, Jarocka-Cyrta, & Kaczmarski, 2009). Interestingly enough, yeast overgrowth, a certain kind of gut dysbiosis, has been associated with sugar craving, depression, fatigue, anxiety, hyperactivity, and irritability.

But what does this mean for little kids? It means that every kid needs to be properly colonized. Proper colonization plays a huge role in the development of proper digestion, immunity, and absorption (Gaskins, Croix, Nakamura, & Nava, 2008). However, the method through which each infant becomes colonized largely depends on the type of birth (vaginal vs. C-section) and whether or not breast-feeding occurs (M'Rabet, Vos, Boehm, & Garssen, 2008). C-sections may delay or alter normal colonization. Also, colonization is significantly altered by the use of antibiotics in breast-feeding mothers and young kids, particularly serial use for chronic infections (especially common with chronic otitis media, a painful infection of the middle ear prevalent in early childhood). Considerable controversy exists about the use of antibiotics for this problem. In Europe this issue is treated conservatively without antibiotics, with similar outcomes.

The second component of good gut health relates to food allergies and intolerances. If a child regularly consumes a food that he or she is allergic to or intolerant of, the gut becomes inflamed and will not function or absorb well. This can create a cascade of related reactions that will pervasively affect the child's body-mind-spirit with a myriad of negative effects. These issues are well explored in Chapters 9 and 15. We now know that celiac patients (with a profound allergy to a component of the gluten molecule found in wheat and rye) have altered brain perfusion and significantly elevated risk for a range of psychiatric illnesses. No one as yet understands how this occurs. The end point of the gut reaction over time may be the alteration of the microbiome so crucial for health.

A recent study points to a relationship between psychosis and gluten allergy. Researchers in Sweden explored blood samples from newborns born between 1975 and 1985 and measured their allergic response to gliadin (the immunologically active component in gluten) as measured by IgG. This material was then compared to the known registry of psychotic (nonaffective) illness. The researchers found that levels of IgG antibodies to gliadin at birth related to an elevated risk for psychosis later in life (Karlsson et al., 2012). Since gluten allergies may predispose patients to psychosis, it may make sense to take anyone with first-break psychosis off gluten-containing products for a 4-week elimination diet, as this intervention carries no risk.

This is one reason why I ask so many questions about colic, infantile reflux, eczema, abdominal pain, constipation, diarrhea, and so on with any child that I treat. If you're to know children and their health, then you have to know the gut and food.

Connection

A newborn enters this world tethered to the mother via the umbilical cord. Quickly, that last physical link is severed and the neonate becomes utterly helpless and dependent. Over the next few years, but particularly from about 6 months to 2 years, the infant attaches to primary caregivers in a process that creates lasting psychological, neurological, and physiological consequences.

Dan Siegel's (1999) towering work, *The Developing Mind*, summarizes the basics of the attachment process: Almost all infants become attached, usually to only a few people, and the earliest attachments form by 7 months. By monitoring a child's behavior via a standard lab measure called the Infant Strange Situation (also called the Ainsworth, after Mary Ainsworth, who developed the test), we can get a good indication of a child's style of attachment. During the test, a 1-year-old child spends time with Mom, Mom and a stranger, just the stranger, alone, and is reunited with Mom. The most useful section of this test is the reunion with Mom. Based on behavior, an infant's attachment is assessed in one of four ways:

1. Secure: Misses parent, prefers parent over the stranger.
2. Avoidant: Doesn't cry on separation from Mom, avoids and ignores the parent on return, and shows little distress.
3. Ambivalent: Uneasy prior to separation, fails to settle or return to play during other steps.
4. Disorganized: The infant seems dissociated or disorganized in the presence of the parent. There is a loss of all behavioral strategies. May freeze up or rock incessantly.

In low-risk nonclinical populations, about 55% to 65% of infants display a secure attachment. About 20% to 30% of children demonstrate an avoidant attachment. In clinical populations, of course, the number of avoidant, ambivalent, and disorganized attachments are higher.

Rather than attributing the attachment style solely to the child, theorists like Mary Ainsworth see the child's behavior as a dyad between the primary caregiver (most often the mom) and the child. The child's behavior is indicative of the quality of care being received from the caregiver. The key point to take away from attachment theorists is that behavior is not based on quantity of time or on specifics of parenting, but rather on the caregivers' sensitivity to the infant's verbal and nonverbal signals.

A variety of barriers can get in the way of the attachment process, including parental depression, addiction, trauma, and loss. These barriers make it more likely for the child to have an avoidant, ambivalent, or disorganized attachment style. Children can, however, change their attachment style. The term "earned secure" has been applied to individuals who experienced insensitive parenting and, in spite of that, became securely attached (Main & Goldwyn, 1994). This makes me think about Henry, our little boy from the Introduction.

Unlike Henry, most children will carry their raw, early experiences forward. In fact, about 70% to 80% of individuals show long-term stability in attachment style (Waters, Merrick, Treboux, Crowell, & Albersheim, 2000). And this can have profound implications for a myriad of behaviors. One study conducted at the University of Minnesota, for example, found that attachment style predicted high school graduation 77% of the time (Sroufe, 2005a). Another found that for prospective parents, the history of the attachment between them and their now older parents will predict the attachment between them and their potential child, with as much as 80% reliability (Van Ljzendoorn, 1995). There's also evidence showing that adults who report a poor relationship with their parents have greater struggles in managing life's challenges, particularly in interpersonal relationships (Shaver & Mikulincer, 2002). The converse is equally true: Adults who report a positive relationship with their folks tend to be more secure and socially competent as they move through life.

Proper Fit

A good fit between a child and a parent is not always a given. Sure, a little boy is just enough like his parents to make him easy to relate to, but he is also just different enough to make some of him a total mystery. This is why fit can be so hard. There's just enough dissimilarity between a child and parent that, sometimes, there's misunderstanding, and trouble.

But there are two factors that can, if properly managed, greatly increase the likelihood of having a good fit: child temperament and parental issues.

Needless to say, a child's temperament is relatively immovable. However, when certain temperaments present in extreme ways—irritability, hyperactivity, insomnia, restlessness, distractibility, withdrawal—it is more likely that they are symptoms. Usually, they are symptoms of some biological imbalance such as food intolerance, nutrient deficiency, or mitochondrial dysfunction. Caley's reactivity, for instance, seemed so extreme in character that I couldn't in all reason just attribute it to her personality. I looked at her physiology and found major imbalances. Keep this in mind when you see extreme presentations.

On the other side of the fit dyad are parental issues. No matter the form, without a doubt, parents' issues will color their style of parenting. In *Parenting From the Inside Out*, Dan Siegel and Mary Hartzell (2003) smartly note that all parents step up to the job of parenting with all the strengths, weaknesses, needs, and gifts of their personality. Indeed, Carl Jung said that nothing affects the child like the unfulfilled life of a parent. That's why anything that negatively impacts a parent's ability to, well, parent needs to be explored and dealt with.

As you look for signs of parental issues and extreme temperament presentations, also be mindful of the fact that achieving a good fit sometimes just boils down to striking a settlement between the struggling parties and, hopefully, finding a shared understanding.

Stephanie

After my colleagues and I heard about Stephanie, we were prepared for the worst. She and her mother argued incessantly and recently their confrontations had reached a fever pitch. Stephanie threatened her mother late one night with a butcher knife. The police were called, and Stephanie was enrolled in our day treatment program.

Stephanie was stocky, a tough 15-year-old who hung out mostly with boys and played sports. She was an average student, but recently her grades had begun to slip. Over the prior 3 years, Stephanie had been in outpatient therapy since she was diagnosed by a social worker as having an attachment disorder. (Stephanie was adopted.) The talk therapy she underwent seemed to help, but when she went home things always got worse. Eventually, she was taken to a psychiatrist who diagnosed her with a mood disorder and put her on medication. She gained weight and her behavior continued to deteriorate. Within a few months, she had the episode that precipitated her visit to us.

Stephanie was willful and stubborn, but she was also playful, energetic, and outgoing. I got the immediate sense that her recent antisocial, violent behavior was out of character. I figured I would get a better sense of what was really going on once I met with her mom and dad.

Marsha was a well-spoken woman who knew what she wanted. She was a high school English teacher, and I had a strong feeling I would have struggled in her class. Her demands in my office gave me an insight into what Stephanie might be experiencing at home. Tom, on the other hand, was relaxed and gentle. "I don't know why Steph and Marsha have always struggled," he told me on the telephone. "Their relationship is like fire and gasoline."

After this conversation, I invited Marsha and Tom to join Stephanie and me for family therapy. We began to meet three times a week, the sessions often tense and volatile. I watched as Marsha and Stephanie were pulled into a dance that brought out the worst qualities of each one, over which neither seemed to have much control.

Stephanie made progress in our program, but at home her issues with Marsha continued. One day, Stephanie told me Marsha had left to visit family for 2 weeks. With Marsha gone, Stephanie was a very different person. I finally understood why Tom got along with his daughter so well. It was also clear during this period that Stephanie did not have an attachment disorder. She had a terrible fit with her mother.

Over the next 2 weeks, I worked to help Stephanie understand how she and her mother were just fundamentally different people with different temperaments. Reserving judgment, I tried to help Stephanie see the ways she could be willful, stubborn, and argumentative. And when Marsha returned, I worked with her on the same stuff, helping her manage and understand her own temperament, and how to navigate Stephanie's.

Mother and daughter began to see how they unconsciously pushed each other's buttons and brought the worst out in one another. I worked with both parties to be more patient and compassionate and less reactive with each other. By the time Stephanie left our program after 8 weeks, she was off all medication and better yet, she and her mother were enjoying a much better fit.

Fit can be improved upon, but not if it goes unrecognized as an issue, as it did in the early years between Stephanie and Marsha. That's why it's so important to think about every child's temperament and how it mixes with the parent and their potential issues.

All too often, an issue of fit boils down to parental depression. The child in this setting is more likely to be aggressive, oppositional, throw tantrums, and exhibit out-of-control behavior. In my experience, in at least 50% of those "unmanageable" cases there is a depressed or highly stressed mom.

The research backs me up. According to one study, a child from a depressed mom has four times the risk of being diagnosed with psychiatric illness (Hammen & Brennan, 2003). Surprisingly, about half of the kids who struggle with depressed moms have behavioral issues and not mood concerns. The researchers noted that severity of maternal depression contributed more to children's risk for illness than did chronicity or timing. Most distressing, children exposed to even 1 or 2 months of maternal depression had elevated risks of illness. The authors concluded, "Exposure to maternal depression at any period in the first ten years equally predicted youth depression if the mother was depressed only once" (p. 253).

Fortunately, according to a follow-up study, if the mom gets treated, 33% of those kids with a diagnosis will remit (Weissman et al., 2006). The authors' conclusions hammer home the point: "Remission of the mother's depression has a positive effect on both mothers and their children, whereas mothers who remain depressed may increase the rates of their children's disorders" (p. 1234). The child's issues are significant and lasting. The 23-year follow-up found more depression, disability, and psychiatric medications, and many fewer friends.

Sadly, this is not an uncommon problem. One large study of 4,398 new moms followed from 39 weeks before pregnancy to 39 weeks after found a 15.4% rate of depression (Dietz et al., 2007). That means that roughly one in seven moms is depressed. Most surprising, the authors noted that many moms of that 15.4% had "high rates of continuity," meaning that the depression was unchanged throughout the study. So we are not just talking about postpartum depression or short bouts of melancholy here.

Social Competency

Relationships are an enduring currency of happiness in our world. So it's important that every kid is competent to navigate the struggles involved. They learn much of this, unconsciously and consciously, from their parents. Attachment and attunement eventually lead to parental role modeling, which sets the stage for the child's early exploration of relationships, under some adult supervision. The teen years, however, are largely autonomous. And there are always bumps in the road. But if the child has a supportive and sensitive parental connection, this bumpy road can also be laden with growth and sophistication. That's why it is so important for parents to help their young kids process and work through relational events.

Luckily, this is not a subject parents will need much convincing of. In a nationwide survey conducted by Mom Central, Inc., on behalf of Hasbro, Inc., of 1,000 parents, 90% of them considered social skills to be crucial to their children's ultimate happiness and confidence as they move through life (PRNewswire, 2008). In fact, nearly 8 out of 10 parents in this survey felt that social skills are more important than academic skills for overall happiness. I agree with these parents, and it's one of the reasons that I support social skills groups and social-emotional curricula in our schools.

Children with poor social competency are more likely to become aggressive and, in turn, more likely to be shunned (Bohnert, Crnic, & Lim, 2003). This locks them in a vicious cycle of social marginalization. Because of impaired development, children with chronic illness (e.g., ADHD, diabetes) struggle with social competency in the same way (Martinez, Carter, & Legato, 2011). Since poor social competency often leads kids to social ostracism, depression, and substance abuse, it's important to intervene and get them the skills they need.

In a healthy trajectory of social competence, a child will migrate from successfully managing a few isolated relationships under adult supervision in his early years to independently managing a number of simultaneous relationships during his teen years. More introverted children will often develop just one or two long-term relationships, but for most kids the number will swell over the years into a web of aquaintances and friends, with a tighter inner circle of more intimate friendships.

This inner circle is key. Social competence means more than just the ability to connect broadly to many people. It also means having the ability to connect deeply—forming intimate and loving bonds—which is vital because it keeps our heart pumping. Famed cardiologist Dean Ornish explains,

> I am not aware of any other factor in medicine—not diet, not smoking, not stress, not genetics, not drugs, not surgery—that has a greater impact on our quality of life, incidence of illness and premature death from all causes. . . . Love and intimacy are at the root of what makes us well, what causes sadness and what brings happiness, what makes us suffer and what leads to healing. (1998, pp. 2–3)

Similarly, a huge host of studies link mortality risk to social isolation across a wide range of common illnesses. For example, women with a strong social support network have less than half the risk of mortality from breast cancer as isolated women (Reynolds et al., 1994). In another study, people with limited social contact had a risk of becoming ill 4.2 times that of people with a robust, diverse social network (Cohen, Doyle, Skoner, Rabin, & Gwaltney, 1997). In fact, research like this is becoming so common and critical to the national discussion of health that it has spawned a new field called social medicine.

Hopefully, results like these will assist health and social service providers, educators, and others in taking the first steps to curb known risk factors and, in the same way, promote protective factors for our kids.

Sleep

Sleep occurs in four stages. In the first three, we move from light sleep (N1) to deep sleep (N3), characterized by slow delta waves. REM (rapid eye movement) sleep occurs at the end of the cycle (90 minutes or so into sleep), and increases throughout the night.

The dire physiological importance of sleep is bared in full in studies on sleep deprivation. When sleep deprived, bodily functions begin to slowly shut down. In fact, rats live only a few weeks without sleep, which is about the time they can live without food. Sleep-deprived humans consistently exhibit a number of sickly characteristics: tremors, sore muscles, yawning, bloodshot eyes, and headaches. And, interestingly, the neuroendocrine sequelae of sleep deprivation look identical to the markers for stress or trauma: increased blood pressure and elevated stress hormones.

These changes in stress hormones contribute to cognitive deterioration and toxic effects on growing neurons. Work with redeployed American soldiers in Iraq demonstrates that sleep deprivation predicts vulnerability to post-traumatic stress disorder (PTSD), depression, anxiety, panic, and suicide risk (Luxton et al., 2011). Perhaps this series of effects is ushered in via the vulnerability created by stress hormone abnormalities.

Loss of sleep also creates a wide range of metabolic issues that can lead to obesity and type 2 diabetes. For example, Esra Tasali, of the University of Chicago, took a group of healthy 20-somethings and restructured slow-wave sleep (deep sleep) for three nights. This restructuring triggered a 25% increase in serum glucose, changes typically found with a 30-pound weight gain (Tasali, Leproult, Ehrmann, & Van Cauter, 2008). It may be that sleep issues, a widespread problem in America, account for some proportion of our country's skyrocketing rate of obesity.

At any rate, it's true that many Americans struggle with poor quality sleep or inadequate sleep. About 6% to 10% of Americans, for example, use hypnotic medications like zolpidem to help them sleep. Unfortunately, according to a landmark study published in *BMJ Open*, adults using hypnotic drugs as sleep aids have a threefold increase in the likelihood of early mortality (Kripke, Langer, & Kline, 2012). There was also a reported 35% overall increase in the likelihood of the development of cancer in hypnotics users—an associated risk similar to that of cigarette smoking. This was the 19th epidemiological study to find an elevated mortality risk with the use of hypnotics. Quite simply, people live longer if they sleep without medications.

And they live better if they sleep well. With sleep deprivation it's not uncommon to see confusion, depressed mood, hallucinations, irritability, psychosis, inattention, poor memory, impulsivity, and agitation. Take your pick of psychiatric disorders; they could just be the manifested side effects of sleep deprivation or chronic insomnia. The reasons for this manifestation are tricky to parse out but some evidence helps to put it in context.

Sleep deprivation creates a disconnection between the amygdala and the prefrontal cortex. With a loss of sleep, the amygdala goes into overdrive and shuts down the prefrontal cortex (needed for planning and executive functions). This cascade of effects results in a more primitive, dysfunctional brain that overreacts and can't modulate itself. This, in turn, can set up mood dysregulation, temper tantrums, and other "bipolar" features. In effect, the brain under the duress of sleep deprivation becomes a primal, volatile version of itself.

Kids and Sleep Loss

As we examine childhood sleep loss, the issues turn more purely developmental. According to neurobiology research, profound sleep deprivation in early life can create a lifetime of debility by decreasing brain volume associated with increased neuronal death (Morrissey, Duntley, Anch, & Nonneman, 2004). An infant sleeps 20 hours a day mainly to satisfy the metabolic demands of its growing brain. If these 20 or so hours are disturbed repeatedly, brain volume can be greatly decreased.

Research shows that childhood is characterized by large amounts of slow-wave sleep, which is crucial in consolidating short-term memory and turning it into long-term memory (Born, Rasch, & Gais, 2006). Still other research links sleep efficacy and sleep duration with working memory performance (Gaylor, 2011). Thus, sleep loss early in life can lead to a decrease in the ability to form, consolidate, and recall memories. Given all this, it should come as no surprise that having a consistent bedtime is the single best predictor of a positive developmental outcome (Gaylor, Burnham, Goodlin-Jones, & Anders, 2005).

Sleep loss, interestingly, looks a lot like ADHD. In 6,800 preschool- and kindergarten-aged kids studied, less sleep predicted worse school performance (Fallone, Acebo, Seifer, & Carskadon, 2005). The researchers also noted, "Some children who are not getting adequate sleep may be at risk for developing behavior problems manifested by hyperactivity, impulsivity and problems sitting still and paying attention" (p. 1561). As little as 1 hour of sleep deprivation created school performance issues detectable by blinded teachers in one study (Steenari et al., 2003). In another, sleep loss was associated with the development or exacerbation of symptoms of ADHD (Mahoney, 2011).

The National Sleep Foundation's first and only poll of children revealed that 27% to 50% of infants, toddlers, and school-aged children do not get adequate sleep (2004). More concerning still, 80% to 85% of parents surveyed thought their children's sleep was adequate. We would hope that physicians would identify such a devastating disconnect. Unfortunately, the majority of physicians (52%) never ask about sleep habits.

Television and caffeine look to be major culprits in this epidemic. Research has linked a TV in the bedroom with major sleep loss (as much as 40 minutes per night) that can endure into young adulthood. And 43% of school-aged kids have a TV in their room. Even more astounding, 20% of infants and toddlers have a TV in their room. Similarly, caffeine has been linked to poor sleep patterns: 26% of children 3 to 10 years old drink at least one caffeinated beverage per day, losing at least 1 hour of sleep per night along the way.

It goes without saying that young ones need sleep to grow, function, and thrive. It's easy to see why sleep disorders have been identified as an early indicator of psychiatric pathology across a wide range of disorders. But it's important for much more than that. As Dr. Emmanuel Mignot, director of Stanford Center for Sleep Sciences and Medicine, said, "Sleep restores not only the brain, but the *whole* body, and sleep disorders have important connections with all medicine" (Mignot, 2012; my emphasis).

Engagement: Good for the Body and the Mind

Kids move. Just think: Words like roaming, exploring, dashing, and playing are all synonomous with a joyous childhood. Activity just comes naturally to children. Somewhere deep inside them lurks a natural spark to move.

Yet, the number of obese children has tripled in the last 25 years. And obese children typically become obese and chronically ill adults, a population that suffers from much higher rates of depression and other psychiatric illnesses. The most potent antidote to generational obesity and its concomitant risks is an active lifestyle. Research shows that an active, fit child in an active, fit family is much more likely to become an active, fit adult and raise active, fit children.

Sadly, the fitness levels of both children and adolescents continue to decline (Tomkinson & Olds, 2007). Considering fitness's importance to short- and long-term physical and mental health, this continuing trend should cause serious alarm (Ortega, Ruiz, Castillo, & Sjostrom, 2007; Malina, 1996).

Numerous studies demonstrate that exercise is as effective at treating depression as our best pharmacological tools, suggesting a close tie between fitness and mental health (Craft & Perna, 2004; Kruisdijk, Hendriksen, Tak, Beekman, & Hopman-Rock, 2012). Moreover, exercise in depression appears effective as a stand-alone or as an add-on intervention. The accumulating evidence from prospective cohort studies and randomized controlled trials (RCTs) also tells us that exercise has proven protective benefits for multiple aspects of mental health beyond just depression. Fit kids are less likely to suffer from anxiety and depression, and more likely to perform well in school (Parfitt, Pavey, & Rowlands, 2009; Grissom, 2005; Castelli, Hillman, Buck, & Erwin, 2007). Not only that, fitness improves children's self-esteem (Ekeland, Heian, Hagen, Abbott, & Nordheim, 2004). The accrued benefit of all these factors is, if nothing else, a call to action. The World Health Organization now recommends 60 minutes of moderate to vigorous activity every day for kids ages 6 to 17.

Physical activity, it appears, also increases BDNF levels, which supports enhanced learning and plays an important role in reducing oxidative stress, a likely culprit in a wide range of psychiatric illness such as bipolar disorder and schizophrenia (Gomez-Pinilla, 2011). If BDNF falls at any time during the critical periods of development, it can cause severe impairment to hippocampal-dependent learning and the development of hyperactivity (Monteggia et al., 2004). By the same mechanism, exercise also improves neuronal repair after injurious illness.

The human body, especially the young, growing human body, has been designed to move, and this design has links to physical health, learning, mental health, and perhaps even hyperactivity. Simply put, children who are vigorously active are healthier and smarter—more whole.

Perhaps just as much so as the body, the mind needs to stay active and engaged. And a strong work ethic is the best way to keep a kid's mind active and engaged in the world. When a kid grows up with a poor work ethic, her mind tends to flag: she participates less in the world, tends to be less optimistic, and feels powerless to change her course. These degenerative feelings invariably lead to depression and mental health issues. As a matter of fact, Martin Seligman (2007) believes that a

deteriorating work ethic is the real source of the progressive generational rise in depression since 1900.

For Seligman, when children grow up with a strong work ethic, they
also inherit a positive explanatory style. Explanatory style is a psychological attribute that indicates how people explain a particular event to
themselves. It is typically set by the third grade and shaped by three factors: the mother's explanatory style; the form of criticism given by adults;
and childhood traumas, events, and crises.

According to Seligman's research, those with a negative explanatory
style (i.e., they explain the events of the world in a negative fashion)
have increased vulnerability to depression. And without the aid of a work
ethic and all that it instills—self-efficacy, resilience, self-esteem—they
are hopeless in the fight. They get caught in a vicious cycle. Conversely,
those with a strong work ethic and positive explanatory style are well
protected against the threat of depression.

The core message from Seligman is to instill work ethic and mental
engagement in every child, and in such a way as to maximize a child's internal locus of control. Armed with the knowledge that they can manage
and change their own lives, kids can avoid despair. They can flourish.

Self-Regulation

Forty-plus years ago, a group of eager 4-year-olds were seated at a small
table in a nursery school in Palo Alto. A researcher, Walter Mischel, entered the room and placed a plump white marshmallow on the table in
front of each kid. Mischel told the kids that they could either eat the
marshmallow sitting in front of them now or, if they waited until he returned in 15 minutes, they could have two marshmallows. A few of the
kids gobbled the treat before Mischel even left the room. But about 30%
controlled themselves and waited for the double bonus (Mischel, Ebbesen, & Zeiss, 1972).

This simple, but illustrative, study of self-regulation (sometimes
called self-control or willpower) showed incredible predictive value for
behavioral issues, attentional problems, and even SAT scores over a
decade later (210 points higher in those kids who chose to wait). Followed into midlife, the delayed eaters had significantly better social, cognitive, and mental health outcomes (Mischel et al., 2011). Studies like

Mischel's show us how important it is to build self-regulation in kids if we're to set them up for long-term success. The ability to self-regulate occurs through a few linked developmental processes: healthy emotional maturation, the honing of executive functioning skills, and growth of character.

Emotional Maturation

When we talk about self-regulation, a lot of what we're talking about is emotionality—the ability to manage emotional states. This is not, necessarily speaking, a given. In fact for many kids it's quite difficult. But, thankfully, it is a developmental process that can be supported.

The first step is to encourage proper brain stem development at a young age by paying close attention to healthy food and sleep. This will help prewire the necessary brain circuitry and prepare the child for a healthy attachment.

During attachment, parents act as the template for emotionality. Infants use the parent's interactions with them to organize their own emotions and behaviors. If the parent is attentive and caring, children mirror this internally, which helps them regulate and control their emotional states. In attachment circles this process is called dyadic regulation (Hofer, 1994). Allan Schore (1994) creates an effective distillation of psychoanalysis and neurobiology by explaining how affect regulation between parent and child becomes critical to who we are and who we become.

After the attachment stage ends, social bonds will dictate the remainder of a kid's emotional development. Learning to deftly navigate relationships and mirror peers' emotions—what might be called empathy—is of particular importance. Building these abilities enhances the child's internal locus of emotional control, which bodes well for the kid having a stable emotional life for the reminder of his or her life.

If this early emotional development is in any way impaired—perhaps via poor attachment or poor social bonding—the child is in for a lifetime of dysregulation. Dysregulation, as Dan Siegel (1999) notes, is impairment in the capacity to organize responses to the internal and external environment. Children are scattered and helpless in their attempt to respond to and control emotions. Without an internal locus of emotional control, they become slaves to their emotions.

Dysregulation may be the result of attachment issues, factors in the outer environment (maternal depression, family conflict, marital discord, or abuse), or factors in the inner environment, such as the child's physical health. In dysregulated kids, I commonly see impaired nutrition, metabolic issues, and gut problems. (As we will see in Chapters 8, 9, and 10, the food and gut microbiome relate to brain perfusion, epigenetic changes, nutrient absorption, and risk for psychiatric illness.) The first is usually the result of a nutritional imbalance, micronutrient deficiency, or toxic overload. The second is sometimes mitochondrial impairment, an SNP, or an issue with methylation. And the third is often dysbiosis, food allergies, or food intolerance. These topics are covered in more depth later. Sadly, most of these issues are missed in the race to medicate.

Executive Functioning

The frontal lobes of the brain are the basis of planning, impulse control, problem solving, inhibition, attention, working memory, mental flexibility, and self-awareness—mental faculties known collectively as executive functioning skills. The most critical time of expansion in these skills occurs during the developmental window from ages 3 to 6, when the frontal lobes increase dramatically in size. Effectively, healthy brain development during this period will help a 4-year-old wait and collect the second marshmallow.

Executive functioning skills are naturalistically developed by parenting, family habits, role modeling, and simple practice—especially in that responsive window from ages 3 to 6. Activities encouraging effort, persistence, inhibition, simple planning, self-assessment, and autonomy build and strengthen these neurological pathways. Television and screen time may play a counterproductive role in development.

In fact, Andrew Weil employs the term "mental nutrition" to describe the power of music, media, news, stories, and images to affect our mental and emotional realms. This flow of material creates a powerful and vastly underestimated influence on mental health by supplying a constant source of building blocks for thoughts and emotions. Jung taught us that symbols are one of the core building blocks of the psyche. We create our world by the choices we make, particularly those that pertain to the flow of symbolic content into our consciousness.

Does this mean we should block all television or violent images from children? We can't deny the negative in our world—as much as we try as parents—but we can emphasize the positive. Nowhere is this more crucial than with children, as the flood of material they are exposed to runs the gamut, from uplifting and inspirational to depraved and disgusting. Parents must aggressively manage the content, and we as professionals must provide encouragement and guidance for this kind of active management.

Poor executive functioning skills have a direct correlation with psychiatric illnesses like ADHD, addiction, behavior issues, and eating disorders. You can see evidence of this in the fact that kids with ADHD commonly have very poor executive functioning skills and, as a result, limited ability to self-regulate. And some research has suggested that kids with ADHD have smaller frontal lobes, which further strengthens the connection.

Luckily, the frontal lobes are plastic, and executive functioning skills can be improved with effort. For example, current research demonstrates success in reducing the symptoms of ADHD through the improvement of executive functioning skills (Klingberg et al., 2005). In a recent RCT, notable improvement in verbal working memory, response inhibition, and complex reasoning in children with ADHD occurred after only 20 hours of executive functioning training (Klingberg, 2010). Training, which included computerized challenges for working memory over a 45-minute session, accelerated healthy changes in the frontal cortex, parietal cortex, and basal ganglia (these parts of the brain are used in planning, organization, complex thought, and understanding), as well as in dopamine receptor density. Not surprisingly, the group whose challenge was constantly adjusted upward showed improvement in executive functions while a lower-intensity group did not.

Character Development

In 2007, Angela Lee Duckworth wanted to see if character building could help kids struggling with self-regulation. Previously in her research she had documented that those people with strong character had strong self-regulatory skills, and as a result also had long-term success. So she was curious to see if character building could function as an intervention for struggling kids. She and her research team came up with a list of seven teachable character traits: zest, grit, self-control, social intelligence, gratitude, optimism, and curiosity (Duckworth, Peterson, Mat-thews, & Kelly, 2007). The goal for Duckworth's group was to integrate these skills and, hopefully, thereby reinforce character. (As an aside, Duckworth is a protégé of Martin Seligman and his valuable work on positive psychology.)

So far it appears to be working. The KIPP Academy Schools, the school system in which the teachable traits were first introduced, had the fifth best middle school performance in New York City in 1999: 90% made it into a private or parochial high school; 80% enrolled in college; and 33% graduated from a 4-year college (Duckworth et al., 2007). This flies in the face of the 8% graduation rate among the other low-income schools in the area (Tough, 2001).

Too many of the children I evaluate come in not so much for psychiatric illness per se as for issues of character. Most of the time it's apathy, poor self-esteem, or a lack of motivation. Usually the harder parents try to intervene in a situation like this, the more the child resists and digs in. Trying to medicate kids in these kinds of cases isn't very successful.

Madeline Levine (2006) has an interesting perspective on this phenomenon. In her book *The Price of Privilege*, she contends that parental pressure and material advantage are creating a generation of disconnected and unhappy kids. Levine contends that the combination of distant, distracted parents and an intense pressure to succeed eventually erodes children's character and, as a result, makes them feel shame and hopelessness.

Character needs to be reinforced and deficits made up for. Think about what might be holding a kid's character back—fear, self-esteem, morale, parental pressure—and treat it as proactively as if it were an affecting disorder. Social-emotional education, such as the Discovery Program outlined in Chapter 11, can be helpful in this regard, as can psychotherapy, perhaps focused on developing Duckworth's seven traits.

Spirituality

For most of human history, health care has been wedded to spirituality. Hospital care, as a matter of fact, was a religious byproduct. In 370 c.e., the bishop of Caesarea, Saint Basil the Great, founded the first major hospital in Western civilization. Inside, physical and mental maladies were treated with the same remedies, as they were thought of as divergent effects of the same cause—spiritual neglect. Hospitals, first and foremost, were houses of spiritual affliction.

Today, we see only a vestige of spirituality left in medicine. Only a handful of medical schools still include spirituality in their curriculums, for instance. But the secular split of health care was never completely decisive. Many hospitals and hospital systems still retain their religous foundation, and integrative medicine, for one, embraces the essential spiritual nature of humanity in the very foundation of health.

Despite the secular predominance of health care, polls consistently indicate that the majority of Americans would like their caregivers to explore the spiritual aspects of their illness (Ehman, Ott, Short, Ciampa, & Hansen-Flaschen, 1999). For that reason, medical educators and researchers have begun to recommend that physicians ask about spirituality or religion when conducting a medical history. And, since 90% of patients believe that prayer sometimes influences recovery from an illness, doctors might do well to employ prayer when appropriate (Ehman et al., 1999).

Increasingly, the literature demonstrates the positive impact of religious engagement and prayer on physical and mental health, in particular substance abuse (Miller & Thoresen, 2003). Harold Koenig, director of the Duke Center for Spirituality, Theology and Health, has published extensively on the topic. His seminal text *Handbook for Religion and Health* documents the vast and growing research on the physical and mental benefits of spiritual engagement (Koenig, 2012).

Dave

A few years out of high school, Dave worked for a large home improvement store in the cabinet department. But the word "worked" can only be used loosely. Going on 6 years, Dave had been suffering from chronic severe depression. Unmotivated and lethargic, he rarely felt well enough to attend to a task or help customers. Medication trials, including 11 different antidepressants and three different antipsychotics, had failed to lift the weight of his heavy mood; thoughts of suicide swam through him constantly.

In our first visit together, Dave wore a Denver Broncos hat pulled low over his eyebrows, obstructing his placid eyes as he looked down and ruminated endlessly over his "worthless life." Tall and long-limbed, Dave moved with unexpected grace, slowly but very carefully—measuring each step and gesture. He immediately struck me as kind and gentle.

Dave was hopelessly alienated from his family. Deep down, he felt he would commit suicide; that it was the only choice left. Depression had finally enveloped his hope. Writer William Styron, himself a sufferer of depression, said that "it is hopelessness even more than pain that crushes the soul" (1992, p. 62). Dave's soul was crushed; he was hopeless, desperate.

Yet another medication trial seemed unlikely to lead Dave out of his darkness. So after a few sessions my intuition led me in an unusual direction. At the next session, I sat down with Dave and told him to flesh out his spirituality. He was caught off guard. I had no specific directions or referral. I simply encouraged him to evaluate and define his own spiritual beliefs.

Obviously this was not a structured treatment, but I could sense that if Dave needed anything it was to connect with something bigger, something that might frame or put his pain in perspective. Often, those suffering from chronic illness become hyperfocused on their pain, and in the process become estranged from their spirit and personal essence of life. Reconnecting with whatever that is—be it religious, philosophical, or social—usually helps recover hope and a sense of purpose.

Dave returned a few weeks later with a much different perspective. He walked into my office, took off his cap, looked me in the eyes confidently, and said he had explored his own spirituality and then met with a spiritual healer, had a few powerful insights, and no longer "needed" his depression. His voice was firm and clear. He also abruptly stopped all his medications in a personal act of defiance. He had, in effect, done it all alone—without agents, without therapy. Through the simple but mysterious act of revisiting his spirituality, Dave altered what some would call "immovable brain chemistry." His new spiritual framework elevated his perspective and also his mood.

Now, 14 years later, we enjoy a yearly visit to update and share. Dave functions well without medication and there remains no hint of his earlier darkness.

Dave's story crystallizes the power of the spirit in mental health. True, it is anecdotal. But that brings up a question worth answering: Is a sense of spirituality beneficial to everyone's mental health?

Yes, it appears spiritual engagement is beneficial to nearly all people. Of 115 articles reviewed in one meta-analysis, 92% showed a strong link between religious or spiritual engagement and better physical and mental health (Dew et al., 2008). This association was strongest in substance abusers but remained steady across all age groups, with clear benefits for adolescents. Further research indicates that the benefits for kids are separate from the external benefits of parental, familial, and community engagement (Mabe & Josephson, 2004), which suggests that some internal mechanism is at work here. This raises the question, how exactly does spirituality support mental health?

It does so by advancing a sense of meaning and purpose. With a strong sense of meaning, a kid is better able to rise above difficult circumstances and process stressful events. A purpose in life helps a young kid set goals; it contextualizes setbacks and pain, as well as successes. Armed with these values, a child experiences less mental anguish, less despair. The child is better equipped to weather the harsh realities of the world. This is more than a medical hunch. Research shows that kids with a strong sense of meaning and purpose have an enhanced quality of life and health, and even live longer (Eriksson & Lindstrom, 2007). Just think of the protective benefits Dave might have enjoyed had he discovered his spirituality sooner.

Spirituality is usually opened up by religious involvement, but not always. Some people prefer to explore their spirituality without religion as a guide. Most kids adopt their spirituality right from their parents. A child who grows up with religious parents will, most of the time, follow suit as he grow up, even if his spirituality eventually takes another form than his parents'. For our purposes, the form of spirituality or religion doesn't seem to be of any real consequence, as long as it reinforces the value of discovering meaning and purpose in life, which most religious traditions and philosophical paradigms do reinforce. Unfortunately, the truth of the matter is that many parents don't have a sense of spirituality in their life. In these cases it is the child we're principally concerned with, because under these conditions the child does not reap the protective benefits of having a well-ingrained sense of meaning or purpose.

Role modeling is the most effective means of instilling spirituality or an independent sense of meaning and purpose in a young kid, so think about mentorship programs if you have identified someone in need. These programs are extremely effective. A school-based social-emotional education program may also be valuable, as it integrates these skills into a viable curriculum without entering into a denominational discussion. Spiritual engagement as found through formal religion can play an important role in this process.

Spirituality makes sure the child is held up by more than just herself. It creates an existential scaffolding that weathers stress and adversity. And that, in so many words, is why spirituality is a core building block of wholeness.

Family

In 1997, the landmark Harvard Master of Stress Study followed 398 Harvard students over 35 years and explored a variety of risk factors, carefully monitoring health and illness for each participant over the duration of the study. Surprisingly, the rating students gave to their sense of parental closeness when they entered the study 35 years earlier turned out to be the single best predictor of illness and health later in life (Russek & Schwartz, 1997). Of those who rated their relationship with their mother and father as highly caring and close, only 25% had chronic illness. Among those who rated their relationship as distant and conflicted, 87% suffered from chronic illness.

Family is the crucible that molds, forms, and sets in place much of what a person is and will be. Not only does family life shape health and social skills, but it also turns out to be the single most powerful determinant of mental health throughout life. Positive or negative, it's vital for a practitioner to find out about a patient's family history. I take special care to ask about the child's relationships with the mother and father, paying close attention to the affect and behavior of the responses. The simple act of asking routine questions about a patient's family can often dredge up many previously unknown or overlooked factors. And if you find something that warrants attention, don't be afraid to suggest family therapy.

To my mind, family therapy is the best, least appreciated treatment model in psychiatry. It has been shown to be effective either alone or as part of multimodel programs for sleep, feeding, attachment, child abuse, child neglect, conduct difficulties (including behavioral issues, ADHD, delinquency, and drug abuse), emotional problems (including anxiety, depression, grief, bipolar, and suicidality), eating disorders, and somatic problems (including chronic pain, diabetes, asthma, and encopresis) (Carr, 2009). Obviously, there is no shared pathophysiology here. Treatment by family therapy is the only connection between them.

And yet it goes largely unused. This is the case for a few reasons. First, it is hard to do well. It's hard with all those people and histories and competing interests in the same room. And most therapists have only the briefest of exposures to it in training. So, naturally, when it's time to start a practice, they drift back to what they know best: seeing individuals. Second, while child psychiatry and family therapy used to be closely linked (Bowen, Minuchin, Whitaker, and Ackerman were all child psychiatrists), the two fields have drifted apart in the neurochemical era (circa 1970 on). Three, parents often prefer to isolate and treat the identified patient—it is less threatening to both the parents and the family unit. And often, individual therapy is just more convenient. There's also the fact that in the typical psychiatric evaluation, family dynamics are often totally overlooked.

At the core of family dynamics is the state of the marriage. If the marriage is functional, assessment and treatment are much easier. On the other hand, if the parents have divorced or if the marriage is strained, everything is much more complicated, both for the child and for the practitioner. The research in this area is clear-cut: Children who suffer through a divorce have worse outcomes across a wide range of health and well-being measures. Judith Wallenstein and many others have well documented the long-term damage. Based on my experience and research, a continuing high-conflict divorce is a greater negative prognostic measure than even the death of a parent. When I encounter a high-conflict divorce, I spend more of my time playing politics than treating the child. Therefore, I typically start the treatment process by giving the parents a harsh but realistic view of how their personal battle harms the child. Only then do I try to inspire a collaborative process between the warring parties.

Because they are the principle agents of the child, parents frame the treatment concerns. And just as personal needs drive many features of parenting, they also color the concerns that bring a child into treatment. That being the case, whenever parents bring a child to be evaluated, a few questions spring up in my head. Why are they coming in now, not last month or last year? Does the child recognize a problem? Does he or she really want help? How do the parents differ in their perception of the problem? How do each parent's personal issues color their view of the problem? What tensions and conflicts in the home have been created or amplified as a result of this problem? What is each person's individual goal for the treatment? Occasionally, some more knotty questions arise: Does this symptom pattern benefit the family or parents in any way? Is there anything in the family that perpetuates this symptom pattern?

Basically, ponder the timing and think about who initiated the process and why. Often what is relevant is not why they are here now, but why they weren't here 2 months ago. With internalized disorders like depression, anxiety, thought disorders, or even PTSD, symptoms can go unnoticed for a long period of time. Sometimes this is because a parent's own issues—depression, divorce, substance abuse, or chronic stress—delay or even prevent recognition of the child's suffering.

The opposite also occurs, when a parent touches off an overreactive treatment. A competitive and ambitious parent becomes convinced that ADHD holds her daughter back from full achievement, and so she demands medication. Sadly, given the very subjective nature of the diagnostic criteria in psychiatry, she will easily locate a psychiatrist or physician willing to medicate her daughter. The problem here is that the issues spurring treatment are never fleshed out. And so a young girl who was perhaps just defying her mother's overzealous demands or simply achieving to the best of her abilities is labeled as ADHD and put on strong medication.

The truth of the matter is that sometimes you have to talk parents into medication and sometimes you have to talk them out of it. Sometimes you need to call attention to the child's suffering; sometimes you need to minimize the child's issue. Often, especially with divorced parents, you have to mediate a shared appreciation of the child's problem, an understanding that backs parents off from reactionary opposition. Whatever it may mean, a thorough investigation and deft navigation of the familial and parental minutiae is necessary.

And to be frank, after all that, addressing and treating the child's issues is sometimes the easier part of this job.

CHAPTER THREE
Barriers to Wholeness

Many times, a comprehensive assessment will reveal barriers to health. Any factor limiting or blocking a child's achievement of health and wellness remains a barrier until overcome. Barriers block health by disrupting self-regulation, harmony, interconnectivity, balance, and the path to wholeness. Once removed, the natural progress toward wholeness resumes unabated.

Barriers can exist on all levels of the child's ecosystem. Barriers can mean an excess in one area (lead toxicity, caffeine, violence) or a deficiency in another (magnesium, sleep, affection). Barriers can be external (bullying) or internal (self-criticism). Barriers can be obvious (obesity) or hidden (food allergies). They can be developmental (early neglect, abuse) or genetic (single-nucleotide polymorphism of the methylenetetrahydrofolate reductase pathway). The barrier can be imposed by the parents (lack of limit setting) or by school (poor fit for learning style). Barriers can be easy to correct (protein-rich diet) or inordinately complex (family dynamics). Whatever the nature of a barrier's composition and makeup, understanding it means understanding the child. And, frankly, there is no shortcut.

The essential logic of wholeness and the building blocks of health reviewed in Chapter 2 dictate that we investigate and address barriers as a first step in treatment. Does it really make sense to diagnose psychopathology and medicate a child's more obvious symptoms if major, albeit hidden barriers to health still exist?

Most of the barriers that we work with are well known as risk factors, but we tend to downplay them or at times ignore them as professionals. "Well, that child has a horrible diet, is quite overweight, drinks a few liters of Mountain Dew daily, plays 5 hours of Halo each day, and fights incessantly with his parents, but I will focus on treating the depression with medication or individual psychotherapy." It may make the most sense to begin a more zealous treatment of those barriers first to magnify the benefits of any evidence-based approach later.

I see a number of common barriers in my practice that shout for attention. First is my list of what I call seven ecological disasters. These are barriers to wholeness that we commonly see in practice and have been well documented to deteriorate a child's mental health. I list them below in no particular order:

1. Poor nutrition/standard American diet
2. Obesity and lack of fitness
3. Poor fit with learning style and school environment
4. Overstimulation by media and video games/poor sleep
5. Parent-child issues of fit
6. Maternal depression (or, more broadly, parental mental health issues)
7. Divorce

All of these are barriers to wholeness and good mental health. This does not mean that no child of divorce will find happiness or good mental health; it just means it has become harder and will require more work and attention. In my current practice, the typical patient will have two or more of these risk factors. These are big problems that should be acknowledged and addressed by each practitioner to support the return to wholeness. Obviously there are more.

One of the most broad and concerning barriers lies in the umbrella term *stress*. I feel that this issue is so crucial to our modern situation that it merits further discussion. Stress and its analogues—trauma, neglect, abuse, and others—are major barriers to health. In some form or other, all people during their lives will experience some degree of them. Unfortunately, the presentations of stress are often largely concealed, kept out of sight, or else camouflaged as some other malady. Trauma in a child, for example, can masquerade as any psychiatric diagnosis, even psychosis.

All things considered, stress is perhaps the most common issue we face as mental health practitioners. Whether it's bullying or trauma or familial turmoil, a lot of things can stress out a little kid's nervous system and lead to all sorts of psychological and biological issues (see Chapter 16 for a longer discussion of trauma and PTSD). That's why it's so important to have a firm understanding of both the biological and psychological effects of stress and how they manifest in the child. In the following pages I describe stress in greater detail—its genesis, body-wide processes, and forms—so that you can better help your kids tackle this barrier to health and once again return to wholeness.

Stress

We all talk about the stress of our jobs, responsibilities, and chaotic lifestyles. It has become such a widely used and applied term, in fact, that it is tough to know what we mean exactly when we use the word *stress*. It functions as a noun, verb, adjective, a process, and even a trend. It is tension, worry, difficulty, pressure, strain—really, any feeling of burden.

The universal utility of the word does not, however, degrade its experience. The suffering is very real. Whatever the meaning ascribed to it, polls consistently document that about 35–40% of Americans experience high levels of self-reported stress. Not surprisingly, parents are the most stressed demographic, with almost 50% reporting high levels of stress. But adolescents and teens are also highly stressed. So it is clear that in one form or another we are all suffering from stress. But what exactly is it?

The word *stress* first entered the human discussion in 1926 when Walter Cannon, a professor at Harvard, used it to describe adverse events that reduced homeostasis. He published his influential book, *The Wisdom of the Body*, in 1932, outlining the self-regulating power of the body's internal chemistry (Cannon, 1963). Hans Selye later built on Cannon's ideas with the general adaptation response, a description of how hormonal responses from the adrenal glands create the natural bodily responses of rest, alarm, resistance, and exhaustion.

Selye identified the hypothalamic-pituitary-adrenal axis as the provenance of stress response. Selye then localized the identification of chronic stress to the adrenal glands. The adrenal glands produce epinephrine and cortisol, two of the hormones responsible for the "fight or flight" response, a term coined by Cannon in 1915. And with this, stress had a name, a function, and a genesis.

Recently, research on stress has moved into a new, novel arena. Scientists are now studying the connections between psychology and the stress response system, including the nervous and immune systems. Much of this work comes out of Ader and Cohen's research while at the

University of Rochester in the 1970s, where they demonstrated the ways in which the immune system could be classically conditioned. In 1981, in the groundbreaking book *Psycho-Neuro-Immunology*, these scientists posited the essential unity of the immune and nervous systems as a single responsive unit of defense (Ader, Felten, & Cohen, 2000). By 1985, National Institutes of Health researcher Candace Pert and her colleagues clarified the links between the two systems by demonstrating the connectivity of emotion, the endocrine system, and neuropeptides (Ruff, Schiffmann, Terranova, & Pert, 1985).

This is why, for example, so many elderly widows and widowers die within the first few months of losing their spouse. The obvious cognitive and emotional responses create abnormalities in the sympathetic nervous system and immune system. Ultimately, this deteriorates the immune response, leading to increased rates of infection, cancer, and premature death from a variety of triggers. In great detail, and with great precision, these studies describe the interwoven fabric of life, the ways in which the body and mind work as one to give balance and order to life. The term psycho-neuro-immunology, by its very composition, highlights the absurdity of the notion of a split between mind and body.

The Mind and Stress

The work of Selye and others firmly established the biological foundations of stress. And by the 1960s, the mental origins of stress became fertile ground for research. In his landmark book *Psychological Stress and the Coping Process*, Richard Lazarus (1966) argued that the cognitive appraisal of stress determined its effect. If a person felt he or she had the resources to manage a stressor, the impacts were minimal. However, if someone felt he or she did not have the ability to manage a given situation and its stress, the event became much more stressful and arduous.

Next, observations about people who seemed better able to manage stress grew into theories about stress resilience. This, in turn, led to research studies about specific personality types that seemed resilient to the toxic effects of stressful events. That thinking, however, was incomplete; personality alone could not account for resilience. Researchers quickly realized that the ability to withstand or recover quickly from difficult conditions had a lot to do with the difficulty of the given situation.

Thus, whereas resilience was previously thought of as a personality trait like those found in E. J. Anthony's (1987) *The Invulnerable Child*, increasingly it came to be thought of as a process in the balance between risk factors and protective factors. The field now supports a more nuanced view, reflecting the ecological perspective of Uri Bronfenbrenner (1979), that incorporates a wide range of protective factors that both promote wellness and protect against risk.

And for good reason: This view is more progressive, more holistic. It is the narrow psychological perspective of personality transformed into a more systems-based view of a child's interaction within an ecosystem. In this model, stress is the interaction of several factors, both internal and external, rather than just the internal state of strain resulting from a situation. And it's not that particular people are simply resilient to stress innately and others are not. It's that there is a fluid spectrum of stress response based on the nature of the stressor and the person undergoing the stress.

Henry and his story of resiliency in the face of incapacitating adversity illustrates the nature of this spectrum and how various factors beyond personality type influence stress response. E. E. Werner began to explore factors of resiliency in kids like Henry in the 1960s and 1970s. She followed a cohort of severely disadvantaged children on the Hawaiian island of Kauai starting in 1955 (Werner, 1992). Most of the children in her study exhibited maladaptive behaviors in response to their environmental challenges, including depression, substance abuse, chronic unemployment, and delinquency.

However, about one-third of these kids rose above all of it and developed into capable and caring adults. Werner and others identified a number of factors (internal and external) that seemed to support resiliency in youth: self-confidence, positive role models, caring relationships, personal agency, and a spiritual sense of the world. Most kids can benefit from such support, and for some it will make all the difference in the world.

Suzanne Kobasa and Salvatore Maddi suggested that personality can be tweaked to help people remain healthy and capable, or "hardy," under stress (Kobasa, Maddi, & Courington, 1981). Hardiness training helps people buffer themselves against the debilitating effects of stressful situations. And whereas resiliency is primarily an assessment of mental, emotional, and social factors, hardiness looks at the whole of health. Physical fitness, for example, plays a large role in protecting against stress, according to these thinkers.

Stress, in every form, deteriorates physical and mental health. That's why the focus of both hardiness and resiliency is to identify factors, internal and external, that enable individuals to digest and metabolize the stress in their lives. What happens in the process is that individuals engage more thoroughly in life and take responsibility for their choices. Consequently, the lessons of resiliency and hardiness make them more positive and able to problem solve in the face of adversity.

Spirituality and Stress

Just after his release from a Nazi concentration camp, where he lost his wife, brother, and parents, Austrian psychiatrist Viktor Frankl developed logotherapy. Rather than power (as Adler thought) or pleasure (as Freud thought), Frankl asserted that striving to find meaning in one's life was the primary motivating force in humans. Logotherapy is based on this principle. Frankl felt that with the help of spirituality, which gives humans meaning and purpose in life, any number of stressors could be endured and any degree of hardship overcome.

He outlined his theories in the seminal book first published in 1959, *Man's Search for Meaning* (Frankl, 1997). In these insightful pages, he shows us how to move out of the mental traps that bind us to stress and pain and how to step into a more sustaining spiritual view of life. In one of his more poignant passages about life in the concentration camp, he wrote,

> If a prisoner felt that he could no longer endure the realities of camp life, he found a way out in his mental life—an invaluable opportunity to dwell in the spiritual domain, the one that the SS were unable to destroy. Spiritual life strengthened the prisoner, helped him adapt and thereby improved his chances of survival. (Frankl, 1997, p. 13)

As well as anyone in modern times, Frankl has given us a path to escape stress and pain. But these are not just adult lessons; Frankl's vision of spirituality can be applied to kids. In fact, I find that supporting the development of a spiritual framework is often a very helpful measure in protecting kids against the stressors of life.

Often, a family's sense of spirituality, whatever it may be, provides a belief system for children, helping them to process stress and pain. Sometimes children modify this religious belief system to create a personalized spiritual framework. Young people may create a unique and individualized spiritual scaffolding as they enter adulthood. Spirit, regardless of form or structure, helps process the various pressures, strains, and hassles of life; it puts them in perspective and imbues them with meaning (or not). For kids, spiritual beliefs help digest the stress of high school, make sense of the death of a friend, or work through a divorce. In this way, spirit, as Frankl and others have noted, is a powerful buffer of stress for every child.

Salutogenesis

In the 1970s, Aaron Antonovsky, a medical sociologist, began to explore the concept of stress in a different way. He studied the factors that contributed to health and well-being rather than the factors that led to the development of disease. He coined a term, *salutogenesis*, which in its Greek origins means "origins of health," to describe the ongoing process of health and well-being.

His concept grew largely from observations about the nature of stress. Antonovsky noticed that while all people experience stress consistently throughout life, only a small number of people experience illness or disease as a result, even under the duress of extremely high stress. Most people and most children adapt and maintain good health in spite of the myriad stressors they undergo on a daily basis. For Antonovsky, this fact reflects the innate human drive to maintain wholeness.

In the salutogenesis paradigm, a sense of coherence supports wholeness and is built from three main components:

1. Comprehensibility: Life is orderly and understandable.
2. Manageability: Confidence that one has the resources needed to take on the stress of life.
3. Meaningfulness: Life has purpose and some greater significance or message.

According to Antonovsky, the earlier people are armed with these three skills, the more functional they will be throughout life. There is no curriculum for this process; however, this broad perspective informs how we care for children, educate them, and most of all how we practice.

Children's Stress Index

The Holmes-Rahe scale was developed in 1967 in an attempt to quantify stressful life events for adults. It is built on four central concepts:

1. Significant life events, both positive and negative, cause stress, although the latter generate more stress (for most individuals).
2. Some life events trigger more stress than others.
3. Stress accumulates and is additive (see glossary entry on allostatic load).
4. The more stress a person experiences, the more likely that the person will become ill.

A wide variety of research supports the idea that stressful life events can trigger medical and psychiatric illness. Depressed teenagers, for example, have significantly more stressful life events prior to the onset of a depressive episode compared to normal control children (Williamson et al., 1998). The correlation between parent and child was between 0.81 and 0.73 for overall comparison (Williamson et al., 1998).

Unfortunately, the Holmes-Rahe scale does not quantify or qualify stressors specific to children. The Wholeness Stress Index that follows, then, is my best attempt to quantify stressful events in children and teens based on my experience, the Holmes-Rahe scale, and the available research. The goal is that the Wholeness Stress Index will help you better gauge the overall burden of stress and the areas of the child's life that need attention and reinforcement.

Instructions and Comments

1. Identify all events applicable to the child in the last year—regardless of perceived level of severity or related stress—and tally up the corresponding stress points. Add them together to reach a total for the

year. (Please be careful to consider that while some events like physical abuse or parental divorce may not have occurred within the last calendar year, it's likely that they still contribute to the child's stress. Thus add those relevant points.)

2. Stress rating (based on Holmes-Rahe): anything under 100 is low stress; 101–200 is moderate stress; 201–300 is high stress; over 301 is extreme.

3. As a general scale, this provides some rough indication of likelihood of physical, mental, or emotional symptoms requiring treatment.

4. A child with factors of resilience, hardiness, a sense of coherence, or spiritual foundation will fare better at digesting stress, at any level.

5. For symptomatic children, addressing the issues relevant on the scale will support recovery and the movement to wholeness.

Issues

1. Family vacation: 15
2. Graduation from junior high or middle school: 17
3. Conflict with teacher: 23
4. Applications to college: 24
5. Loss of a pet: 24–44 (based on how close the child was to the pet)
6. Move to new town or school: 25
7. Move to new home: 27
8. Highly competitive sport: 29
9. Excess TV or video games: 30
10. Violence or sexuality not suited to age: 31
11. No breakfast or high-glycemic breakfast: 31
12. Substance use or experimentation: 32
13. New family member: 32
14. New romance: 33
15. Inadequate sleep: 34
16. Soda, fast-food, and junk food diet: 37
17. Aggressive, demanding curriculum: 38
18. Behavioral issues at school: 38
19. Overscheduled: 39
20. Learning disability: 45
21. Graduation from high school: 46
22. Sick family member: 47

23. Breakup with girlfriend or boyfriend: 47
24. School performance issues: 49
25. Loss of parental income or job: 52
26. Depressed dad: 52
27. Overly critical parents: 53
28. Sibling with developmental disorder: 53
29. Bullied frequently: 55
30. Trouble with the law: 58
31. Obesity: 59
32. Family poverty: 60
33. Substance abuse, significant: 63
34. Alcoholic parent (active): 65
35. Death of sibling: 65
36. High-conflict family: 66
37. Sexual identity or preference issues: 67
38. Chronic illness: 68
39. Divorce (cooperative): 70
40. Depressed mom: 82
41. Unwanted pregnancy: 86
42. Divorce (moderate conflict): 93
43. Death of a parent (ever): 100
44. High-conflict divorce or custody battle (ever): 119
45. History of physical or sexual abuse (ever): 132

The average American child is much more stressed and traumatized than we suspect. Even "normal" stress levels of daily events and demands may be enough to overload the neuroendocrine system for many of our children. Hopefully this list of potential stressors will help all of us to consider the ever-present allostatic load of stress that burdens all of our children. Once appreciated, we can begin to manage and address the related issues that may direct a lifetime of symptoms or illnesses.

CHAPTER FOUR

The Potential of the Child

In beginning to shift our focus to wholeness, we must first recognize the potential of every child to heal and change. Current research in neural plasticity and epigenetics helps us to do just that. From these emerging disciplines we get a glimpse of a changing, dynamic brain and a system of heredity that is responsive and adaptive. This new research not only provides us with cutting-edge tools of science to heal and improve our brains and bodies—it gives us hope to heal.

The Good News of Neuroplasticity

The adult human brain stands as the most complex system in the known universe. It contains around 100 billion neurons arranged in complex networks of interconnected webs. Each individual neuron averages about 10,000 different dendritic connections to other neurons. That means that the average brain establishes more connections than the number of stars contained in 1,500 Milky Way galaxies. The density of the brain can overwhelm attempts to grasp: One thimble full of neuronal tissue contains 50 million neurons, several hundred miles of axons, close to a trillion (a million million) synapses, and a terabyte of data storage. And research at Stanford University suggests that each synaptic connection holds around 1,000 molecular-scale switches (chemical sites capable of turning from on to off based on an outside signal) (Micheva, Busse, Weiler, O'Rourke, & Smith, 2010). The implication of this vast web of information intimidates even the most hardened scientist. It means that the person sitting next to you has more information processing capacity than all of the computers, routers, and Internet connections being used in the world today—combined. These researchers, confounded by their own discovery, were humbled, quietly concluding that the brain's complexity "is beyond anything imagined."

As a thought experiment, imagine a system still more complex. Try to picture a system twice the size, with a much more rapid ability to encode and process data as it speeds through its myriad networks. This system would also have a unique ability to quickly regenerate, adapt, and change form. This sprawling, plastic network operating at breakneck speeds would be without parallel in the known universe in terms of sheer complexity and processing capability. Fittingly, this system would exactly resemble the average 6-year-old's brain.

Beyond measures of size, complexity, and speed, a child's brain also grows at an astonishing rate. It forms 3 billion new synaptic connections per second. And the growth only continues as the child ages, quadrupling in size from birth to age 10. Rate of neural growth, as research shows, is the single best measure of learning capacity. An infant sleeps sometimes 20 hours a day just to keep this system and its metabolic demands in check.

The understanding of the brain 30 years ago was that this growth and molding only took place in early childhood, and after this brief period of development the brain's neurons and neural networks became fixed and rigid. Neurons could be lost, but never again gained. According to this view, the brain's development was finite. In other words, we're stuck with what we got by the end of childhood.

In the 1980s and 1990s, however, a number of groundbreaking experiments showed that the brain, at all ages, continues to change in structure and circuitry. This new understanding of fundamental brain properties was dubbed neural plasticity. This idea, revolutionary 30 years ago, now dominates the core direction and philosophy of neuroscience.

This is good news for mental health. It means that the "hardwiring" of the brain's executive faculties—memory, focus, processing—is indeed pliable, that those suffering from functional deficits can improve with effort. New studies of meditation, in fact, indicate that with 3 months of practice, significant improvements in the brain's ability to attend to tasks and process new information can occur. Findings of this nature promise to transform treatment of ADHD. Toke Klingberg and his associates (2005) at the Karolinska Institute in Sweden have published a series of articles demonstrating rapid improvements in executive function skills through simple but effective training exercises enhancing memory and inhibitory control in kids, both common difficulties in ADHD. They found that in children with ADHD, working memory and inhibitory control could be improved with only 25–40 minutes of training a day for 5 weeks (Klingberg et al., 2005).

These are not trivial gains. These are core changes in brain function. From research like this we're beginning to understand how the brain improves its circuitry and thickness as it tackles new tasks and difficulties. And this is particularly important for struggling young kids, as it means that they are not always stuck with the mental abilities—and disabilities—they were born with, as Norman Doidge (2007) explains in his book *The Brain That Changes Itself*.

"Certain mental characteristics that were previously regarded as relatively fixed can actually be changed by mental training," famed psychologist Richie Davidson wrote. "People know that physical exercise can improve the body, but our research and that of others holds out the promise that mental exercise can improve minds" (Slagter et al., 2007, 138). The more we test, the more potential we continue to uncover about the brain's ability to rewire, rethink, and recover.

This new understanding begs a basic question about mental health: Should we try to improve minds or simply medicate shortcomings? Given the brain's enormous potential for growth and its capacity to learn and relearn, psychiatry might consider revising, say, its approach to treating ADHD. Currently, we diagnose children, place them on rather potent controlled substances, and treat them symptomatically. With the insights of neural plasticity, however, and our better understanding of the developing brain, schools might integrate attentional and other cognitive exercises to strengthen positive adaptation. This much is clear—the earlier these tools are implemented and reinforced in young brains, the larger the gains: less suffering, less economic toll, less educational disruption.

In psychiatry today, our treatment model hinges on the presumption that a fixed chemical imbalance in the brain creates mental illness. But what happens if that presumption is wrong? What if brain chemistry is not fixed but in fact changeable? How can we move forward? We can move forward by integrating the good news of neural plasticity into our understanding of a kid's potential to heal.

Medicated and Unmedicated Brain Change

In 1992, researchers published the first of many studies showing that both medication and psychotherapy altered the caudate nucleus in patients with obsessive-compulsive disorder (OCD) (Baxter et al., 1992). This confirmed the long-held suspicion that psychiatric treatments (talk therapy and medications) change the human brain. The research demonstrated the remarkable powers of medication and psychotherapy to not only perturb normal brain function—as we long knew medication did—but also help the brain compensate for challenging conditions. New tools like single photon emission CT (SPECT), positron-emission tomography (PET), and functional magnetic resonance imaging (MRI) have opened a remarkable window into the living, changing brain. These tools reveal that the very personal experience of psychotherapy indeed alters neuronal structure, remodeling the nervous system at a cellular and molecular level. The researchers concluded that psychotherapy functions as neuro-rehabilitation.

In fact, a variety of psychotherapy techniques—cognitive-behavioral therapy, dialectical-behavioral therapy, psychodynamic psychotherapy, and interpersonal psychotherapy—have been shown to alter brain function significantly in patients diagnosed with a number of disorders, including MDD, OCD, panic disorder, social anxiety, phobias, PTSD, and borderline personality disorder. These therapies share little in philosophy or technique and the diagnostic groups share even less in terms of *DSM* criteria, indicating that a number of psychotherapy protocols can be effective for a range of disorders. This phenomenon seems to hold true for medication therapy as well; antipsychotic medications, for example, are used to treat a number of illnesses. Thus, matching a specific treatment to a specific diagnosis seems somewhat unnecessary, as most illnesses respond to most therapies.

The implication here is that diagnosis and specific technique may not be as critical to treatment as conventional psychiatry would have us believe. Instead, nonspecific factors, like patient-physician relationship or the patient's preference or belief in the treatment, might be of much higher value. If many different therapies alter the brain function of any number of patients suffering from a variety of illnesses, as the research demonstrates, then the individual matching of patient to preferred treatment becomes vital in successful care.

Unlike medicated brain change, however, psychotherapeutic brain change appears to have no potential for adverse consequences. And since a number of patients either don't respond or respond negatively to medication, it's within reason that medicated brain effects are not limited simply to correctly diagnosed patients. Adverse side effects occur in all populations even in healthy control groups or misdiagnosed patients. How much of this response is due to negative placebo response is difficult to measure.

Since 2002, placebo—psychiatry's contentious bedfellow—has routinely been shown to create effective brain change, which suggests that the placebo effect is not only psychological in benefit but also deeply neurological. Helen Mayberg and her associates (2002) studied a group of men with major depression by periodic PET scans of their brains before and after treatment. In this double-blind study, half of the men received fluoxetine, an SSRI antidepressant, while the other half received placebo. An equal percentage of men in both groups responded with remission of their depression. Of those in remission, control and experimental groups showed matching improvement in brain activity. PET scans showed ameliorative effects in cortical (increased activity) and limbic (decreased activity) regions of men in both groups. This experiment has been repeated with similar results.

The implication of this documented effect for both clinical and experimental work is tremendous. It means that any practical employment of medication (correctly diagnosed or otherwise) or psychotherapy must be counted on to alter brain function in some way. Any treatment plan that fails to acknowledge or plan for this effect might need to be revisited.

Epigenetics and the "Biology" of Mental Illness

Each ensuing decade leaves us with a deeper appreciation for the profound intelligence of the human body. In the last few decades, modern science has turned its attention away from a rigid, fixed perspective of human development to glimpse, finally, the fluid, responsive body brimming with its own potential to change and adapt. The old perspective of the central nervous system as physiologically hardwired has now given way to a more integrated vision of how love, culture, environment, learning, physical and mental health, therapy, and family all interface with and change the plastic brain. In the same way, the fundamentals of genetic inertia also seem to be waning. Watson and Crick's inelastic model of inheritance and expression must, at last, reorganize itself to fully consider the new novel insights of epigenetics.

By definition, epigenetics is the study of heritable changes in gene expression by means other than changes in DNA sequence. Basically, the DNA in our cells directs the production of protein, which in turn determines what the cell does. Epigenetics now informs us that this cellular machinery (that constructs our neurotransmitters, for example) responds to a variety of outside signals that can alter production or stop it. This means that nongenetic factors (say, environmental, neuroendocrine, emotional, or nutritional) cause genes to express themselves in a variety of ways. This responsiveness makes perfect sense for survival in a Darwinian paradigm, because it supports the idea that our biology directly interfaces with the environment and changes as a result. However, it deeply challenges many, if not all, of our long-held suppositions about health and illness and the role of pathology and heredity.

Epigenetics also informs a new understanding of how traits and behaviors are passed from parent to child. Rand Jirtle of Duke University grabbed attention around the globe in 2003 with his study of agouti mice and heredity (Waterland & Jirtle, 2003). (Agouti mice are bred to be obese and diabetic—in effect, to have a short life span.) In his study, Jirtle used two identical strains of agouti mice and added folate and B_{12} to the feed of one group. He then bred them. Surprisingly, the experimental group's offspring turned out to be nondiabetic, of normal size, and had a normal life span—all this without any alteration to DNA. Jirtle concluded that the nutritional decisions of a parent impact the life of a child.

In a similar vein, the unfortunate lessons of bisphenol A (BPA), a chemical used in plastics manufacturing, show how seemingly innocuous decisions can send epigenetic shockwaves well into the future. BPA is a building block in polycarbonate plastics and epoxy resins common in a wide variety of goods, from can linings to dental sealants. After decades of reassurance by the plastics industry that BPA was unequivocally safe, recent evidence increasingly shows that it is a metabolic poison and endocrine disrupter. Unfortunately, BPA's impact is felt through multiple generations. Research in mice now shows increased rates of cancer, obesity, and diabetes in the offspring of those exposed (Dolinoy, Huang, & Jirtle, 2007).

Dr. Lars Olv Bygren of the Karlinska Institute brought epigenetic research a step closer to home with his study of Swedish farmers (Kaati, Bygren, Pembrey, & Sjostrom, 2007). In isolated, rural Sweden a poor harvest means little chance of surviving the harsh Scandinavian winter. A bountiful harvest year, on the other hand, fosters a winter of gluttony and weight gain. By tracking family outcomes over many generations in rural Sweden, Bygren amassed convincing data showing that a winter of gluttony for a generation of farmers meant a shorter (by an average of 6 years) life span for their children and grandchildren.

At first glance, results like Jirtle's and Bygren's seem counterintuitive to conventional wisdom. They suggest that expression, rather than simple presentation, plays the largest role in determining heredity, biological development, and disease. Interestingly, the lessons of the Human Genome Project, and its ultimate disappointment, corroborate this kind of thinking, adding impressive strength to the idea that environmental triggers control a much greater array of genetic expression than previously supposed.

In October 1990, scientists began the process of sequencing the entirety of human DNA. Ten-plus years and 3 billion dollars in the making, the Human Genome Project promised to unleash an avalanche of discoveries about the genetic basis of human illness. Many called it the "end of disease." Scientists and politicians were already thinking 20 years ahead, plotting the discovery of an Alzheimer gene or cancer gene. Based on prior research, scientists estimated the discovery of 100,000 human genes, each coding for a specific human protein. Near the completion of the first rough draft, President Clinton announced that the Human Genome Project would "revolutionize the diagnosis, prevention and treatment of most, if not all, human disease" (Travis, 2000, p. 4). Genetics, it seemed, might at last offer the key to a new era of disease-free living.

But it wasn't to be. Ten years later, the Human Genome Project and its hubris have left us with more questions than answers. Instead of the 100,000 genes first hypothesized, they found 22,000—less than in a roundworm. And only 4% of these 22,000 actually code for proteins; the vast majority (previously known as "junk DNA") are unspecified and appear to influence overall genetic expression. Although the Human Genome Project brought many advances in understanding, it has contributed very little to the diagnosis, treatment, and prevention of human disease or mental health issues.

In a relevant coda to the Human Genome Project, 30 scientific papers were published simultaneously in September 2012 detailing the landmark findings of 450 scientists from research labs all over the world. The project, titled ENCODE (Encyclopedia of DNA Elements), provided a major step in our understanding of how the human genome functions in both health and disease. We previously thought only about 2–4% of human DNA coded for proteins and the rest was just "junk." But this new research tells us that over 80% of the genome is active, and that the entire non-coding genome plays an active role in controlling how the 2% to 4% expresses itself (Ecker et al., 2012). "Junk" DNA, it turns out, is actually treasure.

ENCODE tells us that the regulation of DNA activity is much more complicated than we originally thought. The scientists found over 4 million chemical switches active in "junk" DNA. They also realized that the complex three-dimensional shape of the DNA molecule plays a crucial role as the 10-foot strand of DNA is stuffed and coiled tightly within the cell nucleus. In this compressed mode, the way that the DNA folds upon itself creates a specific three-dimensional "rat's nest" of adjacent switches that work to control the expression of our genes. This tells us that most of the changes that affect disease don't in fact lie in our genes but in the chemical switches triggered by the ecosystem that activates them (Ecker et al., 2012). Unfortunately, this kind of complexity means that simple genetic solutions for most psychiatric diseases are unrealistic for the near future.

This understanding is borne out in the literature. In 2009, for example, three separate articles published in the prestigious journal *Nature* (Stefansson et al., 2009) compared the entire genetic sequence of 10,000 patients with schizophrenia to that of 20,000 unaffected controls in a method called genome-wide scanning. The reseachers hoped to find a few common abnormalities that would translate into some possible treatments, or at the very least a few diagnostic tests. What they found instead were over 10,000 rare and isolated genetic variants. The researchers all concluded that both diagnostic tests and treatments are unlikely to be found in the near future.

If we take these lessons of genetics and apply them to our understanding of mental health, a few implications become immediately clear. First, although mental illnesses such as autism and schizophrenia tend to run in families, there's no real clinical relevancy to such claims. Arturas Petronis, head of the Epigenetic Lab at the Toronto Center for Addiction and Mental Health, crystallized this sentiment when he said, "After thirty years of molecular genetic studies we can explain only about 2% or 3% of inherited predisposition to psychiatric disease," and from this flows little to no clinical utility (Miller, 2012). Second, the vast majority of disorders such as anxiety, depression, and ADHD arise from environmental factors, not genetic predisposition. Clearly genetic heritage is a factor in these illnesses—it's just not the determining factor.

Twins, interestingly enough, offer some clarity on this new view of genetics and its implications for mental health. Certain differences arise when you study a large sample of identical twins and compare them to fraternal twins. Some illnesses appear in both twins; they are called concordant diseases. Since identical twins share the same DNA while fraternal twins do not, studies of twin concordance ratios give us the best evidence of how illnesses like schizophrenia express genetic factors.

Numerous studies cited in biological psychiatry show a 50% concordance of schizophrenia in identical twins compared to 15% in fraternal twins. According to these data, schizophrenia looks like a predisposed illness, which backs up biological psychiatry's broad claim of biological predominance in mental illness. If we dig a little deeper into the statistics, however, a slightly different picture emerges.

Two issues challenge biological psychiatry's claim. The first is the nature of the numbers. Even though these concordance rates (50% and 15%) have been cited for decades, a number of statisticians and researchers have recently called them into question. The numbers date back to the 1940s when research methods and data collection were, in a few words, less rigorous. The rate from one large study in 1946, for example, showed a concordance rate of 86%, wholly out of line with all the studies since. If one eliminates these earlier "less rigorous" studies and instead pools the data from the nine most recent studies, the rates look much different: 22.4% and 4.6% (Joseph, 2003). This is still a significant difference, but dramatically less so. What's more, the three most recent studies report even lower rates. The well-respected psychiatrist and schizophrenia expert E. Fuller Torrey (1992) estimates the concordance rate at about 25%.

The second issue challenging this claim is the basic problem of controlling for environment. Part of the rationale for biological predominance rests on the assumption that twins have the same environmental influences (i.e., all of their genes express in the same way). Yet, as common sense would suggest, as twins age they develop different identities, different food preferences, different belief systems, different habits. In short, they come to have different lives. By the time one twin develops schizophrenic symptoms, he has created his own micro- and macroenvironment, one totally different from that of the other twin. Actually, the chance of two twins sharing identical gene expression is, in mathematical terms, pretty slim.

In July 2011, the *Archives of General Psychiatry* featured an article examining the genetic factors of autism, another very "biological" illness. The study was designed to examine environmental factors as compared to genetic factors in the causality of the illness. It looked at 192 pairs of identical and fraternal twins. Mathematical modeling indicated that 38% of the cases could be attributed to genetic factors, while shared environmental factors accounted for 58% of the cases (Hallmayer et al., 2011). These numbers appear in spite of the 77% concordance in these twins. One shared environmental factor implicated in the development of autism was the use of SSRI antidepressant medication by mothers of twins in the year before delivery (Croen, Grether, Yoshida, Odouli, & Hendrick, 2011)—which sounds eerily reminiscent of some of the epigenetic studies previously discussed.

Currently, autism and schizophrenia are understood as the most biological of mental illnesses. Yet, as these studies and others indicate, that might be more of a stretch than the science allows. In fact, it appears environmental factors might play a larger role in expressing these illnesses than does genetic predisposition. Once we step outside the most biological of disorders and move to the type of problems that we most commonly encounter as practitioners (depression, anxiety), the influence of genetic predisposition drops even further.

The Slow Erosion of the Chemical Imbalance Theory

The chemical imbalance theory posits that once triggered, psychiatric illness represents a permanent imbalance in neurotransmitter function. Medication rights this imbalance, stabilizing neurotransmitter function in the ill brain. But since medication only stabilizes the imbalance and does not cure it, the affecting chemical imbalance must be continually treated, with patients sometimes remaining on drugs for the rest of their lives in order to regularly modify the brain's disproportion.

This theory, then, is founded on two basic suppositions. One, there's a biological predominance in mental illness (internal factors alone cause a chemical imbalance). And two, the nervous system is hardwired (once triggered, a chemical imbalance is enduring). But as I've just shown in the last few pages, both of these notions need to be retooled (or even thrown out) in light of emerging discoveries in epigenetics and neuroplasticity. We can't rest on these suppositions anymore. The proverbial rug is being pulled right out from under the chemical imbalance theory.

But, as the supporters might point out, the theory still has empirical support.

Unfortunately, despite widespread cultural support, the bulk of emerging evidence does not support a chemical imbalance as the culprit of mental illness (McHenry, 2006). If there is, in fact, a specific chemical imbalance for a particular mental illness—say, depression and depleted serotonin—then reason holds that exacerbating that imbalance should exacerbate the illness, like injecting a hypoglycemic person with insulin. However, in major clinical trials, drugs that increase and drugs that decrease serotonin levels fare equally well in quelling depressive symptoms, as we noted in Chapter 1. In fact, no category or compound seems to fare any better than another. In the STAR*D study, for instance, the largest and most comprehensive study of depression ever untaken, patients who switched categories (SSRI vs. SNRI, selective norepinephrine serotonin reuptake inhibitor) or specific agent experienced no benefit and no worsening of symptoms (Rush, 2006). And agents that treat one category of chemical imbalance appear to work just as well as those treating two or three different types of chemical imbalances. The pharmaceutical industry even reluctantly admits that for depression, placebo is often comparable and sometimes more effective than experimental agents.

None of these data fit very nicely in the logic of the chemical imbalance theory. In fact, it contradicts its basic thinking. David Healy, past secretary of the British Association of Psychopharmacology and author of 13 books on the subject, described it this way: "The serotonin theory of depression is comparable to the masturbatory theory of insanity" ("The Case Against Antidepressants," 2011). A significant review of antidepressant research published in the *New England Journal of Medicine* concluded, "Numerous studies of norepinephrine and serotonin metabolites in plasma, urine, and cerebrospinal fluid, as well as postmortem studies of the brains of patients with depression, have yet to identify the purported deficiency reliably" (Belmaker & Agam, 2008, p. 55). The chemical imbalance theory limits our understanding of the patient and his or her specific malady. It also limits the available treatment options, which limits the possibility of recovery.

In my experience, a typical family that enters a doctor's office with, say, a hyperactive kid will typically walk out of the office 45 minutes later with a *DSM* diagnosis of ADHD and a prescription for a stimulant medication (and no other advice or direction). Pathology is all psychiatry can see anymore: diagnoses and medications. In effect, the chemical imbalance paradigm has strapped the blinders on us. We can't see the short distance past pathology to the child sitting in front of us. In clinical practice, more attention needs to be paid to assessing and treating each child's unique condition or needs. One of the unfortunate side effects of this kind of solitary focus on pathology is that after 40 years of treating ADHD with the same agents, we have little practical information about what causes it, what the other effective treatments are, and, more important, what could prevent it.

This is why it is so important to peek outside the blinders and assess atypical features, get to know the child personally, and be on the lookout for potential culprits everywhere. Little Josh's story makes at least this much clear.

Josh

Josh bounded into my office followed by his sluggish mom, Jenny. At 7, Josh looked and acted a few years younger. Thin and endlessly moving, he explored every corner of my office, poking around in my desk and digging through my papers while I talked to Jenny. She told me that after holding on for a few years, she and her husband needed help. Teachers were complaining; friend's parents were exhausted; Mom and Dad were tired of keeping up with their supersonic son. Josh, on the other hand, displayed a devilish smile and not a care in the world.

He met all of the criteria for a *DSM* diagnosis of ADHD—combined type including classroom feedback. However, some atypical features drew my attention. Josh was colicky as an infant and had severe reflux— vomiting frequently. He developed chronic ear infections and required more than 10 courses of antibiotics and the surgical placement of tubes in his ears. Chronic constipation and abdominal pain plagued him. I had to sit and wonder—were some other underlying issues responsible for this particular combination of symptoms? I knew that numerous studies had found a link between a history of ear infections and later ADHD (Loe et al., 2008; Adesman, Altshuler, Lipkin, & Walco, 1990; Hagerman & Falkenstein, 1987). So I looked a little deeper. I wanted to correct all these metabolic problems before assessing his baseline—I wanted to see him healthy and pain free, first and foremost.

I instructed the parents to make significant changes to Josh's diet. They were to remove all dairy products so that his gut might get a well-deserved break, as I suspected a food allergy. We also added probiotics to help his GI health and talked to him about eating healthier. Three months later, Josh was different in some ways. He was not as wound up, agitated, impulsive, or out of control. And, oddly enough, he had also stopped wetting the bed. Josh no longer met the criteria for ADHD. He was back. His parents were thrilled with his progress. He was still a handful, but his parents could better manage him. They could see the light at the end of this challenging tunnel.

We will explore the exact research and thinking behind Josh's treatment later in this book, but needless to say, solid clinical evidence supports his recovery and suggests that others like Josh can benefit from nutritional approaches to mental illness. With Josh, I tried to respect the wisdom of neural plasticity, epigenetics, and the emerging lessons of psychopharmacology. In this way, I was afforded the chance to readily expect Josh's brain and behavior to change and adapt for the better, and, more importantly, we didn't have to rely solely on some powerful medication for symptomatic control of his problem. Josh instead learned life-long coping skills and proper nutrition by dealing with his illness and nutritional imbalance. In practice, Josh doesn't make any sense according to the chemical imbalance theory. No agent intervention; no long-term medication required; and yet, a happy and healthy little boy sat calmly before my eyes.

CHAPTER FIVE
The Role of the Therapist

How do we actually apply the principles of wholeness? It's tricky, of course, as it requires daily awareness and insight, not just adherence to some step-by-step program. Nevertheless, let's start by breaking down our job into a few identifiable pieces. This will help us see exactly what's required of us in our job and where the potential trip-ups lurk. This will also hopefully show us the places where we need growth and work. In the simplest terms, the process of evaluating and treating young people with mental health complaints requires the ability to:

1. Connect with the young person in the face of presenting issues
2. Connect with parents while managing the relationship with the young person
3. Assess the body-mind-spirit of the young person and the surrounding ecosystem
4. Develop a treatment plan and manage engagement from all involved parties

The first two abilities are covered in some detail—including some guiding principles and the professional utility of various methods—in the following pages. The latter two are not covered in as much depth in these pages, however, as they are the subjects of their own respective chapters (Chapters 6 and 8).

Experienced mental health practitioners often ask me if it is difficult to connect with kids as compared with the more typical adult patient. The connection is basically the same, I tell them, but the mechanics of getting there are a little different, a little more precarious. Connecting with kids takes more trust and respect than it does with adults. Adults, most often, are in the psychiatrist's office under their own agency. They're there on purpose. Kids, on the other hand, usually are not. So naturally they are a little more suspicious of what's going on, a little more guarded in the first few meetings. Honestly, a lot of the time a kid won't have the first clue as to why he is sitting in a psychiatrist's office, or what a psychiatrist does exactly.

A good first step in establishing a connection with a kid is to get a sense of what brings this kid to your office to begin with. This will guide the development of the connection. If you think the parents are over-zealous, for instance, and are spurring an overreactive treatment, let that guide your interaction with the kid. Reassure him about how well he is doing and the pressure he is under. On the other hand, if the parents seem unconcerned or apathetic, reach out to the kid. Reaffirm her struggle and her ability to overcome.

Once you have a sense of what brings the kid to treatment, it's important to adapt to each kid as quickly as possible if you're to make the relationship comfortable. That is, you have to appraise and dial in each kid's individual maturity, anxiety, motivation, and communication style in order to begin a healthy dialogue.

Respect and trust are paramount in beginning a dialogue. So remember to frame the presenting issues in terms every kid can understand. This will ensure that the office exudes an atmosphere of safety and respect. It's never beneficial to preach to the child or sound off in tricky terminology. It will put a wall between you and the child.

The second part of building respect and trust is making sure to allocate one-on-one time for each kid. Time alone fosters respect and trust; it lets kids know that you are there for them, not just for their parents. So get the parents out of the room for at least part of each visit. All too often I hear stories about younger patients not getting a chance to meet with their psychiatrist alone or not getting a chance to ask questions about their care. And it's easy to see why this would make kids feel angry and disrespected. The trouble is, this mistake is commonly committed by less experienced practitioners. And when it happens, all the possible respect and trust between a practitioner and child is sucked out of the room.

On the other side of the coin, I hear of a large number of kids who meet with a therapist who spends almost no time working with parents. A rough rule of thumb: with kids 6 and younger, spend most of each visit with the parents, and at 16 and older spend most of each visit with the teen. For kids in between, slide the scale accordingly. Of course, family dynamics and maturity can change this dramatically.

As I've mentioned, the most challenging aspect of working with kids is often managing the dual relationships of child therapist and parent therapist. In many cases, this means moving two very different treatment plans forward simultaneously: one for the child and one for the parent. Take, for example, a beaten-down, depressed child and a critical, overbearing parent. In this case, a lot more is accomplished with separate sessions for the parent and for the child, since they probably would not be able to collaborate in a healthy way in their current state. Later on, however, once they are a little more amicable toward each other, you might be able to move them into dual sessions where you coach them together.

Once you reach a place of safety and trust, it all comes down to building rapport. There are as many ways to do this as there are kids. In general, though, I try to be as frank as I can with my young patients. It sets up an atmosphere of candor and lets them know they can talk about anything. Some kids will prefer a more indirect approach, something less invasive and threatening. Whatever the method, make sure it is modeled on the child you're trying to approach.

Relationship Over Technique: What Matters in the Therapeutic Connection

People often ask me what style of psychotherapy I practice. My response is usually vague or extemporaneous: "a form of eclectic problem solving" or "something like pragmatic existential exploration." Ultimately, there are interesting and useful techniques in a variety of different modalities, so I don't place too much stock in any one school. Certainly, I respect and employ the techniques showing a good evidence base (i.e., CBT and DBT), but my primary concern is what's best for a particular kid. Rather than trying to think about what technique might get a kid better, I think about what technique (or facet of a technique) might help me better connect with a kid.

As it turns out, therapeutic outcome with a kid is based less on technique than on the kind of connection developed between the therapist and patient, according to research in psychotherapy. T. B. Karasu, previous chairman of the Department of Psychiatry at Albert Einstein College of Medicine, is an expert on psychotherapy and has written extensively on the factors responsible for positive outcomes in therapy. Karasu has explored an expansive inventory of contributing factors in his research, but he's concluded that "nonspecific factors" such as the quality of the relationship between the patient and therapist and the therapist's background are the best predictors of healing. (Specific factors would include technique and treatment style.)

Research like Karasu's shows us how our emotional tone, mental attitude, and spiritual beliefs do indeed impact those with whom we work. Our age, our gender, our experience, our struggles, and our intentions all add to the nonspecific factors dictating a kid's therapeutic outcome. "In fact, the therapist's skills are contextually tailored manifestations of his or her personality," says Karasu (1999, p. 155). That's why for true healers it is tough to find a clear demarcation between "the therapist" and "the therapy." They meld into one, connecting to the little kid in need.

Two researchers in psychotherapy, Strupp and Hadley, have taken Karasu's work one step further to contend that positive changes in psychotherapy can be solely attributed to "the healing effects of a benign human relationship" (1979, p. 1132). In fact, these two have gone as far as to suggest that the therapist-patient relationship is the supraordinate therapeutic influence (Strupp, 1970, 1974, 1975; Strupp & Hadley, 1979). M. D. Smith, in his comprehensive analysis of the benefits of psychotherapy, sums this point up well: "The weight of the evidence that now rests in the balance so greatly favors the general factors [patient-therapist relationship] in the interpretation of therapeutic efficacy that it can no longer be ignored" (Smith, Glass, & Miller, 1980). In other words, you're more important than your therapy.

Credentials and methodology may be important for some issues, particularly in complicated cases, but most research shows that these factors have poor predictive value for the efficacy of the therapist in psychotherapy. To frame this in another way, there is very little evidence that the type of training, special technical skill, professional discipline, or theoretical orientation corresponds to therapeutic outcome (Frank et al., 1978; Hogan, 1979). Or as Karasu says, "Too much attention is often paid to the professional training of therapists and not enough to their personal formation" (1999, p. 145).

Even if psychotherapy is not the focus of treatment, the strength of the interpersonal connection between practitioner and patient is still paramount to success. Nonspecific factors play a role even if the practitioner is only providing medication or psychological testing. Think about the therapist's presence as a positive reinforcement of success. The very nature of the healing relationship—one-on-one—inextricably ties healer and patient together, no matter the treatment.

The Wounded Healer

Training for traditional healers, shamans, and medicine men has always focused on two areas: the outer world and the inner world. Outer-world training consists of remedies, techniques, and rituals. Inner-world training, often characterized by an initiation rite, involves a path of pain, transformation, and exploration. Inner-world training is so vital to the success of a healer, in fact, that elders of a particular tradition often select healers at a young age based solely on their personality and temperament. These future healers are usually groomed simultaneously in body-mind-spirit, as healing for many traditions is a sacred rite.

Part of the reason for this drawn-out process is that many cultures believe that the personality, thoughts, and emotions of a healer color his or her ability to heal. Also, since healers always carry wounds, they must be well on their way through their own inner journey if they're to be a guide to others. Psychiatrist Viktor Frankl seemed to have this in mind when he mused, "What is to give light must endure burning." Interestingly, psychiatry recognized the importance of the healer's own inner journey early on and encouraged residents in training to be involved in their own psychotherapy or analysis. This was common practice all the way up through the 1970s. At the time, it was the only field of medicine that acknowledged a healer's own personal healing journey. With the ascendancy of biological psychiatry, however, this tradition has largely been lost. Perhaps it is time to revive this old tradition.

As healers, we inevitably bring our own experience and pain to the healing partnership. But the more present we are in our own vulnerability, the deeper the connection we can offer. Mentally, we can sympathize; emotionally, we can empathize; spiritually, we can feel compassion. The availability of these states lets us fluidly move beyond the self and into a deeper resonance with the other. In its fullest expression, this transcendence of self is a spiritual, sacred experience, which heals both parties. In ancient Greek, the word *therapy* means service to the gods. And, indeed, therapy is a sacred service—to all parties involved. It is transformative, giving strength and calm to those it connects. As Carl Jung once said, "The meeting of two personalities is like the contact of two chemical substances: if there is any reaction, both are transformed" (1933, p. 49).

In pursuit of this kind of therapeutic ideal, each encounter with a kid must be thought of as a valuable opportunity for personal and professional growth, not merely a one-way exchange of information or remedy. Growth like this comes from daily awareness and self-examination, from listening to your patients and your intuition. And hopefully, as you grow—personally and professionally—you'll be more accepting of those little kids you work with and more receptive to new learning experiences. The healer's own growth cannot be ignored, as it is a major factor in creating a positive therapeutic outcome for children. Without personal growth, the practitioner can end up trapping both parties in a therapeutic dead end.

> Traditional approaches eventually reach an impasse, a place where the therapist himself resides and in which he and his patients can become irretrievably trapped. This invariably occurs when the confident clinicians, regardless of their respective schools, present themselves as prototypes of health and salvation for their recipients to emulate. Alas, they are limited by an inherent constraint: they can take their patients only as far as they themselves have come. Then the question—and the quest—remain: How does the therapist get beyond this barrier; more aptly, how does he venture toward, and eventually attain, a soulful and spiritual experience? (Karasu, 1999, p. 143)

The more we acknowledge our humanity, our wounds, and our intrinsic spirituality, the more that we can heal others. Existential psychologist Rollo May sums this up well: "The therapist is assumedly an expert; but if he isn't first of all a human being, his expertness will be irrelevant and quite possibly harmful" (1958, p. 82). We must step out from behind the desk and the padding of credentials and look to connect, human being to human being. By examining the self and addressing our own wounds, we can become more fully available in the therapist-patient relationship and thus become more empowered as healers.

The healer is, in a very real way, healing itself. Procedure and technique are most effective when they are used merely as a framework to direct the individual healer. In fact, research from the Spindrift Foundation and other investigators suggests that healers are most beneficial when they remain totally free of specific technique and clear all personal directives from thought. "An understanding heart is everything," said Carl Jung; "warmth is the vital element for the growing plant and for the soul of the child" (1939, p. 284). That's why we need to hold the non-specific factors of the healer (connection, intent, belief, acceptance, and affection) in as much, and perhaps higher, regard as the specific factors of technique or method.

To be truly helpful to our little patients, we need to address our personal issues and needs, those factors potentially limiting the healing relationship. This path of personal and spiritual growth can only deepen our capacity for caring, understanding, and sensitivity, which in the end only helps us better care for the little kids in our practice.

Surrender

In moments of true healing, we reach down and touch the pain of the other. They bring forth this experience in order for us to better connect and understand. In return, we must meet their courage and vulnerability with our own empathy and compassion.

Both parties actively participate and benefit in the journey. But for this to occur, both parties need to bring an expectation and desire for change to the table, as well as a willingness to surrender to the process. Surrendering means removing personal agendas and clearing away specific intentions. Surrendering replaces the personal with the shared hope of healing.

In order to surrender, both parties must release themselves from any internal attachments that may limit the healing process. This means that both patient and practitioner need to emancipate themselves from selfish preoccupations, from ego, from pretense. The therapeutic relationship can act as a vehicle to move both parties to this place, because while it is certainly possible to surrender to a remedy or a belief, most humans find it easier to surrender to another human being. In its most pure form, Karasu calls therapeutic surrender "two persons mutually confirming each other's underlying sense of common destiny without blame or debt"

(1999, p. 150). He continues, "It is the rescue of self . . . an emancipation from the confinement of ordinary human attachments and entanglements, and deliverance from the imprisonment of mind and body without soul. It is a peaceful and restorative union."

Surrendering means trusting the other in a confiding relationship. (To confide means literally to speak "with trust.") When we do so, we engender the confidence of the other party. Confiding, in this way, is also a type of complete surrender; it allows us to release our self, as we are, to the possibility of who we might become. That's why it is so important for the practitioner to establish a confiding relationship with the patient if there is any hope of moving forward. In fact, the confiding relationship is one of the two central criteria of Jerome Frank's (1961) therapeutic factors in psychotherapy. I find that a direct, respectful, and honest relationship with a child has the best chance of creating an atmosphere of openness. That's why I always meet with kids alone first, so that I can ask about their concerns, hopes, and ideas. Obviously some of the younger kids will not step up to the plate as willingly. (If a kid seems particularly reticent to talk, I don't force her. I'll just get out a board game or play with some puppets or stuffed animals and wait for her to get comfortable with my presence.) Respect and a willingness to listen go a long way.

The acceptance of one's condition is also vital to the process of surrendering. For many patients, simply accepting the condition they are in can help them move beyond their pain. Dr. Andrew Weil, who has written extensively on the nonspecific factors of healing, is convinced of this: "The most common correlation I observe between mind and healing in people with chronic illness is total acceptance of the circumstances of one's life, including illness. Often, it occurs as part of a spiritual awakening and submission to a higher power" (1995, p. 100).

Many of the therapies outlined in this book do not follow the traditional psychotherapy model. Some of these techniques are wordless (EMDR, meridian psychotherapies, and spiritual healing), instrumental (acupuncture, herbal medicine, nutritional supplements), or autonomous (meditation, creative arts). Regardless, all these approaches create the same opportunity for healing that psychotherapy does. The individual experiences a moment of surrender to vulnerability. Whether we are meditating, talking with a therapist, taking a supplemental remedy, or having someone lay hands on us, we surrender to something beyond us. This transcendence forms the essence of healing: an extension outside our being lending strength, correction, or healing.

Boundaries

We walk a razor's edge as we strive for an ever deeper connection with our little patients. Without healthy boundaries, a therapeutic relationship can easily descend into the inappropriate. I am reminded of one caring physician who would overextend herself to care for her patients, often visiting them in their homes when they called in distress. In her desire to heal, she lost sight of healthy boundaries. In the end, she was mentally taxed, physically drained, and often irritable with her office staff. Her well-intentioned actions certainly soothed her subliminal need to please, but they didn't really help her young patients. With their doctor available round the clock, her patients simply became dependent on her and less capable in their own lives as treatment moved forward—an outcome none of us want.

I can think of another practitioner who passionately cared for his clients—so much so, in fact, that they became his friends and confidants. During sessions, he ended up spending more time sharing his troubles and issues than his patients did. And gradually, his young patients felt increasingly burdened with their practitioner's woes. No doubt he was a talented practitioner, but, sadly, he used his patients to comfort himself. In the end, his needs trumped his professionalism.

On the flip side, I see practitioners who hide behind professionalism, fending off connection and vulnerability in favor of distance and detachment. As we know from psychotherapy research, withholding personal information and amity from a patient can often be very helpful, but be careful not to withhold all intimacy and warmth. When this happens, the patient is never moved to trust or respect the practitioner. And the therapeutic relationship—and outcome—suffers as a result. On top of that, practitioners working in this way miss out on opportunities to widen their professional palate and deepen their personal growth. We must set one foot into our patient's circle of pain, but never two. We must join them on level, but not lose sight of our objective.

The central challenge for the practitioner working with kids, then, is how to connect on the deepest level possible while also maintaining appropriate boundaries. This is the razor's edge we walk.

As my prior examples illustrate, teaching proper boundaries to a therapist who has significant, unattended personal issues is pointless in some ways. That's because boundaries in therapy are for the most part intuitive and reflective of personal awareness, and when a practitioner has unresolved personal issues it clouds intuition and awareness. Someone with good intuition and a sense of awareness will naturally feel out most boundaries without prior instruction and will be able to put personal issues on hold in the office. On the other hand, a well-schooled psychotherapist with unresolved personal issues that cloud intuition and awareness will remain an ongoing risk, overstepping boundaries and stepping on toes. Therapy and the active resolution of personal issues is a good step for any practitioner learning to navigate the razor's edge.

Given the vulnerability and immaturity of kids, boundaries are a heightened concern on both sides of the dialectic. The power differential between an older authority figure and a young kid puts these kids at a potentially threatening disadvantage. That's why it is so important to respect the kid's boundaries and proceed into the intimate space of therapy with heedfulness.

Obviously with kids, physical touch can be one of the most severe boundary violations. Traditional psychotherapy appreciates this and strictly admonishes against physical touch. In fact, in some states it is illegal for a practitioner to touch a patient. For the most part, this is a prescient decision. Shared physical touch between a patient and practitioner can open all sorts of thorny issues.

But children also have a real need to be touched, particularly those recovering from trauma or abuse. Many are desperate for appreciation and yearn for the experience and warmth of appropriate human relationships. There is solid evidence supporting nonsexualized touch from a practitioner as a positive therapeutic experience. Innovative psychotherapies such as Hakomi and process work commonly employ touch. Fortunately, in order to make it safe, these therapies aggressively train for the complicated personal issues involved.

The Value of Intuition

Carl Jung (1971) popularized the idea of intuition in his 1921 book, *Psychological Types*. He labeled intuition an irrational function because it bypassed the rational thought process, arriving directly from the machinery of the unconscious. A rational function tends to be linear and impersonal, whereas intuition is always nonlinear and derived from the minute details of experience. According to the Myers-Briggs Type Indicator, which employs Jung's four dimensions of the psyche—introversion-extroversion, thinking-feeling, sensing-intuition, and judging-perceiving—intuition is a sense of the big picture, an attunement to the broad strokes of the potential and patterns.

Intuition is neither validated nor understood in psychiatric training, and for the most part it is denigrated. Particularly for rational types—including most physicians—the very idea that this latent, uncontrollable sense could steer professional decision making is threatening. It undermines the rational decision making we champion in the sciences. Ironically, the most rational and left-brained thinkers tend to be the worst psychiatrists and psychotherapists. Assuredly, analytical thought is helpful in mental health care, but without a balance of intuition and social skills, it's just not enough to be effective in clinical practice. Given the complexity of the brain and the many influences on mental health—be it behavior, social systems, or culture—a purely logical approach to care has grave limitations. A practitioner working in mental health needs the ability to synthesize broad fields of personal information and patterns quickly—which takes intuition.

The challenge for us is polishing and honing intuition, allowing knowledge and clinical experience to complement and color this addition to our professional palette. Intuition in treatment and assessment must be aimed at doing the best for the person currently in front of you: getting a sense of who he is and what he is here for.

Luckily, people attracted to the field of mental health tend to be more intuitive, so the groundwork is already laid. In fact, evaluation of the Myers-Briggs Type Indicator in counseling students found 76% had an intuitive predominance, by far the highest for any field of study or occupation group (Briggs Myers, 1990). Given these numbers, we'd expect the mental health care system to make good use of its people's intuition, sharpening and enhancing this skill for clinical practice. And yet, nowhere in training or practice is intuition even validated as a skill, let alone taught.

This is wrong. Considering that intuition probably brought you into this field to begin with, trust it. Trust your intuition in your professional life the way you trust it in your personal life. It will help you reach more kids on a deep, personal level, which, as we've learned, gets more kids better, faster. Meditation and mindfulness practices are great tools to hone your clinical intuition. These skills clear away the personal clutter and agendas that distort subtle perceptions.

The only thing I know that truly heals people, particularly kids, is unconditional love. Our ultimate task, then, is to employ our professional skills and wisdom in such a way that they become a deep, personalized expression of commitment and love. That's how kids get healthy; that's how they get whole.

CHAPTER SIX

Assessment Is Key

A clinician cannot and should not rely on a single system of thought, such as the *DSM-IV* or neuropharmacology, to understand the patient. As it happens, the *DSM-V* is moving to dimensional descriptions of criteria in an attempt to broaden its understanding of the patient. This has value, but in the end it does not tell the clinician anything about the core imbalances that any given patient has or why the patient is troubled in the first place. On top of that, *DSM* diagnoses—in any form—often promote medication management as a first line of defense, which is almost always too narrow a treatment plan.

A new model of assessment is needed, one that makes provisions for the ongoing roundtable discussion that is mental health. The model should be broad enough to encompass the myriad influences on mental health (e.g., environment, biochemistry, heredity, relationships) and malleable enough to take advantage of advice and reasoning from the many theories of mind and mental health (e.g., family systems, attachment, object relations, neurochemistry). It should be simple and easy to apply.

Here is a model of assessment that takes these factors into account.

The Wholeness Model of Assessment

The Wholeness Model of assessment moves away from a narrow algorithmic evaluation and instead makes room for the potential use of any and all methods and theories that might inform an assessment. Instead of focusing its attention on specific technique and rational-scientific thinking, the Wholeness Model of assessment brings attention to the nature of the patient-practitioner relationship and the use of clinical intuition.

For those reasons, the Wholeness Model is a set of six guiding principles instead of a structured step-by-step practice. (I'll go into more detail on treatment approaches to specific disorders in Part II.) They will show you what to assess, how, and why. I'll also be providing you with some example evaluation forms in order to give shape and color to some of the principles. Think of these principles and example forms as merely a representational system through which to structure your own thinking in the office. Don't hesitate to break with some of the principles, rearrange them, make new provisions, tweak an evaluation form, seek guidance from another existing model, or tailor something to fit your practice or your patient.

These six principles of assessment were developed and revised over the course of my 30-odd years practicing medicine and psychiatry in a variety of forms and environments. But I'm just one doctor. I have my own style and approach. And so do you. So I encourage you to use these six principles simply as a guide in the drafting of your own assessment process. If it helps, just think about them as helpful tips.

Let's take a closer look.

1. Assess the Six Realms

The child's world can be divided into six realms: environmental, physical, mental, emotional, social, and spiritual. The practitioner should inquire about all six realms in order to create an overview of the child's ecosystem. This helps provide a more holistic picture of what's really going on with the kid, where the imbalances are, where the issues lie. This means you need to explore most areas of the child's life, trusting your clinical intuition about what the child and the parents say, but also what they withhold. Partly, this thorough exploration is for information. Partly, it is for the therapist-patient connection. But most of all, it meets the child's need to be heard and understood. This kind of comprehensive assessment also makes it easier to hone in on what potential models or theories or techniques might be helpful in treating your young patient.

In no particular order, assess each of the child's six realms:

1. Environment: Look at the physical environment in which the person lives—issues of beauty, noise, air quality, water quality, light, and so on. The patient's environment includes a wide range of issues, including environmental toxins like mercury, lead, air pollution, and pesticides. Also take into account the amount of sunlight and time in

nature that the patient experiences. Physical crowding and the actual physical environment of the home are other contributing factors. Is the house cluttered, dirty, and noisy? Is it clean, pleasing, and calm? Think about potential travel or commuting issues that can have an impact.

2. Physical: Take a careful survey of the biological family history of mental and physical illness; this provides the best overall insight into genetic predisposition. The diet and ongoing nutrition of the patient also factor in here. Both micronutrient and macronutrient patterns are the biochemical foundation for proper brain development, in children and adults. Ask about the child's personal history of illness. This offers a critical understanding of physiological predispositions and past episodes. The amount of sleep, exercise habits, and relative fitness of the kid create the basis for proper stress management, so factor these variables into the equation. Examine the child's use of supplements, medications, herbs, and homeopathic remedies and how these may be impacting physical health. In addition, think about issues of strength, flexibility, ideal body weight, energy, illness, resistance, and recurrent patterns of physical symptoms as measures of physical health.

3. Emotional: Study the current emotional tone (positive or negative) of the child, as well as the emotional range and regulation. How well regulated are his or her emotions? Also important here is the patient's ability to fully experience pleasure, love, grief, anger, and joy. What is the trauma history and current impact? A history of chronic abuse or neglect will impact the liability of any child or adult in the emotional realm. Every patient has a different pattern of ambient mood and affect. Is there freedom from chronic fear or sadness? What is the patient's capacity to forgive and accept, particularly himself or herself? How expressive is the patient at a healthy baseline? Also of concern here is the emotional tone between the parents, and the general emotional tone, supportiveness, and acceptance found in the household. If divorced, are the parents supportive of each other or still at war?

4. Mental: The mental realm includes many factors commonly considered in the psychology of resilience, for example, the presence and strength of mental traits such as perseverance and grit. Are there supportive mental attitudes? Weigh the balance of opportunity versus threat, self-confidence versus self-doubt, optimism versus pessimism,

internal locus of control versus external locus of control, active engagement versus passive avoidance, and acceptance versus resentment. Is the balance between work and play level or weighted heavily to one side? What is the role of humor and the degree of intellectual stimulation and challenge in the kid's day-to-day life? Consider issues related to learning style in school (e.g., auditory, visual, kinesthetic). You must understand the learning preference and classroom challenges of every child. Also assess the goodness of fit with the child's school. Very often, a poor fit with school will lead a child to failure, despair, and psychiatric symptoms. General consideration of cognitive capacity and formal learning disorders is also included here. Review the stage of cognitive development, educational background, and level of intellectual stimulation. Finally, the level of perceptiveness, self-awareness, sensitivity, memory, and processing speed also factor into the mental realm.

5. Social: Ask the kid about the number, variety, and depth of his or her relationships. Are they intimate, confiding relationships or mere acquaintances? Does the kid feel isolated or well connected? The degrees of trust and openness with friends are good barometers of social skills. In older teens, consider the degree of sexual satisfaction and expression. Is it healthy and appropriate? It's also important to probe for the level of emotional stability, safety, and satisfaction in any primary relationship. Question the family and extended family dynamics. Parents with many children are aware that their connection, comfort, and ease of interaction vary from child to child. Most parents are more drawn to one child than another, and this is perfectly normal. Fit becomes a practical concern only when there is a conflict between the parent and child. Also ask the kid about relationships with neighbors, family friends, coaches, teachers, and pastors. In an era when extended family plays less of a role in a child's life, these other adults can make all the difference in the world.

6. Spiritual: Ask children about their sense of meaning and purpose in life, if they have a spiritual practice, if they feel connected to a higher power, and if they pray. What is the patient's sense of life purpose or inner guidance? Consider whether a child's actions are congruent with personal spiritual beliefs and values. The specifics of the belief or value system do not really matter. The crucial factors here are regular participation or attendance as well as the active practice of the family.

Role modeling may be the most crucial step for parents. Many kids and parents will be initially intimidated or uncomfortable with the topic of religion, but push on. Many kids will feel negative about their early experiences of religion. Or they may even believe that they are neither innately spiritual nor "good enough" to have a personal spirituality. Whatever the circumstance, I find it helpful to explain that we are all spiritual beings, in many varieties of form and expression, and that we need spirituality to be healthy. It's also important to think about whether kids practice tolerance and acceptance of other spiritual perspectives, and how they experience transcendence.

2. Appreciate the Individual

Perhaps the most important part of any assessment is getting to know whom you are working with. This might seem like a given, so obvious that it does not even merit mention. However, this part of the assessment is increasingly absent in conventional psychiatry. At a typical medical office visit, the doctor has a working diagnosis within 6 minutes. It may take slightly longer for a psychiatrist, but not much. Only a cursory pattern of symptoms can be collected in that time frame. The person, unfortunately, goes largely unnoticed. In the Wholeness Model, ample time should be taken for you to familiarize yourself with each kid and appreciate his or her uniqueness.

This section offers some guidance on how to explore and get to know the individual child. Any assessment should evaluate the child's individual strengths. Focus on talents and gifts, in particular. Each child's talents and gifts represent the ideal path for developing self-esteem and self-confidence. If a 13-year-old finds a talent in dance and poetry, she has a strong sail to pull her through one of the most difficult crossings in life: adolescence. Create a map of the person's strengths and talents. And have the kid help you design it in session.

Often, talents and gifts come in the form of intelligences. Harvard University professor of education Howard Gardner (1993), in his book *Multiple Intelligences*, describes seven types of intelligence that humans possess: bodily kinesthetic (dance, movement); visual-spatial (architecture, design); intrapersonal (introspection); interpersonal (social skills and emotional savvy); musical (a grasp of rhythms, sounds, and pitch); linguistic (words and language); and logical-mathematical (numbers, reasoning, calculating). A child may be gifted in any of these areas but it may escape detection. Sometimes one has to probe and explore to find these gifts. If you find a hidden talent, encourage the child to develop it.

Likewise, explore what the child loves to do. What are his or her passions and interests? At times, these things can be hidden—even from the child. But it's important to flesh them out, as they help to keep children engaged in the world and give them a daily sense of satisfaction. This is especially important for kids with depression, as they typically have low self-esteem, low engagement, and a basic lack of zest. Passions can also help save teens from less positive uses of their time: video games, lethargy, drugs, and delinquency. Help the child find his or her passions.

Provocative questions may help to open this discussion up. What do you do best? What is your special gift? What are other kids jealous of in you? If you could do just one thing for the rest of your life, what would it be? What is your secret wish? What would you really like to be when you grow up? Sometimes outsiders see this most clearly; have the child ask grandparents, teachers, and coaches about his or her talents and passions. This can be a really fun area to explore. Enjoy. The basic goal here is to get to know what makes this person unique and different. Once you have a grasp of these qualities, it's easier to understand a person and what is needed for wholeness.

The next step is to ask about the child's temperament in early childhood, elementary school, and preteen and teen years. This will give you a sense of the kid's arc of temperament and basic disposition. Think about whether or not the child is reactive or staid, effusive or closed off, energetic or slow moving, fearless or apprehensive, and how these characteristics have changed over time. I find asking whom the child is most like—Mom or Dad—helps to clarify the child's temperament.

I also like to think about inborn vitality. This is hard to define exactly, but it's obvious to anyone who works with sick kids. Children differ greatly in their ability to recover and heal. In the same way, they differ in their predisposition to illness. Some of this may relate to factors of geography or socioeconomic status, but some portion of it also just appears to be inborn. Assessing a kid's inborn vitality will give you a sense of whether or not a kid is generally healthy or generally unhealthy, which will inform how you understand the current issues (chronic or sporadic?) and how to tackle them.

Next, cover learning style. I tend to explore this topic only for children who have struggled in school. Have they significantly underperformed? If this is true, then I begin to look at learning style and learning differences. Learning disabilities like expressive and receptive language disorders can create disarray for children and derail their entire school experience. These issues are significantly underappreciated and under-remediated. In children with ADHD, for example, as many as 20–50% suffer from a comorbid learning disability, especially speech and language disorders. And these issues put a child at a heightened risk for future depression, school failure, substance abuse, and delinquency.

Ask parents and teachers questions about processing: Does the child seem to misunderstand instructions or need more repetition than other children? Does the child struggle to share a story or relate questions? Was the child late in learning to speak? Does he or she like to read? Does the child seem frustrated when writing or require more time than peers to complete written work? If any of these questions raise concerns, then the kid should be aggressively evaluated with an Individual Education Plan (IEP) or neuropsychological evaluation to pinpoint the issue and develop a remediation plan. If you can identify a receptive or expressive language issue early on, you can save the child years of frustration and declining self-esteem.

Although the scientific validation of the link between learning style, instructional technique, and school performance remains far from clear, it seems reasonable to explore for individual patterns if the child has repeatedly failed to succeed in school. Think about whether the child is a visual, auditory, or kinesthetic learner. Does he prefer to learn via a hands-on approach that has limited instruction or does he like someone guiding him through the whole process? Assess and intervene accordingly.

Also, think about if the child seems right-brained in her approach to the world. Is she a nonlinear thinker? Does she have more of an artistic or creative approach to situations? The book *Right-Brained Children in a Left-Brained World* is a great guide for parents trying to understand a uniquely creative child (Freed & Parsons, 1998). Stop and think about this before labeling a kid with ADHD.

I also like to look at a kid's character and think about how it impacts his or her experience in the world. It's tough to define character precisely. It has become synonymous with that unique imprint of personality, values, and style that makes a person memorable. It's also often used to describe a system of values and behaviors. For the purposes of assessment, character is simply the mix of values and enduring traits that help define an individual. Obviously, these change over time. As you assess children, begin to create an image of their character. Think about what makes them unique and different. What patterns of behavior do you see that define them? What is their value system or worldview?

This section highlights the need to spend a lot of time with each kid. Be ready to spend the duration of each appointment exploring and opening yourself to the unique young person that you are assessing. I spend 90 minutes with a kid during the initial assessment, and anywhere from 30 to 60 minutes during regular appointments. The more you can appreciate the whole child, the better you can relate, the better you can understand, and, most important, the better you can heal.

3. Identify Patterns of Imbalance

As you explore the six realms, you'll naturally intuit areas of imbalance or concern. "His nutrition looks pretty poor," or "He seems to have some issues with his dad." This is an example of how important intuition becomes in identifying the patient's ills. A computer program or diagnostic guide cannot do this. Your gut can. So trust your perception. I find it very useful to explore my intuitions with the patient and the parents as I summarize my findings: "Seems like your diet is pretty poor," or "It sounds like you and your dad have been struggling." Most often I will see nods of agreement. Most parents and older kids will have some intuition of their own about what's imbalanced. This mutual understanding will also help create a bond of trust.

Since every kid has unique strengths and weaknesses, different kids can tolerate imbalances better than others. For example, someone with no family history of depression may tolerate inactivity better mentally or emotionally than someone who carries a genetic predisposition. Thus, a person in the latter scenario may need to exercise more regularly than a person in the former scenario to avoid the onset of an imbalance in mood.

Think about which areas are strong and balanced and which are weak, ignored, or depleted. Are there patterns of excess? For example, a kid may be very successful in schoolwork, but is that all he or she does? This kid may not have much of a social or recreational life, and this may indicate an imbalance. In the same way, a young athlete may be strong and vital but have no inner life, no spiritual awareness. A smart teenager may be intellectually vital but have a sagging, neglected body. Obviously, each kid has an individual pattern, but is it excessive or imbalanced? For children, this may be less obvious but no less worth exploration. Trends and patterns are often set early in childhood and often by parents. So look at the patterns of imbalance in the parents' lives, as it might give a good indication of potential imbalances in the child's life.

4. Evaluate Barriers to Health

Barriers block the path to wholeness and limit health. So the identification of potential barriers is a make-or-break step in any assessment of a symptomatic child, teen, or young adult. Otherwise we fall into the all-too-common path of pathologizing the child and the brain. As we remove barriers the innate power of wholeness will pull the child back to health, reducing symptoms along the way.

Barriers are found in many arenas of life. So as you move through each of the six realms of the child, remain alert for anything that stands out as a barrier to health. Here are some common examples of barriers in each of the child's six realms.

1. Environmental: Too much TV, overstimulation from electronics, too much lighting in the evening, mercury in the food, pesticides causing poor concentration, lack of time in nature, or a lack of sunlight.
2. Physical: Lack of sleep, lack of exercise, inadequate protein in the diet, food allergies, caffeine, obesity, processed foods with dyes and preservatives, hydrogenated oils, high glycemic load, sugars and highly processed grains, lack of breakfast, chronic symptoms of any kind, or chronic illness or fatigue indicative of mitochondrial issues.
3. Emotional: Poor self-regulation, attachment issues, trauma, abuse, overstimulation, divorce, a depressed mom or dad, an alcoholic parent, a disengaged parent, a critical parent, or a hostile marriage.
4. Mental: Too much pessimism, poor executive functioning skills, a pat-

tern of impulsiveness, poor planning, chaotic organization, poor self-control, problems with concentration and sustained attention, learning disabilities, poor working memory, dyslexia, difficulty relaxing, or a lack of motivation.

5. Social: Poor social skills, social isolation, excessive introversion or extroversion, poor attachment, unhealthy family or friend relationships, or a lack of role modeling.

6. Spiritual: Lack of meaning or purpose in life, insufficient spiritual practice, too much or too little engagement in religious activities, self-absorption, or self-serving behavior. (Obviously, spiritual issues are a bit more mercurial, but no less vital to health. Just keep a close eye on the vitality of the kid's spirit. It is often a seemingly insignificant spiritual conflict that leads to a full-blown existential crisis and suicidal ideation. Also, be wary—teens that are mired in an existential crisis with suicidal ideation do not respond well to medications.)

5. Fit: How Is the Match?

During an average assessment, I spend a good deal of time thinking about fit. Fit is a broad term for the nature of the interaction between two different components: to be suitable with or in a state of harmony. The nature of fit with each parent and child should be assessed. But you should also think about fit as it relates to different spheres of the child's ecology. Chess and Thomas, famed experts in child temperament, offer a good insight into this thinking:

> Stated briefly, there is a goodness of fit when the person's temperament and other characteristics such as motivation and levels of intellectual and other abilities, are adequate to master the successive demands, expectations, and opportunities of the environment. This formulation stems from the conviction that normal or pathologic psychological development does not depend on temperament alone. Rather, it is the nature of the interaction between temperament and the individual's other characteristics with specific features of the environment, which provides the basic dynamic influence for the process of development. If there is a goodness of fit between child and environment, the foundation for a healthy self-concept and stable self-esteem is laid down. If there is a poorness of fit, a negative, denigrated self-evaluation begins to crystallize. If, in latter childhood or even in adult

life, a poorness of fit can be altered, such as by the emergence of new positive capacities or a favorable change in the environment, then a negative self-image may be transformed into a positive one. (1977, pp. 15–16)

It's important to ask how the child fits with each parent, and how the child fits with the family, extended family, neighborhood, school, and church. School is a particular area of concern, though, as every school has a particular culture, focus, and style that can support a child's needs or, conversely, clash with them. For example, a playful, active, and somewhat immature 9-year-old may not fit well in a rigid, discipline-oriented prep school. Moreover, the fit between specific teachers and the child must be considered, especially in elementary school. Sometimes the style or expectations of one teacher may create an ideal setting for a child or, on the other hand, they can make school a living hell for the little kid. This is rare, but it does happen. If the child is struggling in school, inquire about the child's various teachers and their teaching styles.

In addition to school, assess how well the child meshes with the many environments in which he functions. How is he with his parents, peers, and extended family? His neighborhood? His church? The alternative to assessing these environments and relationships invariably involves labels, pathology, and medication. Instead of that, explore how the child and his many environments must change or adapt in order to improve the fit and the child's health and happiness. R. M. Lerner sums this up well in *Concepts and Theories of Human Development*:

> The child's individuality, in differentially meeting the demands of the context, provides a basis for the feedback he or she gets from the socializing environment. That is, just as the child brings his or her characteristics of individuality to a particular setting, there are demands placed on the child by virtue of the social and physical components of the setting. First, these demands may take the form of attitudes, values, or expectations held by others in the context of the child's physical or behavioral attributes or others in the context with whom the child must coordinate, or fit, his or her behavioral attributes for adaptive interactions to exist. (1986, p. 101)

As you begin to explore the child's many environments and interactions, you'll notice the many "demands placed on the child by virtue of the social and physical components of the setting," as Lerner puts it. You will begin to better contextualize the child's behavior and mental attitudes. This is a good first step in creating change in those contexts where the kid is suffering. More specific questions will surely arise, but the most basic question will always be, is this situation a good fit for the child?

6. Remember to Assess the Family

When you assess a child, you must also assess the family. Parents are the predominant role models for children and their primary support system. Children attach to parents and create important bonds to their siblings. Values and character typically form in the family crucible, as it's the main environment in which they function. I could go on and on, but needless to say family plays a central role in the development, health, and happiness of a child. For that reason, it needs to be scrutinized in the assessment process. Doing so will give you a good idea of the context out of which the kid's issues spring. In my experience, if the clinician possesses a depth of understanding about a family, it creates a solid foundation for success in treating that family's child.

Here are 10 key reminders to keep in mind during the family assessment process:

1. Parents act as agents for the child, and their own needs and issues may overlay the presenting issues.
2. Everything reflects in some manner the nature and quality of the parents' marriage.
3. In a family, a lot is hidden.
4. When all else fails, think of family therapy.
5. Aggressively screen for and address maternal depression and anxiety.
6. Behavioral issues create parenting issues and vice versa.
7. The younger the child, the more parental involvement is needed.
8. Build a bond with both parents; involve both even if one does not attend sessions.
9. Explore parental attachment and relationships with grandparents.
10. Parents, in general, are hungry for education and support.

I find it helpful to think of the family as a big tent. Every tent is different. Some tents are protective and can withstand the worst gales and weather. Other tents get torn up and collapse in a strong wind. Think about what kind of tent each child lives under and how you might be able to patch or reinforce its weaknesses.

Intake Form

At Wholeness Center, prior to the first session we use an intake form completed by parents (see Appendix A). This provides some overview of the child's history, the family, past treatments, and the issues at hand. Obviously, it's easy to create a massive, cumbersome form that asks every possible question, but this is an undue burden on parents and usually fails to replace a thoughtful discussion. Over time, at the Wholeness Center we have reached a compromise between brevity and completeness. The key here lies in creating a broad enough overview of history. The form should highlight concerns and direct your attention to areas that might otherwise be missed. It doesn't need to be conclusive. It just needs to open up new areas for further exploration.

The Psychiatric Interview and Patient Preference

To begin the psychiatric interview, start by meeting with both parents (as appropriate and possible) and the child all together in the same room. This will give you a chance to watch the interactions of each party in the room and hear everyone's take on the problem. I typically start with less threatening topics like interests and recreation, moving into school information, family background, medical history, and early development. It is useful to take note of how much sensitivity, support, and criticism come up as parents talk about their child. Only after moving through these topics do I go through a typical medical review of systems: sleep, appetite, headaches, stomachaches, mood, and so on. As one of the final steps, I ask why the family is here and try to get everyone's perspective. While this is central to the assessment, I move to it later in the interview in order to build rapport and ease the inevitable stress of the first encounter.

Finally, ask what each person is hoping to get from your involvement. This will give you a better understanding of each party's expectations and hopes. After this, inquire about prior treatments: Why it didn't work or why they moved on. As one of the last steps in the conjoint interview, ask the family about their belief system as it relates to treatment. Document the discussion and record their preferences. Usually, I present the basics of conventional care (e.g., medications, psychotherapy) and holistic care (e.g., natural approaches, skill-building techniques, mind-body approaches, nutrition, supplements) and explore their beliefs. My basic philosophy here is to start with the safest options, saving medications for later if backup is needed. But always make sure to explore the patient and family preferences. For example, the parents may have little interest in complementary modalities or they may adamantly refuse psychiatric medication. Generally, most parents prefer some mix of the above with a preference toward the safest options.

Like me, most parents are leery about using psychiatric medications in a developing nervous system. In fact, about 95% of parents I meet with feel relieved that medications are not the first step. And about 30% of the families I encounter indicate that their preference is to totally avoid psychiatric medications if at all possible. Make sure to ask the family about their preference and the rationale behind it. It may be that the family has diminished faith in medications after numerous failed trials and odious side effects. Or the family may simply want to delay the use of psychiatric medications until totally necessary. Some families just don't believe in drug treatment at all. Whatever the case may be, listen to the family's preference and make note of it. An all-too-common complaint I hear is that the child's previous psychiatrist did not listen or understand the family's treatment preference. That's why this kind of discussion should occur prior to any diagnosis or the development of any treatment plan. Try to understand the belief system of the family and match it to your treatment plan. This simple act of consideration can aid health in profound ways.

It is widely recognized across all cultures and health systems that a patient's belief system is a central factor in healing (Frank, 1961). Dr. Astin of Stanford has documented similar findings. His research reveals that people seek out complementary and alternative medicine (CAM) approaches not because of efficacy but because the treatment options better fit with their worldview and overall philosophy of health (Astin, 1998). CAM represents an emerging paradigm of health care, with anywhere from 30% to 60% of people now endorsing some practice of it. As practitioners, it is incumbent upon us to assess the underlying world-view of our patients and honor it to the best of our ability.

People are not always forthright with their belief system or treatment preference during a session. However, I find that if you ask enough of the right questions, you can usually get a good sense of what kind of treatments the patient and the family are comfortable with. Focus on asking positive questions, such as, What do you think can help you become well? Do you believe that medications, psychotherapy, herbs, acupuncture, or prayer will help? Why do you believe that? It's well documented that belief can alter the response to all kinds of treatments. In cross-cultural psychiatry, this premise is a given. So be mindful of it. Each individual creates an internalized microculture of personalized beliefs that must be addressed and validated if the person is to heal.

At this point in the interview, after assessing the family's belief system and treatment preference, excuse the parents and meet with the child alone. In my practice, I offer the kid the opportunity to direct the interaction: Sometimes we play games, just sit and talk, or maybe go for a walk. This makes the exchange less formal and eases the tension of seeing a shrink. The only agenda for the first meeting is to get to know the child and take in what you can, trying to make her as comfortable as possible. The style should be relaxed, the conversation light, touching on her interests and skills. Humor is a wonderful ingredient for new encounters. Make a real effort to listen and present opportunities for the child to express concerns, fears, hopes, wishes, and goals.

Make sure to take detailed notes of the child's responses to the various questions you ask and behavior during your meeting. (Often, it's helpful to use a structured series of topics or questions to explore the child's world, but don't be afraid to stray from it as necessary.) But also make sure to pause and put down your notes at various intervals so you can just absorb the general atmosphere of the interview.

Only once the kid seems to be pretty comfortable with you and your initial questions is it okay to ask more probing questions about his view of the presenting issues. Try to get a sense of how he thinks about these issues and where he believes the issues stem from. Some details of the family and parent-child dynamics will usually emerge unsolicited from this kind of talk. Near the end, make sure to turn the tables and ask what questions the kid has for you. If he has the capacity, inquire about how he might like to see the treatment go and what treatment approaches seem appropriate or interesting to him. The fundamental atmosphere, of course, should always be one of respect and caring curiosity.

The remaining time in the first session is with the parents alone. Here, inquire about the marriage, stress levels, and other concerns that have cropped up over the course of the interview. At this point, it is pretty common for parents to further elaborate on their observations of the presenting issues. Take careful note here: Do they save more negative material for this private conversation, or do they share more in front of the child? This will give you a good indication of the level of parental involvement and their style of parenting. Are they overcritical or detached? During this conversation, allow ample time for the parents to ask you questions. Listen to their concerns and explore relevant topics.

In the wholeness approach, the first-session interview takes over an hour, often 90 minutes. Unless it is a true crisis of safety, I never diagnosis, treat, or prescribe in the first session; it is fully devoted to gathering information. For insurance purposes, my diagnosis on the superbill (the document signed by the practitioner and given to the patient indicating date of visit, location, diagnosis, and CPT code for insurance billing purposes) is almost always general after the first interview: mood NOS, anxiety NOS, disruptive DO, or even disorder of childhood NOS. I take the time between the first and second sessions to get collateral information (e.g., information from teachers or other practitioners) and order labs. The second visit is devoted to exploring a possible treatment plan. This takes away the urgency to identify the right treatment while you're still getting to know the patient.

First Session

At the beginning of the first session, I meet with the child and parents together. I ask about what they enjoy and love to do. Hopefully this gets them talking. From there we go on to explore school and family life: what's up with siblings, pets, and patterns of interactions. As they talk, I try to get a sense of the relationship between the parents and child, as well as their patterns of communication. I go over developmental history, medical history, and family psychiatric history with parents and notice the transition the child makes in terms of attention and engagement. Sleep and nutrition are my next topics. Finally, only after I have developed some rapport do I inquire about the chief complaint and why they are here.

After the chief complaint has been articulated, I meet with the child or teen alone. First we explore topics of ease and interest to the young person, perhaps over a game or a walk down the running path near my office. I ask about his or her home life and concerns. I treat the child as an equal and give respect. I also provide the chance for the child to ask me questions. Here is where internalizing disorders such as trauma, depression, and anxiety must be ruled out. But be careful about asking questions about these things directly; if the child seems nervous or scared about a subject, move on to something low-impact. It is important to ask the child's opinion about meeting with a therapist. Does he or she think that something is wrong? If so, what is it? At the end of this time, if appropriate, I share my observations and sense of who the child is and what matters to him or her. If I have a sense of where treatment might go, I explore the child's willingness to participate and offer my thoughts on how treatment might help the child reach his or her goals.

Third segment: Meet with just the parents. This is time for parents to share difficult or uncomfortable information. We explore the marriage and household stresses in more depth. I ask about belief systems and preferences on care. Parents are free to ask questions, and we may discuss some treatment options. I share my view of the child or teen and see if that matches up with what the parents see. This is crucial: Everyone has to be on the same page if the child is going to succeed.

Take the time between the first and second sessions to reach outside the confines of the office and gather outside information. Survey teachers, other practitioners, and anyone else you believe can give you a more exact, multidimensional picture of what's going on. This is a crucial but underutilized step in assessment.

With rare exceptions, I survey the school of every kid I see. I use a standardized form (such as the Vanderbilt) for attentional and disruptive issues. However, I've also created a simple open-ended teacher feedback form that I use for every child, preschool to high school senior (see Figure 6.1). In this prepared form, the teacher shares his or her perceptions and observations. This simple bit of outside feedback provides a lot more useful information than any of the standardized forms. Sometimes it merely reinforces perceptions about the child or teen, but at other times it sheds light on some previously unknown facet of the

Pupil's Name: _____Grade:_____Date:_____

School:_____Teacher's Name:_____

Do you have any problems or concerns about this child in the classroom? ___
_____
_____
_____

What are this child's strong points in the classroom? _____
_____
_____

What are this child's weak points in the classroom? _____
_____
_____

How does he/she get along with peers? _____
_____
_____

Is attention or distractability a major problem? _____
_____
_____

How does this child respond to discipline? _____
_____
_____

How is this child's mood? _____
_____
_____

Other comments: _____
_____
_____
_____

If you need more space, you may continue on the back.

Figure 6.1. Teacher Feedback Form

child, unlocking some vital clue to the form or root of his or her issues. Either way, I want to hear from people who see this kid every day before I diagnose or initiate treatment after knowing him or her for only a few days.

Next, I like to reach out to current or prior therapists to hear their impressions and concerns. Given the difficulties of modern professional life, sometimes this means trading curt voice mails. One of the joys of working in the same region for over 20 years is that I've been fortunate to develop relationships with most of the other professionals working nearby. Because of that, when I need to reach out for collateral information or a referral, I have a good sense of various practitioners' skills and styles of work and how a kid might mesh with them.

As a final step in outside assessment, I like to engage significant others in the assessment and treatment process by checking in with them and asking about the presenting issues and any other concerns I should be aware of. Beyond that, youth ministers, coaches, and friends often have helpful perspectives. Also, I always let the young person know who I am talking to and ask if he or she thinks I should be talking to anyone else. If the kid has any ideas, I make clear that he or she is welcome to sit in on any of those meetings.

I also take the time between the first and second sessions to order labs. Lab tests are a wonderful window into the human body. Very often they help pin down physiological problems contributing to mental health issues. For most folks, I order a basic group of eight standing items:

1. Thyroid-stimulating hormone (TSH): If there is a family history of thyroid disease or symptoms that match thyroid dysfunction (fatigue, lethargy, anxiety, or restlessness), I will order T3, T4, and thyroid antibodies. TSH should be around 1. Anything over 3 is a concern, and I have also found that elevated TSH corresponds to gluten sensitivity. Gluten is an immunologically active molecule that seems to be related to low-grade Hashimoto thyroiditis, the most common cause of hypothyroidism—an epidemic concern.

2. Vitamin D (25 hydroxy vitamin D): This a good general health indicator related to mood and cognitive well-being. Vitamin D levels have also been linked to seasonal affective disorder, schizophrenia, and depression. In one study, psychotic features were observed in 40% of

mentally ill teens with low vitamin D levels, compared to 16% of teens with normal vitamin D levels (Splete, 2011). I like to target 40 to 45 ng/ml. Most kids I test in sunny Colorado are deficient. Those people living in less sunny areas should monitor and supplement their levels.

3. Ferritin: This is the best indicator of total body stores of iron, which plays a crucial role in the production of dopamine needed for attention (the target of stimulant medications such as Ritalin and Adderall). My target is 40 ng/ml. Anemia is a late indicator of iron deficiency.

4. Homocysteine: This indicates the health of the methylation system in the body, which produces all neurotransmitters. Should be in the range of 5 to 7. Elevated numbers indicate failure of methylation and a need for B vitamins.

5. Cholesterol: This is the mother steroid hormone molecule crucial to the maintenance of mood and physical recovery. Recent evidence correlates low levels with increased risk of depression and suicide. Target 150 mg/dl. If low, diet support is needed to augment good oils.

6. C-reactive protein: This is one of the best measures of inflammation within the body. Depression and many other psychiatric illnesses are, at their core, inflammatory diseases. I like to see this measure under 2. Fish oil, diet, and other supplements can help to reduce high levels.

7. Methylenetetrahydrofolate reductase (MTHFR): This is one of our few useful genetic tests in psychiatry. It tests for single-nucleotide polymorphisms (SNPs) of the enzyme that activates folic acid in the body. A child who has both C alleles is at a heightened risk for depression and anxiety disorders. B vitamins and activated folate are the ideal treatment. I do not get this all the time, but consider it for chronic cases.

8. DHEA (dehydroepiandrosterone)-sulfate: I use this test for anyone with chronic illness or extreme fatigue. It is a useful indicator of adrenal function. I treat to the average level of a healthy young adult.

Depending on the symptoms, I will select other lab tests as well, including tests of mitochondrial function and status, gut dysbiosis, urine for organic acids, plasma amino acids, liver panels, or serum levels. (These are covered in greater depth in Part II.) I typically order labs on the first visit and request prior outside labs and other evaluations for the purpose of review.

Second Session

I meet with the parents and the child. We go over labs, school forms, and other new material. I offer my observations about common presenting issues and my ideas for treatment and why it all makes sense to me according to what I found in the history, the interview, the new evidence, and their concerns. I offer lots of time for questions and I write notes and instructions for treatment for them to take home. If needed, I spend time with the young person alone to see if he or she endorses the plan, if we have not already done that in the first session.

Third Session (and Beyond)

I meet with parents and child to check in on treatment and to make adjustments to any facet of the treatment plan not working or yet to be administered. If needed, I meet with the kid alone to see how he or she is holding up with the treatment, and if we need to make any quick adjustments according to the kid's preferences.

CHAPTER SEVEN

Common Presenting Issues

One day in 1973, eight totally sane people walked into different psychiatric hospitals across five states. During the evaluation process, all eight people gave an accurate personal history, with only one exception. They all lied to the evaluators, saying they occasionally heard their own name being called out at night. And with that, all eight were admitted to a hospital, given a range of psychiatric diagnoses, and started on treatment for their "illness."

Ironically, the only people who knew these eight pseudopatients were "sane" were the patients inhabiting the hospitals. The psychiatrists and nurses never figured it out, despite the fact that those eight people continually expressed their sanity and desire to be released. (Which perhaps only further confirmed their insanity.) In fact, all eight people were forced to admit their insanity and had to agree to take antipsychotic medication as a condition of their release.

Later that year, the psychologist behind this famous experiment, David Rosenhan (1973), published this story in *Science* under the title "On Being Sane in Insane Places." Suffice to say, the validity of what we do in modern psychiatric diagnosis remains an open and contentious discussion. Many people, most prominently Thomas Szaz, have come forward to openly question the validity of our diagnostic system (1984). At a very basic level, given the complexity of the human mind, the enormous number of outside variables, and the extremely reductionistic nature of modern psychiatry, it should come as no surprise that the validity and reliability of our diagnostic system is in question. Rosenhan confirms at least that much.

I suspect you've noticed by now that there is no "diagnosis" section in this book. (I did, however, devote Part II of this book to disease and disorder protocols, since it's sometimes helpful to organize one's thinking according to known categories of care.) This is because, like Rosenhan, Szaz, and others, I have fundamental objections to the system of psychiatric diagnosis, particularly as it relates to children. To tell the truth, I do not place much value on labels in my clinical practice. There is a host of reasons for my position (experiments like Rosenhan's being one), but for the sake of concision, I have provided a list of just a few of the most relevant ones. They can be roughly broken into three categories: concerns over reliability, concerns over validity, and other practical concerns.

Concerns Over Reliability

1. In clinical practice, the reliability of diagnosis is poor. (Only with structured interviews in an academic setting is it somewhat reliable. But only research scientists use structured interviews.)
2. There is no way to definitively confirm any psychiatric diagnosis.
3. Diagnosis depends on the personal judgment and opinion of one person.
4. It's easy to develop idiosyncratic perspectives that can dramatically color your opinions (e.g., a psychiatrist can begin to "prefer" certain diagnoses).
5. Because primary care physicians are usually the front line of defense for kids, they make the majority of psychiatric diagnoses and they often have insufficient training for this very difficult process.
6. Children are much harder to diagnose than adults.
7. The average child comes out of a psychiatric evaluation with over three *DSM* diagnoses.
8. As many as one-third of children outgrow a given diagnosis in a year or two.

Concerns Over Validity

1. Psychiatric diagnoses are the only medical diagnoses not based on verified tissue pathology.
2. Psychiatric diagnoses are designed and voted on by a committee.
3. Psychiatric diagnoses are a mix of theoretical paradigms (e.g., behavioral, psychodynamic, biological, family systems) without a consistent foundation.

4. A poorly trained volunteer can simulate most any psychiatric diagnosis and even merit involuntary hospitalization (à la Rosenhan).

5. Psychiatric diagnoses morph over time and vary in different cultures. Where are hebephrenia and neurasthenia now? Homosexuality?

6. Our diagnostic system carries little treatment specificity for our medications.

7. Human genetic studies and the Human Genome Project have poked holes in a perspective based solely on biological psychiatry.

8. The emerging sciences of epigenetics and neuroplasticity dramatically weaken our current biological perspective of fixed illness.

9. Long-term (5 years or more) outcome studies of conventional psychiatric treatment provide very little evidence of consistent benefit.

10. Psychiatric research has been heavily influenced by the pharmaceutical industry, thereby tainting the research base.

Other Practical Concerns

1. Psychiatric labels are often incorrect.
2. A psychiatric label carries a stigma for most people.
3. Labels do not empower people, nor do they convey the appropriate steps that lead to action.
4. A psychiatric label will often prevent future insurance coverage or job eligibility.
5. Labels often needlessly lead to medication.
6. A negative label can convey a nocebo or medical hexing effect, associated with a negative outcome and diminished expectations.
7. Our current system creates inappropriate expectations of precision.

Rather than offering a diagnosis, I prefer to identify common presenting issues and treat them appropriately.

Common Presenting Issues

Proper identification of personally limiting issues is the first step in healing. By accurately breaking down a child's particular limiting issues, a clinician can better understand and manage a child's health. Below is a list of 23 of the more common presenting issues affecting kids.

It's far from exhaustive, but this list covers about 98% of the issues typically encountered in a busy clinical practice. Think of the list almost as a mental health checklist. It can help direct your thinking about what potential issues could be affecting the child and causing suffering: "Does she have focus and attention issues? Pain? Issues with behavior cooperation?" And unlike diagnosis, this checklist breaks down the patient's issues into amenable subtypes, making the issues more manageable. It also accurately individuates the patient and his or her health, instead of just stuffing all the potential issues under a blanket term like depression or anxiety.

Here is the current list of our common presenting issues:

1. Sound sleep
2. Proper diet
3. Stress management
4. Weight and fitness
5. Mood and self-regulation
6. Family harmony
7. Relationships and social skills
8. Joy and self-esteem
9. Peace and serenity
10. Behavioral cooperation
11. Gut health
12. Inflammation and toxic overload
13. Trauma
14. Focus and attention
15. Learning difficulties
16. Addiction
17. Obsession and compulsion
18. Thought clarity
19. Pain
20. Eating habits
21. Metabolic concerns
22. Spirituality
23. Other health issues (medical illness and chronic conditions)

Each and every one of these issues can have a hand in the development or manifestation of any number of mental illnesses. For example, major depression in one of your patients might really just be a troublesome mix of issues like sound sleep, gut health, inflammation and toxic overload, addiction, and spirituality. Identifying and resolving these issues one at a time gives your patient a better chance of returning to health and wholeness than does medicating more superficial symptoms of depression or anxiety.

One way to think about these common presenting issues is as subtypes of the seven building blocks of wholeness (see Chapter 2). If a little boy is struggling with sleep (building block number 3), for example, one or more of these common presenting issues is likely a factor. Thus, identifying and correcting the issues will naturally restore balance and strength to his building block of sleep and restore him to wholeness. In the same way, a little boy who shows no common presenting issues during evaluation would, necessarily, have strong and well-balanced building blocks of wholeness. In short, that little boy would be healthy and whole.

Typically, I wait until the second or third session to run through this list with the patient and the parents. I do so for two reasons. One, you're going to need some sense of the kid and parents if you're going to single out any of these issues. Two, it's important to wait so that you can consult labs, teacher forms, and past practitioners' feedback (these should be back by the second or third session). These forms and outside feedback often offer crucial insights not otherwise available to your eyes and ears. For example, you may be able to identify gut health as an issue only after you review the child's labs. Or it may be that you identify relationships and social skills as an issue only after a teacher writes back with some abiding concerns.

You can certainly make note of any issues you notice as you're working through your initial six realms assessment (see Chapter 6). (In fact, since each of the 23 common presenting issues corresponds to one of the six realms—sound sleep and gut health fall under the physical realm, for example—it might be helpful to break the issues down according to assessment realm. That way, as you work through each of the six realms, you'll also be working through an initial impression of the 23 common presenting issues.) I only advise that you hold off on your final assessment of the child's issues until you've seen the child a few times and you've reviewed the outside feedback.

Over the course of the next few pages, I discuss each of the 23 common presenting issues in greater detail, showing you how to recognize when problems exist and the various ways in which they can be ameliorated. Each common presenting issue section is broken into two succinct subsections. The first subsection, What to Look For, reviews questions for the patient and identifying factors. The second, What to Do, details potential remedies and treatments to resolve the affecting issue.

Sound Sleep

What to Look For

How well do you sleep and for how long? Do you wake up? Nightmares or bad dreams? Sleep terrors? Is the child afraid of sleeping in his own bed? Any problems going to sleep? Does the child snore, gasp, or have irregular breathing? Leg movements? Family history of sleep apnea? Any daytime fatigue, problems with concentration or mood?

What to Do

Sleep hygiene, dedicated sleep schedule, take electronics out of room, decrease lighting in the room or home, sleep psychologist to do cognitive behavioral counseling for sleep, actigraphy (low-cost, less invasive diagnostic tool), formal sleep study, melatonin (low dose: 0.5 mg or at most 1 mg), lemon balm or valerian, magnesium glycinate, hot bath, nighttime routine, treat underlying anxiety if present (see Chapter 12).

Proper Diet

What to Look For

I ask everyone about what they like to eat and drink. Do you drink caffeine? How much protein do you eat? How healthy is your diet? (Parents and teens have an honest sense of how good their diet is.) Skipping breakfast is a major concern, and so is lack of appetite. If blood sugar issues (hypoglycemia) are present this can be a significant concern as well, as it can affect focus and mood regulation.

What to Do

If I have a concern over diet quality, blood sugar issues, dysbiosis (see Gut Health), or food allergies (this is the case with at least 30% to 40% of the kids under 10 that I evaluate), I refer them for a nutritional consultation by a naturopath or nutritionist. Otherwise, I provide basic nutritional education. I instruct them about the importance of protein, a regular breakfast, the need to eliminate all soda and caffeine, the need to decrease processed foods, and the need for whole grains and whole foods. No single tool has helped my practice more than having a solid nutritional resource available for kids and parents. The conventional hospital-based registered dietician may not work well for these needs, as these practitioners tend to be more focused on macronutrient balance and typically do not have the appropriate background to address the gut and dysbiosis issues that so often accompany dietary issues in this population. I prefer to work with naturopaths, given their medical background and comfort with gut health, supplements, and related medical issues.

Stress Management

What to Look For

I ask people (kids and parents) if they feel overwhelmed with demands. I ask about what stresses them. Do you feel like you are going to explode and that your mind is always racing? Do you always feel rushed? Do you always feel behind and have too many things to get done? Do you feel like you can't do all that you need to? Do you have a hard time relaxing and letting go of it all? Having someone rate their stress level on a 0 to 10 scale can be helpful (see the Wholeness Stress Index in Chapter 3). This concept is typically more of a teenage, young adult, and parental concern. Younger kids do not usually conceptualize stress. Examine the child's behavior, sleep, and perceived anxiety to assess for stressors. Perfectionistic traits will tend to magnify the sense of pressure and anxiety. If you suspect something might be out of whack, order labs to check for abnormal adrenal stress index and diurnal cortisol pattern, as well as low serum DHEA-sulfate level.

What to Do

The single best stress management tool is focused counseling examining stress triggers and exploring resources and coping tools. Additional treatments include biofeedback, yoga, meditation, exercise, inositol and B vitamins, acupuncture, massage, retreats, time in nature, more sunlight, long walks, time with animals, sleep, and better food. Caffeine makes even the regular user experience more stress in a typical day. I ask everyone with anxiety, stress, or mood issues to consider a 2-week trial cutting out caffeine. Ideally, patients should identify the tools best suited to them and try each one on for size. Create a schedule and plan for practice (see Chapter 16).

Weight and Fitness

What to Look For

Overweight or unfit body. Ideal weight is easy to screen for. Body mass index (BMI) scales and charts are readily available. Simple scales and growth charts are helpful assessment tools. But your eyeball is also a fairly good tool. Ask kids with a concerning profile if they are themselves concerned. They may recognize an issue and worry about it (often, others tease them about it). Ask how much exercise they get, how much time outdoors they get, and what they like to do. The President's Challenge Fitness Test has been around since 1966 and provides a pretty good basic assessment of fitness. Active parents tend to have active, fit kids. Ask about what they do together as a family. Ask about the parents' activity levels. A healthy child should be able to play hard for hours.

What You Can Do

It might seem obvious, but the first step is to get the problem out in the open. A study of 3,665 children and teens in Canada found that 70% of overweight or obese kids had an unrealistic appraisal of their weight and body (Parker-Pope, 2012). According to the study, the kids with the heaviest peers and parents had the least accurate self-appraisal, whereas those kids with peers and parents of normal weight had the most accurate view. Document the BMI and talk to the child and parents about it. If you're concerned, send them to a nutritionist or dietician. Create reasonable weight and fitness goals with them, keeping track of the child's progress. Prescribe exercise and limit screen time. Studies show that when you limit screen time, inactive kids get more exercise. For this to be most successful, you need to get the parents moving as well. Make it a family-wide adjustment. Explain this to the parents. The term *exercise* may be a turnoff for parents and kids, a holdover trauma from gym class or childhood. So mask the exercise: Prescribe hiking or biking, use the word *activity*, not *exercise*. It can be anything that gets everyone to move. Make it part of the family routine, and most of all see if you can help them make it fun.

Mood and Self-Regulation

What to Look For

Mood swings, irritability, rages, explosive temper, reactive mood, lack of self-control, impulsiveness, or aggression. Mood and self-regulation issues are often difficult to separate from oppositional defiant disorder (ODD). Take care to remember that the issues in ODD kids mostly stem from limits set by parents (also see Behavioral Cooperation). When I identify mood or self-regulation issues, I like to know if the behavior applies only to the parents or if it occurs in all settings. If it occurs in all settings, it is much more likely to be an issue related to biology and self-regulation. If it occurs only with parents and there is a good deal of self-control in all other settings, family dynamics and parenting are probably the culprits.

What to Do

If the kid is older, try dialectic behavioral therapy (DBT). If the kid is younger, try executive skills training. Explore diet for food allergies. Supplement with magnesium, EMPower Plus, omega-3 EFAs (EPA), martial arts training, neurofeedback, or choline. Reduce stimulation, limit violent videogames and screen time, reduce medication load, and improve sleep schedule. Explore for hypoglycemia and mitochondrial disorders. For ODD issues, I have found the Nurtured Heart Approach by Howard Glasser to be most useful (I explore this in more detail under Behavioral Cooperation; for more on mood regulation see Chapter 13).

Family Harmony

What to Look For

I ask about tension in the family. How often do you fight? How do you get along with your parents and siblings? Is there ever any aggression or physical fighting? Do people yell? Teens are usually good about relating this kind of stuff. But it can be much more difficult with younger kids. Parents will usually tell you what's going on if you set the question up right: How difficult is your son to manage? Does he ever push you until you lose your cool? How bad do things get? An important subset of this line of questioning involves the marriage: How are you two doing with each other? How has this stress affected your marriage? Do the two of you fight?

What to Do

The obvious solution here is family therapy. Sometimes it makes more sense to start with marital work first, however. With younger kids, parenting support may also be a good first step. I recommend Howard Glasser's Nurtured Heart Approach (see Behavioral Cooperation). This approach provides parents with management tools and insights that help to shift the attitude and atmosphere in the home. If parental tension is high following a divorce, then mediation or structured family therapy may help to reduce the ambient anxiety. Sometimes one family member needs to be referred for assessment or treatment as part of the family systems solution. If either parent is abusing a substance or dealing with depression or anxiety, this must be addressed (see Chapter 11).

Relationships and Social Skills

What to Look For

I ask about the child's friends. Do others seek you out? Do you lose friends easily? How many friends do you have? What do you do with each other? Is there a lot of fighting or drama? Do you have controlling friends? Do you feel lonely and isolated? Ask the parents questions, too. Are you concerned about your son? Does your son prefer to be alone? Does he avoid social situations? Here, it's important to separate out social anxiety (fears and anxiety about being with new people or groups) from problems reading social cues. Also, try to parse out whether the kid is poor at navigating social settings or just has poor self-control and self-regulation. Don't just lump social skills together. Identifying the exact issue is paramount to finding a solution.

What to Do

Social skills groups, group therapy, recreation (e.g., sports, clubs, Boy or Girl Scouts), church groups, individual therapy, or more family time.

Joy and Self-Esteem

What to Look For

Does the young person lack the typical joy and spontaneity we find in children? Does he or she seem weighed down? What is the nature of that weight? Is it serious debilitating depression with vegetative features? Or is it related to peer criticism and parental limits? Look for sadness, hopelessness, negative attitude, depressed mood, poor sleep, low appetite, weight loss, low self-esteem, lack of confidence, suicidal thinking, tearfulness, low interest, or lack of motivation.

What to Do

Individual therapy, group therapy, exercise, St. John's wort, DHEA, SAMe, chromium picolinate, acupuncture, yoga, meditation, light therapy, singing, EPA, service, dawn simulation, mental stimulation, pets, dance, art, family therapy, nature, medication, body work, activated folic acid, diet quality, B vitamins, gluten-free trial, elimination diet, and neurofeedback (see Chapter 10).

Peace and Serenity

What to Look For

Many kids I see don't have enough peace and serenity in their life. They're hyperstressed or anxious and can't slow down. Sometimes it's a shy, cautious child who's anxious or afraid in most situations and has trouble sleeping alone for years past the usual age. Sometimes it's a kid with a brooding style who's pessimistic and overthinks everything. Another common presentation is a child who seems at first to be ADHD but is actually just disorganized in social or school settings because of anxiety and tension. Obviously, there are a variety of presentations; the important thing here is to look at how much stress and anxiety kids are under and how well they are able to relax and unwind. Also, look at a child's apprehensiveness, insomnia, fears, worry, tension, separation issues, controlling style, and a variety of somatic issues like headaches and migraines.

What to Do

Biofeedback, inositol, yoga, relaxation training, meditation, kava, acupuncture, L-theanine, medication, 5-HTP (5-hydroxytryptophan, the intermediate between L-tryptophan and serotonin) (see Chapter 12).

Behavioral Cooperation

What to Look For

Oppositional kids, often 5 to 12 years old, show great resistance to parental limits and explode with defiant rage. These kids are often hard to distinguish from kids with mood regulation issues. These days, this pattern of behavior tends to be quickly labeled bipolar and heavily medicated. The most typical pattern of behavior cooperation issues that I encounter is a basically cheerful child who explodes when a parental demand is made or limit set. Often, the parent is too nice or is depressed and can't set firm, consistent limits. In my vocabulary, these kinds of parents lack the necessary fierceness to manage young children, who then quickly learn that they can up the ante and get their way by intimidating the adults. These tantrums are often extreme and explosive. This presentation can sometimes include a kid who is meek at school. But some kids will be difficult in almost every setting. These kids tend to be less socialized and come from more difficult and contentious homes.

What to Do

Parenting support or family therapy. The Nurtured Heart Approach, developed by Howard Glasser (Glasser & Easley, 1998), is my favorite recommendation for these families. It is a parenting intervention that reorients parents to build a stronger and more positive parent-child bond. This program can then be followed by a behavior reinforcement system to sustain the responses and take the parents out of the police role that they may dread or overemphasize. Sometimes mood issues such as extreme irritability coexist with this pattern. The outcome is best if you treat both simultaneously. Often with these kids self-regulation is poor. And they are usually immature. These shortcomings can be aided in therapy and parental guidance. Group therapy can be a wonderful tool for some of the older kids, if available (covered in depth in Chapter 11).

Gut Health

What to Look For

Kids with a history of food allergies and dysbiosis. If there's no known history, screen with a lab test. Also ask about the child's history of infantile colic, reflux or GERD (gastroesophageal reflux disease), ear tubes surgically placed, repeated courses of antibiotics, chronic constipation or loose stools, chronic abdominal pain, chronic headache, long bone pain ("growing pains"), insomnia, bad breath, bad foot odor, sugar cravings, narrow diet preferences (e.g., noodles, bread, macaroni and cheese), and chronic irritability. I ask about a strong sweet tooth and sugar cravings, as this often points toward dysbiosis. Anything that might fit the category of irritable bowel syndrome qualifies here. It may be a pattern of malabsorption with low levels of nutrients such as vitamin D. A comprehensive digestive stool analysis may be helpful to characterize a pattern of the problem—pathogenic bacteria, yeast overgrowth, absence of beneficial bacteria, inadequate digestive enzymes, and so forth. Some of these kids have a pattern of low cholesterol (often near 100 ng/dl), which can be associated with depression and suicide. This can also be a genetic disorder, like an SNP. Address it with a high good-fat diet.

What to Do

Review the patient's history and symptoms and order lab tests accordingly. Often, a treatment will entail the use of digestive enzymes (in cases of elevated stool fat, undigested food fibers, poor absorption markers, or decreased enzyme markers). If there are indications of dysbiosis or bacterial imbalance, supplement with probiotics. Typically, however, food allergies are the source of a chronic imbalance in the gut. If so, this needs to be addressed first by removing the offending agent from the diet. If yeast overgrowth is present, it must be treated as well. If severe, an antifungal such as nystatin or diflucan should be used. In more mild cases, use an herbal agent such as olive leaf extract or oil of oregano.

Inflammation and Toxic Overload

What to Look For

Increasingly, scientists and physicians are coming to the conclusion that most chronic illnesses are inflammatory in nature. Depression is clearly a chronic inflammatory illness with abnormal prostaglandin and leukotriene patterns. Bipolar disorder also looks to be related to a reactive, inflamed brain. Alzheimer's is clearly a disorder of excess inflammation. I routinely screen for inflammation by looking at high-sensitivity C-reactive protein and sedimentation rate. These two markers give me some sense of the inflammation in the body. In terms of toxic overload, high levels of heavy metals impair the body's detoxification pathways. Testing for heavy metals like lead or mercury as well as the adequacy of the detoxification pathways makes sense for some patients with chronic conditions. Studies continue to demonstrate a link between pesticide exposure and chronic learning issues, for example.

What to Do

For inflammation, I emphasize an anti-inflammatory diet supplemented with fish oil, alpha-lipoic acid, and more sleep. For toxicity, I recommend an organic diet. In one study, following the initiation of an organic diet the pesticide metabolites in children's urine fell off significantly within 2 weeks (Lu et al., 2006). Also try filtered water. Support the detoxification pathways with broccoli, garlic, turmeric, and vitamin C. Oral or IV chelation may be needed for elevated heavy metal levels.

Trauma

What to Look For

Anxiety, depression, sleep issues, chronic pain, fibromyalgia, flashbacks, nightmares, endometriosis, poor focus, hypervigilance, dissociation, morbid visual hallucinations, extreme aggression, or irritability. Trauma can masquerade as most any psychiatric illness in childhood; keep this in mind during evaluations.

What to Do

Trauma often requires a broad-based approach. I am a big proponent of EMDR and almost always recommend it. Trauma-focused cognitive behavioral therapy (CBT) is also valuable. To calm the body and mind, I typically recommend biofeedback, neurofeedback, yoga, meditation, the elimination of caffeine, acupuncture, inositol, 5-HTP, lemon balm, magnesium, or kava. Medications may help, especially alpha-agonists like guanfacine or clonidine. Over the last few years, I have become increasingly impressed with body-oriented psychotherapies such as Hakomi or Somatic Experiencing (Chapter 16).

Focus and Attention

What to Look For

Poor focus, impaired concentration, or an inability to attend to tasks. If the child is in school, teacher feedback is a must, as this will help to identify and isolate the problem. Focus and attention issues have a complicated differential because their presentation is similar to those of anxiety, learning disabilities, poor diet, poor mood, food allergies, toxicities, and trauma (see Chapter 9).

What to Do

Neurofeedback, dimethylaminoethanol (DMAE), bacopa, pycnogenol, centella, iron supplementation (if low), zinc supplementation (if low), executive functioning skills training such as CogMed (a proprietary computerized cognitive training program), whole-foods diet, correct food allergies, add a high-protein breakfast, reduce overstimulation and video games, or set an earlier bedtime.

Learning Difficulties

What to Look For

Was the child late to read or late to speak? Is there a difficulty in understanding instructions or telling a story? Is there a family history of dyslexia or learning issues? Are there problems retaining and following through on two- or three-step commands? Poor coordination? Is there a strong dislike of school starting at a young age? A dislike of reading? Test phobia? Also make sure to evaluate diet quality.

What to Do

Often, kids with learning issues have a high level of anxiety in a school setting. This has to be addressed first. It's helpful for parents to read with the child and set a regular reading time. Storytelling can also help get kids excited about reading. Try supporting executive functioning skills training, as well as supplementation with omega-3 EFAs, DMAE, bacopa, or iron (as needed). Proper school fit is crucial: Look at getting a 504 Plan (educational modifications and accommodations for the child, as specified by the Rehabilitation Act and the Americans With Disabilities Act), IEP evaluation, or neuropsychological evaluation (see glossary for more information on these programs). You can also try remedial instruction, tutors, identification of primary learning style, and verbal games. Think about an elimination diet to test for food allergies and testing for gut dysbiosis (see Chapter 9).

Addiction

What to Look For

Substance abuse (e.g., nicotine, opiates, alcohol, cannabis, amphetamines), workaholism, sexual addiction, shopaholism, or the like. The key thing to look for here is if there appears to be an unhealthy relationship with an agent or process.

What to Do

Twelve-step program, acupuncture, better diet, exercise, neurofeedback, rational recovery, full-spectrum free-form amino acids for withdrawal, B vitamins, IV nutritional program (if severe), vitamin C, multivitamin, multimineral, caffeine-free diet, body work or psychotherapy (see Chapter 14).

Obsession and Compulsion

What to Look For

Obsessions, compulsions, repetitive behaviors (hand washing, ordering, checking), rigid and inflexible routines, stereotyped routines, or recurrent violent images. The Yale-Brown Obsessive Compulsive Scale is a good measure of this behavior.

What to Do

For me, the first line of attack is exposure and response prevention. SSRI medications seem to work well for some kids. Try supplementation with inositol, magnesium, or 5-HTP (not in combination with SSRIs). Gluten-free and caffeine-free diets show periodic success. Reduce video game and television exposure (see Chapter 12).

Thought Clarity

What to Look For

Signs of psychosis, thought disorder, thought blocking, inability to abstract, severe agitation, hallucinations (visual or auditory), paranoia, extreme suspicion, inability to comprehend, delays in response, aggression, inability to make sense, or loose associations. When in doubt, consider using a projective test such as Rorschach.

What to Do

Supplement with omega-3 EFAs (EPA), choline, inositol, EMPower Plus, or glycine. Think about social support, cognitive training, heavy metal testing, gut assessment and correction, substance abuse assessment and correction, acupuncture, and low-dose medications. It's also important to work on diet and family conflict.

Pain

What to Look For

Complaints of pain, restricted mobility, headaches, abdominal pain, prior injury, motor vehicle accident, crying, distress, irritability, or restlessness.

What to Do

Assess and correct for inflammation and gut imbalance. Think about massage, body manipulation, antioxidant therapy, fish oil supplementation, acupuncture, somatic psychotherapy, correcting food allergies, and improving social and family support. Explore history for psychological trauma or abuse.

Eating Habits

What to Look For

Preoccupation with weight or calories, preoccupation with body image, binging on food, purging, excessive use of laxatives, yo-yoing weight, weight loss, preoccupation with food or diet, loss of enamel on teeth, soft downy hair, excessive exercise, fear of eating in public, loss of menstruation, going to the bathroom immediately after meals, skipping meals, only wearing baggy clothes, refusal to eat, or complaints of always being cold.

What to Do

Psychotherapy, assess and correct gut health, nutritionist consultation, group therapy, behavior program, family therapy, inositol and zinc supplementation, massage or other body work, somatic psychotherapies, art or other expressive therapies, meditation, or spiritual work. Also make sure to assess and correct for a history of trauma.

Metabolic Concerns

What to Look For

Family history of psychiatric issues, mental retardation, or autism. Also look for significant developmental delays, fatigue, and mood and behavioral issues that start before age 4, or consistent cognitive delays.

What to Do

Assess for metabolic issues by testing urine for organic acids. Also assess mitochondrial function with carnitine levels and EFA profiles. Make sure to check for MTHFR gene abnormality, serum cholesterol, homocysteine, serum amino acid profile, and thyroid antibodies. Treat any abnormality symptomatically as needed. Think about diet work, hyperbaric oxygen, acupuncture, and massage.

Spirituality

What to Look For

Sense of defeat, lack of effort or investment, lack of hope, preoccupation with death, cynicism, overwhelming resentments, apathy, materialism, preoccupation with violence, victimhood, depression, anxiety, somatic preoccupation, lack of joy or humor, or absence of life purpose. Chronic illness is a relevant indicator of spiritual strain and the hopelessness that can wear people down. The longer they have been plagued with any illness, the more closely I explore the spiritual arena.

What to Do

Spiritual reading, philosophical exploration, meditation, prayer, retreat, service, dream analysis, shamanic journey, existential psychotherapy, religious engagement, or mission work.

Other Health Issues (Medical Illness and Chronic Conditions)

What to Look For

I always make sure to ask about ongoing medical care or past diagnosis and the child's history of medication use. If anything of concern comes up, I ask questions about the child's engagement with treatment, acceptance of diagnosis, understanding of diagnosis, physical symptoms, weight loss or gain, fatigue, and progressive loss of function. Assess self-esteem and coping mechanisms.

What to Do

Refer for medical evaluation and care and talk to past practitioners. Pay close attention to diet, sleep, relaxation, stress management, emotional distress, and spirituality.

Remember, just as some mental health problems can be hard to diagnose, some common presenting issues can be hard to recognize. You may need to review these issues with the patient more than once in order to accurately diagnose where the issues lie. If appropriate, share your preliminary findings with patients and see if they corroborate or repudiate what you've found. Not only will this substantiate your conclusions, but it will also develop rapport between you and your patients and give you a sense of how they view their issues.

Once you've assessed a child and identified his or her common presenting issues, you'll need to develop a coherent approach to treatment. The next chapter will guide you through the process of weaving your findings into a treatment plan.

CHAPTER EIGHT

Facets of a Treatment Plan

The Wholeness Model includes five facets for creating a successful treatment plan:

1. Prioritize key issues.
2. Understand the interplay between safety and effectiveness.
3. Match patient preferences and belief system.
4. Facilitate full engagement and expectation.
5. Create an effective treatment team.

As with the list of common presenting issues in Chapter 7, I will move through each of these facets in turn, detailing their importance to the success of a treatment plan and how they can properly apply to a range of cases.

Prioritization of Key Issues

Functional medicine always starts with the gut. For children with mental health issues, though, the gut is often fine. So where to start? Unfortunately, there's no step-by-step template for treating mental health; there's too wide a range of potential contributing factors. Sometimes it's poor nutrition affecting a kid's mental health; sometimes it is high levels of innate anxiety; sometimes it is family conflict; sometimes it is a history of trauma; and sometimes it is a poor fit for learning style. Really, it's dependent on the particular child and circumstances. In psychiatry, there's just no good template for step-by-step intervention.

The truth is, the conventional neurochemical template for treatment struggles with treating children because the primary problem is not always located in abnormalities of neurochemistry. A neurochemical intervention can be a weak or limiting treatment if it does not align with the issues most affecting the child. Take Henry and Caley, our kids from the

Introduction, as examples. They were treated with neurochemical interventions for problems that were not, in the end, neurochemical. As a result, they continued to struggle while being treated solely with medications. Treatment must focus on the realms of the child's life where the major imbalances exist, where the issues really lie.

A child coming in to see you may have one of the aforementioned common presenting issues or six. Doesn't matter; you need to address each of them as clinically relevant. Obviously, it's beyond the scope of clinical ability to treat each of these common presenting issues simultaneously with any efficacy. Some need to be prioritized over others. Thus, the first step in designing treatment is to recognize which of these common presenting issues are of more immediate or heightened concern and which are only minor.

So, after you assess the child and look for common presenting issues, begin by identifying where the greatest areas of imbalance and deficiency are located—where you sense the child is the most imbalanced—and focus your treatment there. If, for example, the major imbalance is in the social realm, work on that. Conversely, if the major imbalance is in the physical realm—the child is severely overweight and not sleeping—tackle that first. If you identify an issue with family harmony and it appears to be wreaking havoc in the child's life, tackle that issue first. Clinical intuition and experience will tell you where to act first.

It's important that the intervention match the dysfunction. Many depressed kids are unfit and overweight, so exercise is a simple and applicable first intervention. However, if I evaluate a depressed 20-year-old who also runs marathons, I wouldn't think of exercise as an effective recommendation. The intervention in this case doesn't properly reflect the dysfunction. Some of the children I evaluate have an ideal diet, the result of extremely conscientious parents. Telling these families to work on diet is a waste of time. However, the recommendation of dietary change or exercise makes perfect sense for the many overweight and sedentary families I evaluate.

Rather than all or nothing, think about allotting proportional treatments. For example, a child's diet may be horrible, his gut extremely unhealthy, but he might also have some minor family dysfunction and a learning issue. In this case, I might focus 70% of the treatment effort on diet and gut intervention and the remaining 30% spread over the issues with his family and learning.

In the long run, a broad treatment plan is better than attempting a single, silver bullet intervention. A medication may alter some variables for 6 weeks or even 6 months, but over 6 years or 6 decades there's little proof of lasting success. This is why so many psychiatric visits for chronic patients involve the continual readjustment of medications. They work for a short time, and then the bodily system—because of its chronic imbalances—is pulled back toward the prior instability. A simple intervention that fails to correct the myriad underlying issues affecting a child will ultimately fall short of getting the child healthy. A successful treatment plan must acknowledge the power of various underlying imbalances and issues and attempt to correct all of them. Furthermore, a successful treatment plan must address these imbalances and issues in proper order and proportion.

Understanding the Interplay Between Safety and Effectiveness

Two factors dominate medical decision making: safety and efficacy. Very often, however, these two factors are in direct tension with one another. In fact, it is almost unheard of for a treatment to be both completely effective and perfectly safe. A major quandary for all health care providers, then, is how to juggle safety and efficacy and in what proportion to weigh the two factors against each other.

Since there's no way to automatically select the single safest and the single most effective treatment (it might not exist), a practitioner often has to come down on one side or the other of this philosophical divide. Most of the time in conventional medicine, efficacy wins out; practitioners usually select treatments solely based on clinical trials and perceived efficacy. Rarely if ever does safety dominate the selection process; it's usually a second-tier consideration.

Regardless of the current trend, the balance of safety and efficacy must be weighed impartially. Further, since the vast majority of psychiatric medications have inadequate evidence for both safety and efficacy, and since psychiatric medication has never documented both long-term safety (5-plus years) and long-term efficacy in children, the real decision makers must be the patient and the parents, not the practitioner. The patient, after being properly informed of the degrees of safety and efficacy of various options, must make this choice.

The need to inform the patient of safety in addition to efficacy looms larger as serious reports emerge challenging the safety of psychiatric medications. For example, we now have short-term studies that document serious biochemical abnormalities and even full metabolic syndrome (the immediate precursor to type 2 diabetes) in many kids placed on antipsychotic medication (Dori & Green, 2011). Similarly, increasing reports of sudden cardiac death and growth retardation in children using stimulants must give us pause to consider the long-term safety of these medications, and must generate some discussion of beginning to inform patients of concerns over safety. A 2005 ban of a popular stimulant by the Canadian government (over cardiac concerns) and the FDA's contentious debates over the safety of certain medications and whether or not to have a black box warning on stimulants should raise serious concerns in the health community about weighing efficacy over safety.

Simply put, we do not have sufficient research to support the extensive use of medications in young persons. In fact, most psychiatric prescriptions for kids are considered off-label, meaning the FDA has not yet approved the use of the medication for that specific condition. Worse still is the fact that off-label prescriptions don't really have any medical backing. In 96% of cases of off-label use in psychiatry, the agent had little or no sound scientific evidence for the condition for which the drug was prescribed (Radley, Finkelstein, & Stafford, 2006).

Sadly, this seems to be a pervasive phenomenon. A few studies have found that the amount of indicated (FDA and evidence-supported) use in pediatric mental health is quite low: anywhere from 9.2% to 24% (Lee et al., 2012; Leslie & Rosenheck, 2012). This means that the vast majority of medication use in child psychiatry does not have the support of the FDA or carry adequate evidence. This is probably because many doctors like to prescribe combinations of psychiatric medications, which are almost always considered off-label. At this point, we just don't have adequate safety studies to reassure us that these medications, alone or in combination, are safe in a pediatric population. If nothing else, these reports and information should prompt practitioners to properly inform patients of their options and the risks. (For a comprehensive discussion of safety and efficacy and how they relate to medical decision making, see Shannon, Weil, and Kaplan [2011].)

Patient Preference and Informed Consent

A frequent complaint I hear from patients about mental health care providers is that they don't listen to the patient's preference for treatment; they seem too intent on pushing their own preference (usually more medications). This kind of open disregard for a patient's choice is disrespectful, and in effect opens up a yawning therapeutic divide between patient and practitioner. When this happens, the patient becomes less involved in his or her treatment and the practitioner's ability to heal suffers. If the treatment process is going to go smoothly, practitioners have to understand, and ultimately respect, the patient's belief system and treatment preference.

A sound treatment plan must equally reflect the issues facing the patient and his or her preference for treatment. The first layer of this process represents the ability of the clinician to identify the deficiencies, excesses, issues, and imbalances of the child, such as inadequate sleep or a need for more family harmony. The second layer of this process reflects the practitioner's ability to ask about, listen, and consider the preferences of the patient while drawing up a treatment plan. This two-layer process represents the practice of informed consent.

At its core, medical decision making is about informed consent. The doctor must, with some level of objectivity, inform the patient of the various treatment options, while at the same time making recommendations tailored to match the individual's needs and belief system. Really, the true challenge of developing a good treatment plan is balancing the efficacy of the treatment (your belief) with the comfort of patients (their belief). This is the most important expression of therapeutic alignment.

Randomized controlled trials often dictate medical decision making, but judging treatment options based on RCTs poses a few basic problems. In psychiatry, most RCTs are short term—6 to 12 weeks—and sponsored by the pharmaceutical industry. And, because the studies have so many exclusions for concurrent conditions, they often have limited external validity. For example, Mark Zimmerman evaluated 346 patients that showed up for treatment of depression at his clinic and pretended that he was screening for eligibility for an antidepressant trial. Only 29 out of 346, or 8.3%, qualified (Zimmerman, Mattia, & Posternak, 2002).

The patients studied in RCTs do not look like the patients that you provide care for. Basically, since most patients have multiple conditions—the typical child evaluated has three *DSM* Axis I diagnoses—and your typical RCT excludes patients with multiple conditions, the information gathered from RCTs can be largely irrelevant to your clinical practice. RCTs are also enormously expensive. The typical pharmaceutical evaluation process costs hundreds of millions of dollars, with a Phase 3 clinical trial costing over 15 million dollars. The high cost of testing creates an inherent bias in the system in favor of conventional commercial products, such as medications, that are able to quickly earn back the money invested in trials. This means that alternative medicine is all but excluded from the discussion of efficacy, since there are very few commercially viable or patentable interventions in alternative medicine capable of earning back such a huge sum of money. This high expense also adds to the temptation to alter data. This has become more of an issue over the last few decades as big pharm has taken over the majority of the research funding previously supplied by the federal government. But perhaps the biggest drawback to RCTs is the fact that they alter only one treatment variable in a closed system. Basically, they are built to evaluate narrow interventions like medications, not systemic interventions, like psychotherapy or educational reform.

Patients will at times make treatment choices based more on practicality than belief or efficacy. Patients may choose antidepressant medication, for example, simply because they have some real-life urgencies (busy job or child care) and they feel the perceived speed of medication is just their best option given the circumstances. Some patients in intense pain will wave off other options and just choose the treatment with the best chance of quickly ameliorating their suffering.

Whatever the motivating force behind the patient's preference, the role of practitioners in medical decision making is to guide and advise, putting in their two cents as experts but also respecting the preference of the patient. In the best of cases, the process of medical decision making should look something like this: The practitioner offers the actively engaged patient an honest, unbiased overview of the safety and efficacy of all the appropriate treatments. The patient then declares a preference for one treatment over the others according to his or her beliefs and advice from the practitioner. This kind of open collaboration allows us the best chance to fully and appropriately serve our patients.

Facilitating Full Engagement and Expectation

Treatment plans have little value if no one follows them. The difference between a good practitioner and a great practitioner very well might be the ability to get a patient to follow and fully engage in the treatment plan. I encounter many professionals who struggle to get their patients, young and old, to follow through on treatments. This is a huge problem in conventional child psychiatry. In one study examining medication adherence in children and adolescents, only 21% of them complied across both acute and maintenance phases of treatment (Fontanella, Bridge, Marcus, & Campo, 2011). In my experience the closer the treatment plan is to the patient's belief system, the higher the compliance. The establishment of a well-bonded therapeutic relationship creates trust, a trust the patient will most often carry over into the application of treatment.

I employ a fairly simple strategy to bond with my young patients. Near the end of every session I sit down with the child alone and try to summarize how I see and understand him or her up to that point. I'll usually say something like, "You are a caring, sensitive teenager who worries about how others think of you, and you struggle to make friends. Your parents push you hard and have high expectations. Sometimes you collapse into a spiral of despair if something goes wrong, feeling like your world will never be right." Sure, it might be crude and curt, but a little summary like this works wonders to open up the relationship to sharing. It shows the child I am paying attention, and it lets her know I am first and foremost thinking about how to help her. From here, I share my vision of what treatment might look like and we discuss her preferences. As mentioned previously, I usually withhold the treatment plan (unless the patient is in true crisis) until the second or third visit. This serves two goals: It gives me more time to think about the treatment plan and it builds expectation in the patient.

When you do broach the subject of treatment, make sure to choose your words carefully. The manner in which you set up a treatment plan and the statements you make about specific interventions may turn a potentially successful tool into a waste of time. Conversely, your enthusiasm may convert a placebo into a cure. Consider the difference between these two practitioner comments: "I heard this could be useful—you might as well give it a try," versus "I am very impressed with this tool—I think you will experience good results." The first sets the patient up for failure; the second engages the patient with an expectation of success. Milton Erickson, a master of communication and the father of modern medical hypnotherapy, enjoyed creating a positive expectation of success in his patients. One of his favorite things to say to patients was something to the effect of, "Imagine how pleased you will be when you notice these positive changes."

Engage and create an expectation of healing; it is perhaps the most powerful tool that the mental health (or any) clinician possesses. Steward Wolf, a medical researcher from Cornell University, created the basic foundation for our understanding of the placebo effect and expectation in the 1950s. His first set of experiments involved giving people medications that acted against the patient's medical need. For example, he gave ipecac (used to induce vomiting) to a pregnant woman with intractable vomiting and told her that it would cure it. And it did. In 1955, H. K. Beecher published a groundbreaking article called "The Powerful Placebo," summarizing the ability of patient expectation to override normal physiology (1955). In its pages, Beecher detailed how sedatives could wake sleepy patients and stimulants could put them to sleep, if only the patient was set up with that expectation. The dumbfounded author concluded that patient belief and expectation could be predicted to override or induce any medication effect.

Here's a quick, and potent, medical anecdote reaffirming the expectancy of success. The 1950s was an era before coronary bypass surgery for angina. The surgery of the day was called mammary artery ligation. This involved cutting open the chest and sewing closed an artery on the chest wall with the understanding that it improved blood flow to the heart. Multiple studies demonstrated about 70% improvement with this invasive surgery. Following the Beecher article, two researchers evaluated mammary artery ligation versus sham surgery. (Thankfully, this would never pass an institutional review board today.) Half of the patients had the real surgery. The other half had their chest cracked but did not have the artery tied off. The success in the real surgical group was 73%. The success in the sham group was 83%.

This is the beauty of the placebo effect at work. Andrew Weil (1983) has written extensively on the placebo effect, arguing that practitioners should try to maximize the placebo response in patients since it elicits the healing power of the body without any of the risks of medications.

But the placebo response can work on medicated people, too. In fact, despite antidepressants' weak inherent biological effectiveness, often they can be very effective if the prescribing physician remains confident in their success. Why not take advantage of this effect? Engage the patient and create the expectation that the drug will help. Based on recent data, the window for our current antidepressants may be closing, as we are now witnessing a steady decline in the public's perception of antidepressant's potency—so engage the expectation of success while you still can (Fournier, DeRubeis, & Hollon, 2010).

Creating an Effective Treatment Team

I have worked in every possible clinical setting: private practice, psychiatric hospital, academic university medical center, medical hospital, group mental health practice, residential treatment center, nonprofit agency, community mental health center, integrative medical clinic, hospital-based holistic center, day treatment center, and now an integrative mental health clinic. Working in these varied settings has made one thing abundantly clear: I can provide better care when I work side by side with other talented practitioners. Developing a list of on-and-off collaborators in the community is a step in the right direction. Even better, if you can, is to develop a team that works together closely. One study found that collaborators worked well together if they had offices less than 32 feet from each other. Further away and the quality of collaboration fell off progressively. In any case, if you're to provide your little patients with the best care possible, you'll need to seek out and collaborate with the best clinical providers in seven key medical specialties:

1. General health care: An open-minded primary care doctor.
2. Psychiatry: Someone comfortable minimizing medication use and working collaboratively in the Wholeness Model.
3. Psychotherapy: People skilled in individual, family, group, and child therapy.
4. Nutrition: Someone knowledgeable and comfortable working with general diet issues, food allergies, gut issues, and specific diets.
5. Psychoeducation and stress management: In this area, you may have to seek out a variety of classes, school settings, or individual session

providers. Also, find someone familiar with mind-body skills like yoga, biofeedback, and meditation.

6. Acupuncture: Someone familiar with mental health.
7. Body work: Someone who can do a variety of soft tissue work as well as energy work. Cranial manipulation is also a useful skill set.

Set up appointments and meetings with possible professionals in your community, so you can get to know one another and learn about each other's practices. Arrange a professional development seminar once a month for all the people in your local cadre and teach each other your different practices. Make sure you all share the same basic or underlying philosophy; get to know the ins and outs of each other's practices, building reciprocal trust and communication. Finally, start sharing complex patients and begin learning from each other's perspectives.

Common Mistakes

Think of this common scenario: After a nasty breakup with her boyfriend, a previously well teenage girl expresses some suicidal thoughts to her friend; the friend tells the girl's parent; and the girl gets admitted to the local psychiatric hospital. Two or three days later, she leaves with a prescription for an antidepressant. Now, what's more reasonable, that this kid became upset and despondent because of a nasty breakup or that she has a neurochemical imbalance?

Whatever your answer, what's clear is that this kid could have benefited from somebody addressing her breakup. For teens in this situation—and I see scenarios like this all the time—an SSRI does not really solve any of the key issues that brought them to despair and suicidal ideation. Perhaps the antidepressants might help stabilize her later (if she responds), but if that breakup goes unresolved and she never works through the origins of that pain or her responses, we can reasonably expect her suffering to continue for quite some time and perhaps expect to see her back in the hospital. I see it all the time. This kind of silver bullet treatment is an all too common mistake of practitioners. But it's easily avoided by making a proper and thorough assessment.

Another common mistake is something I call the "ivory silo." In this scenario, the practitioner falsely assumes that his or her expertise alone is sufficient to treat a complex kid. When this happens, and the practitioner fails to seek outside help or resources, chances are the patient will continue to suffer or further deteriorate. Medicine does not have to be a solitary burden. And no practitioner's pride or feeling of satisfaction is as important as getting a child healthy. So if you're unsure or confused, as I suggested, reach out and collaborate with other practitioners.

PART TWO

Disease & Disorder Protocols

CHAPTER NINE

ADHD

Although I avoid labels as much as possible, sometimes they're clinically useful. General diagnostic categories, for instance, can often be very helpful when considering hypothetical treatment protocols. However, these kinds of protocols can also have drawbacks. Using a cookbook treatment, no matter how holistic or well intentioned, recapitulates many of my concerns with conventional psychiatry and its over-reliance on diagnostic labels and one-size-fits-all treatments. So, please consider the illness-specific protocols found in the following chapters as a reference to be individualized to the child in front of you. Each protocol offers an overview of the reasonable options to be considered as you care for the whole child.

In child psychiatry, attention-deficit/hyperactivity disorder (ADHD) is the problem of our time. It represents one of the strangest and most edifying phenomena in health care. It is exploding in both prevalence and incidence, and child psychiatry has no clue what causes it or how to prevent it. The only thing we know clearly is that stimulant medication sometimes effectively reduces the symptoms, at least in the short run.

In this chapter, we'll discuss the history and thinking behind the discovery of this "illness" and what we currently know about stimulants. We'll talk about whether or not ADHD is really a disorder or disease or what. And finally, I'll offer a new vision of how to think about ADHD and the ways in which this vision frees psychiatry to treat more children more effectively. Once we have a better idea of the underlying process that leads to these common symptoms, we can move to eliminating triggers and providing supports. In order to expand our current narrow and limited perspective, our first step must be to envision these symptoms in the most comprehensive manner possible.

The recordable history of ADHD begins with George Frederick Still, who first described the condition in 1902. He observed a distinct pattern of defiant behavior and poor inhibitory control in 20 children and adolescents, a pattern he later termed a deficit of moral control. The typical treatments, as has often been the case in the prior history of psychiatry, were lashings and other physical abuse. Still's work was later picked up by Kahn and Cohen in 1934 when the two researchers published an article in the *New England Journal of Medicine* titled "Organic Driveness." In the article, they described a formal pattern of hyperactive, impulsive, and immature behavior in young kids. Around the same time, Charles Bradley took a bold step new step in treating these kids: He gave them Benzedrine and, surprisingly, found it had the paradoxical effect of slowing them down. Ritalin formally entered the market in 1956 to treat this population, who were given the formal label MBD, or minimal brain dysfunction.

In the late 1960s, MBD was renamed hyperkinetic syndrome of children. And by 1970, about 150,000 kids were identified as suffering from this disorder, most of them medicated with Ritalin or Cylert. The best estimate was that hyperkinetic syndrome represented about 0.2% of American children. Then, in the early 1980s, the third edition of the *DSM* came out, renaming hyperkinetic syndrome attention-deficit disorder, with a hyperactive subcategory called ADHD. By the time I entered psychiatric training in the early 1980s, the number of diagnosed kids was estimated to be at around 2–4% of the childhood population. Until 1987, the diagnostic criteria were pretty specific and the rates of diagnosis remained low, the disorder hovering under the national radar. However, when the *DSM* criteria were revised that year for the *III-R* version, a simple change in one group of criteria resulted in a 14% spike in the number of children diagnosed (Lahey, 1990). And so began the breakneck cascade of kids diagnosed with ADHD. The federal Individuals With Disabilities Education Act (IDEA) of 1990 further opened the floodgates by providing a school-based incentive to carry the label when ADHD was added to the eligibility list in 1991.

Four and a half million American children were diagnosed under the criteria in 2003, and over two and a half million were put on a stimulant. Today, somewhere between 5% and 16% of American children meet the criteria for ADHD, with the best current estimate between 6% and 7% (Barbaresi et al., 2002, 2004; Willcutt, 2012). We see huge variation in the regional numbers of ADHD, with a 4:1 variation from state to state and an 11:1 variation from community to community (Jensen et al., 1999). By all accounts, boys outnumber girls 4:1. In some locations, one out of every three or four boys is being treated for this "illness." And most are being treated with stimulant medication. To make this even more confusing, one study demonstrated that the majority of children receiving treatment in one region do not meet ADHD criteria, and a significant number of afflicted children are not treated (Angold, Erkanli, Egger, & Costello, 2000). We use about 80% of the world's stimulants here in America. In more ways than one, this is an American illness—inextricably tied to an American business: pharmaceuticals.

And that business is taking a hefty economic toll. A review of 19 studies on the total economic burden of ADHD symptoms and treatment in the United States estimated that $38–72 billion are spent each year on children, with the largest chunks of change coming from education ($15–25 billion) and health care ($21–44 billion) (Doshi et al., 2012). In adults the numbers are significantly greater: $105–194 billion, the majority of which is related to productivity and income loss ($87–138 billion).

As these numbers and that 14% spike in incidence from 1980 to 1987 illustrate, each ensuing revision of the *DSM* has the potential to sway health care and indeed economics. That's why every 5 or so years during the revision of the *DSM*, a great deal of public and private discussion goes on. The expansion or revision of diagnostic criteria is understandably contentious: Very often many years of work and ideology are on the line, not to mention money. Currently, a very public debate over the criteria of ADHD (and other disorders) for the forthcoming *DSM-V* has erupted and gained a great deal of attention.

Most of this debate stems from concerns over perceived corruption in the committee process. A study revealed that 70% of *DSM* committee members have direct ties to the pharmaceutical industry (Cosgrove & Bursztajn, 2010). And many folks are concerned by the committee's secretive process. Because nondisclosure agreements were required for participation, the committee process is not transparent, and with almost three-fourths of committee members already in the pocket of big pharm, many people fear the worst. In June 2009, Allen Frances, head of the *DSM-IV* task force, issued strongly worded criticisms of the committee's process and the risk of "serious, subtle, . . . ubiquitous" and "dangerous" unintended consequences such as new "false epidemics." Frances didn't pull any punches: "The work on DSM-V has displayed the most unhappy combination of soaring ambition and weak methodology."

This semipublic spectacle of disorder design has been instructive and off-putting to many. Certainly the road to the newly designed ADHD has been rocky. On the *DSM-V*'s own Web site, the new proposed definition of ADD includes a list of pros and cons. The cons for one considered option was blatantly honest: "Little empirical or experimental data available to define pathology of this diagnosis" (American Psychiatric Association, 2010, p. 4).

ADHD: Illness, Syndrome, or Disorder?

Without much evidence to define pathology, can we even call ADHD an illness? Let's examine the evidence base.

ADHD, like all other psychiatric "illnesses," is not determined by verifiable tissue pathology. Rather, the diagnostic label describes a group of symptoms that commonly occur together. Therefore, it's more accurately a syndrome, or a group of symptoms that consistently occur together, or else a condition characterized by a set of associated symptoms. Like many syndromes, this does not tell us much about the nature of the illness—neither the cause nor the ideal method of treatment. It simply isolates a group of diagnostic criteria.

The symptoms that consistently occur together in ADHD include inattention, impulsivity, or hyperactivity. But these symptoms are not exclusive to ADHD. In fact, this group of symptoms consistently occurs together in the presentation of other syndromes, disorders, and diseases. Irritability, for instance, is prevalent across all diagnostic categories and is a poor differentiator (Massat & Victoor, 2008). We have documented evidence, for instance, that this group of symptoms can also occur with thyroid abnormalities, lead toxicity, depression, closed head injury, parental divorce, food additives, fetal alcohol syndrome, psychological trauma, pesticide exposure, Fragile X, anxiety, food allergies, and even cancer. If you look at this list, you will see there's no single shared pathological process. So what do they share? It appears, merely the end point of a common expression of dysfunction in an extraordinarily complicated process of focus, attention, and learning.

Given this, I think about ADHD expression in the same way I think about fever: a final, common expression of a problem in the body. Fever is always nonspecific. A fever's cause can be trivial or life threatening:

allergic reaction or viral infection, medication reaction or bacterial abscess. It does not tell us what is wrong with the body. When we treat fever, we never think that we are treating an illness. That is, when a physician observes a fever in a patient, he has not diagnosed an illness. It strikes me that ADHD represents a similar phenomenon: a common pathway that indicates some problem within the human body. A dashboard warning light, if you will. Let's examine whether current science supports this view.

The National Institutes of Health (NIH) convened a panel of experts from a variety of fields (neuroscience, neurology, psychiatry, psychology, etc.) to examine the question of ADHD's qualification as an illness. After investigating the evidence base and conducting their own research, they reached an interesting conclusion: "It is unclear whether ADHD is at the far end of the spectrum of normal behavior or if it reflects a qualitatively different behavioral syndrome" (Ferguson, 2000). They finished by saying, "We can't conclude that ADHD represents a disordered biological state."

Since this last NIH consensus panel issued its report, the data have become much more clear. Shaw and his colleagues at the National Institute of Mental Health published a landmark study in December 2007 in the prestigious *Proceedings of the National Academy of Science*. This was the largest and longest study of pediatric brain scans ever completed. They followed 446 kids for many years. These children were divided into two groups: those diagnosed with ADHD and controls. After repeatedly scanning the brains of these children over many years, they concluded that in the ADHD group there was "no evidence of abnormality, only delay in brain development" (Shaw, Eckstrand, & Sharp, 2007). Shaw found that children with ADHD lag behind their peers by about 3 years in proper brain development. Interestingly, he found the ADHD group often demonstrated precocious motor cortex development.

If ADHD is not, strictly speaking, a "disordered biological state" and there is "no evidence of abnormality" in those affected kids, we can't in all reason call ADHD an illness. We can't even say that ADHD represents a particular pattern of symptoms, as a score of other diseases and disorders share similar symptomatology. What we can say is that, like a fever, ADHD is an increasingly common collection of symptoms that can arise as the result of a host of different triggers. The symptoms are real—we just need to address them in a different manner.

The high rates of comorbidity in kids affected with ADHD add further weight to the idea that this "illness" is really just a heterogeneous collection of symptoms. Rates of depression in ADHD, for example, run as high as 30%, while conduct disorder (20% in boys, 8% in girls), oppositional defiant disorder (62% of boys, 32% of girls), and anxiety disorders (20% to 30% of boys and girls) are also quite common (Spencer, Biederman, & Wilens, 1999). According to one study, kids with both ADHD and anxiety tend to be more inattentive, less impulsive, and have longer reaction times (Schatz & Rostain, 2006). Findings from one study indicated that as many as 73% of kids with ADHD also have sleep problems, and 45% of those have severe problems (Sung, Hiscock, Sciberras, & Efron, 2008). The comorbidity data just keep coming. Studies suggesting a bidirectional relationship between bipolar disorder and ADHD, for example, continue to surface. In one review, 85% of those with bipolar disorder also had ADHD, and bipolar disorder occurred in as many as 22% of ADHD kids (Singh, DelBello, Kowatch, & Strakowski, 2008). What these comorbidity data tell us is that ADHD symptomatology cannot be easily isolated from other disorders and syndromes, and that its symptomatology is probably directly connected to other syndromes and disorders.

Learning disability data are perhaps the strongest evidence in this argument. In community samples, the rates of learning disabilities in ADHD populations run between 25% and 70% (Willcutt & Pennington, 2000), while in populations of kids with learning disabilities, the rates of ADHD range between 15% and 40% (Willcutt & Pennington, 2000). Overall, the rates of comorbidity in ADHD run between 50% and 90% (Wilens et al., 2002). It's tough to look at these numbers and not speculate about whether ADHD symptomatology is directly connected to learning disabilities, and vice versa. It's also hard to put one's finger on what symptoms arise from what syndrome. What these numbers do tell us is that there is an incredible array of ADHD expression. It seems there are as many subtypes (anxiety with ADHD or learning disability with ADHD, for instance) as there are kids.

Perhaps, then, the best course of action is to think about ADHD presentation as a dashboard warning light, a sign to look under the hood and treat individual concerns manifesting as the symptoms of ADHD.

ADHD and the Placebo Effect

One of the most interesting facets of ADHD is the placebo effect. Children with ADHD typically express little placebo effect as they hold little expectation about the intended response. Multiple studies have failed to find a placebo effect with the cognitive impact of stimulants in children. It appears, however, that there is a placebo effect in medicated kids' parents. A meta-analysis confirms it. Parents and teachers express a placebo effect when children are given stimulants, because the adults hold a clear expectation for the medication's effects (Waschbusch, Pelham, Waxmonsky, & Johnston, 2009). Parents and teachers evaluate a child more positively if they believe that the child has been medicated. They also tend to attribute positive changes to the medication even when no medications have been given (Waschbusch et al., 2009). This finding diminishes the reliability of parent and teacher reports in evaluating kids for ADHD—the core of the diagnostic process.

ADHD and Stimulant Effectiveness

After nearly 60 years, stimulant medication remains the cornerstone treatment of ADHD. But its time may be drawing to a close. Increasingly, studies are challenging the long-term effectiveness of stimulants. Let's explore the science surrounding the long-term use of stimulant medication and try to summarize its efficacy.

The Multimodal Treatment Study of Children With ADHD (MTA) remains the largest and most important study of children's ADHD ever undertaken. This was a NIMH cooperative agreement involving six clinical sites around the United States that followed 436 children over 14 months (in the initial phase of the study). The children were placed in four different treatment groups and compared to local controls. As anticipated, the medication groups fared significantly better than behavioral management and controls, but the combination of behavioral support and medication had the best outcome of any group for internalizing symptoms (depression and anxiety), social skills, reading scores, and parent-child relations (MTA Cooperative Group, 1999). When it first appeared in 1999, the study was widely cited as an endorsement of the widespread use of stimulant medication.

The endorsement, however, proved to be premature. Follow-up studies at 22 and 36 months as well as 8 years revealed concerning data. In fact, in spite of retaining the majority of the kids on medication, by 10 months fully half of the benefits of the agents fell away (Molina et al., 2009). By 22 months, all of the benefit for the medication groups fell away completely. To quote the authors: "These long-term follow-up data fail to provide support for long-term advantage of medication treatment beyond two years for the majority of children" (Molina et al., 2009). More startling still, the use of medication, which early in the study had predicted a positive outcome, by 36 months predicted worse functioning, the need for more school services, and greater symptoms (Jensen et al., 2007). In a nutshell, the medications had a deteriorating effect.

Interestingly enough, the 8-year follow-up study came to a conclusion very similar to mine about the need to identify individual markers and subtypes: "Our results also lend some support to the idea that indicators of functioning (beyond symptoms) may be crucial, if not more important than measurement of symptoms, in the design and study of treatments for ADHD" (Molina et al., 2009). The authors also noted that this study period occurred in the time frame when the medical community witnessed the release and widespread acceptance of long-acting stimulant formulations with escalating treatment doses. A few other details to note from this crucial but often ignored study: Only 30% of the ADHD children met the criteria for this disorder 8 years after they met the strictest of criteria to merit the label (Molina et al., 2009). It's tough to know the exact mechanism behind this phenomenon, but it seems as though those 70% just outgrew their ADHD. The question I have is, do we need to create another disorder for those 70% or do we simply need a better understanding of why they struggled in those earlier years? It seems like identifying individual markers and subtypes might indeed be the way to go.

The Oregon Study was a broad overview of ADHD research commissioned by 15 U.S. states to explore the support for ADHD treatment efficacy and safety. These states had no commercial axe to grind. The exhaustive 731-page report was published in 2007 by Oregon Health

Services University (McDonagh, Christensen, Peterson, & Thakurta, 2007). It analyzed virtually every study on ADHD medication treatment ever done (2,107) and found 180 studies that met criteria for quality. The meta-analysis came to a number of conclusions. First of all, it found that most studies were too short: "Analysis severely limited by lack of studies measuring functional or long term results" (McDonagh et al., 2007). (Remember, most pharmaceutical-sponsored studies are 6 to 8 weeks.) The Oregon Study also found that as a result there was no decent evidence to support the long-term value of stimulant medications: "Good quality evidence on the use of drugs to affect outcomes relating to academic performance, risky behaviors, social achievements . . . is lacking" (McDonagh et al., 2007). On the whole they found the quality of data poor.

The Raine Study was a prospective government-sponsored study in Australia that followed a large population of children (2,868) in Western Australia over many years, tracking outcomes for children from birth to 14 years old. This is the longest and most comprehensive examination of health, educational, and social outcomes for youths taking stimulant medications available. Of these children, 131 were diagnosed with ADHD at some point. When evaluated at age 14, the kids were placed in four groups: never medicated, consistently medicated, inconsistently medicated, and previously medicated but now off. A comparison at age 5 prior to the use of medications showed no differences among these four ADHD groups in terms of severity or other relevant factors (Smith, Jongeling, Hartmann, Russell, & Landau, 2010). This study found that use of stimulant medication in the children diagnosed with ADHD increased the odds of performing below school level 10-fold over the non-medicated children with ADHD. The children who had received medication exhibited a 950% increased incidence of school failure compared to the other kids with ADHD. The authors could find no evidence to support the long-term value of stimulant medication in the treatment of ADHD.

The results of these three big longitudinal studies show that there's really no long-term benefit to stimulant medications in children diagnosed with ADHD. As a matter of fact, there may be deteriorating effects.

It seems we're already in the middle of an economic epidemic. The incremental cost of treatment per child with ADHD is on average $14,576.

That's a lot of money—a lot of money that many American families increasingly cannot afford. This cost includes the cost of treatment and education as well as crime and delinquency. It does not include the cost to the family in terms of stress, heartache, lost time, and conflict. The cost to society in North America is $7.9 billion a year for treatment, $13.6 billion in educational costs and $21 billion in crime and delinquency. This amounts to $42.5 billion, which approaches the annual cost of depression at $44 billion. As the costs continue to escalate, so too does our need to shift our thinking and approach to this problem. We need to find new, safer, more financially sustainable options.

What's a Clinician to Do?

Let's review what we know. ADHD represents a common group of symptoms affecting education, impulsivity, attention, behavior, and so on. It's a brain-based issue exceedingly complex in its biological expression and, at the same time, not really a true illness. It might even be tough to call it a syndrome, because so many other disorders and diseases have similar groups of common symptoms. On the treatment side, we have some evidence that stimulants work in the short run, but it appears they offer no benefit in the long run. In fact, they may cause deterioration over time and carry some very real health risks.

But what's a clinician to do? If one accepts the final common pathway premise that, like a fever, ADHD symptomatology represents a dashboard warning light that something's amiss in the body, then the real challenge in treating ADHD is detective work to uncover the underlying cause or causes. This kind of detective work holds the promise of true effective treatment and, ultimately, perhaps true prevention. Making the ADHD diagnosis is the easy part. It's not hard to document a fever. What's tough, what a doctor's real job is, is figuring out what's causing it. And fixing that.

As we're learning, ADHD comes in a lot of forms. And it's tough to make differential diagnoses, as ADHD shares so many common symptoms with other disorders and diseases. So, one way to make the detective work of uncovering underlying causes easier is to identify common clusters of symptoms in the child. That is, break down the child's issues according to subtypes of ADHD. This way, there's added specificity in both the assessment and treatment. This will help narrow your focus and, hopefully, weed out the exact underlying causes of the symptomatology, and in turn focus you on what adjustments need to be made in order to get rid of them. I have found that there are at least seven common subtypes of ADHD in kids:

1. Anxious and overfocused
2. Food allergy and gut imbalance
3. Mitochondrial issues and developmental delays
4. Classic ADHD
5. Angry and oppositional
6. Environmental issues
7. Apathetic and disengaged

The Seven Subtypes of ADHD

As I did in Chapter 7, I will go over each of these seven subtypes in turn, breaking them down according to what to look for (assessment) and what to do (treatment).

This list of subtypes will help you identify common patterns of ADHD presentation. Thinking about where a particular kid fits on this list of subtypes will, hopefully, help you better sort out a specific method to evaluate and treat him or her. Sometimes, a child will have a mix of features from different subtypes. A little girl may have features of 1, 4, and 7, for example. Take lessons about presentation and treatment from each presenting subtype and let them inform your understanding of the child and how you might heal her.

Anxious and Overfocused

What to Look For

The typical children in this subtype have the ability to hyperfocus. They can read a book or explore a topic on the Internet for hours. They often have a hard time falling asleep and have some undertones of anxiety. These kids appear scattered in school and can easily get overstimulated in groups. They are often hyper and silly. They are typically immature, on the nerdy end of the spectrum, and may struggle socially.

One parent may be an engineer or technically oriented. These kids are usually cautious in many areas of their lives.

What to Do

Treat the anxiety with inositol, L-theanine, and magnesium. To improve social skills, think about reduction of electronic overstimulation. Remove TV from the bedroom. Also, support physical activities and get these kids outside to play. Neurofeedback also works well for these kids. Stimulants are usually not effective in the long run and cause excessive sleep issues and growing anxiety, not to mention the added social stiffness that comes with stimulants. These kids get mechanical and robotic.

Food Allergies and Gut Imbalance

What to Look For

Assess for a history of colic, reflux, ear infections or tubes, multiple antibiotics courses, constipation, abdominal pain, and eczema. If any of these issues are or were chronic, the child probably also has some sort of food allergy. Also, if the child has a limited diet (just macaroni and cheese, for instance), sugar cravings, a high-carb diet, low protein, poor skin color, low levels of nutrients (ferritin, vitamin D), or chronic loose stools, there is a chance that a food allergy is the culprit. These kids are often anxious or explosive, or both. Look for a brittle and unpredictable mood, often with OCD components.

What to Do

Work with a naturopath, nutritionist, or the like. Elimination diet can be helpful to test for food allergies. So can food allergy testing (IgE and IgG). Test urine for organic acids and/or comprehensive digestive stool analysis. Supplement with digestive enzymes, glutamine, and probiotics. Suggest a whole foods diet and the reduction of processed and junk foods. Think about a gluten- or dairy-free trial.

Mitochondrial Issues and Developmental Delays

What to Look For

Multiple developmental delays (e.g., 16 months to walk). Kids slow and late in all categories of development that don't like to move around much, stay less active, need more rest, tire easily, and sleep a lot (potentially sleep apnea). Look for inattention but not necessarily hyperactivity. These kids will be better in the morning and slow in the afternoon.

What to Do

Test free and total carnitine levels; test urine for organic acids. Supplement with CoQ10, acetyl-L-carnitine, EPA/DHA, coconut oil, and medium-chain triglycerides. Ginkgo, ginseng, and DMAE can be helpful as well. Low-dose stimulants work in the short run. Think about a sleep study, as sleep apnea is sometimes a problem here.

Classic ADHD

What to Look For

Consistent high level of energy, walked early, positive mood, sleeps well, loves to play, daredevil attitude, ebullient personality, and impulsivity.

What to Do

Support more structure in the home, exercise before school, martial arts, reduce video games, and high-protein diet (especially at breakfast). Supplement with EPA, pycnogenol, or DMAE. Allow child to move in school. Sports, behavior management plan, and neurofeedback can all be helpful as well.

Angry and Oppositional

What to Look For

Tantrums and meltdowns, high energy and frenetic pace, poor sleep, positive family history for mood disorders, labile mood, erratic behavior, conflicted relationship with parents, depressed mom, history of abuse, and family conflict. These kids are usually worse at home than in school.

What to Do

Family therapy, Nurtured Heart Approach, supplementation with EPA, magnesium glycinate, EMPower Plus, or inositol. These kids benefit from a structured routine, exercise, improved diet, parental education and support, individual counseling, and a reduction of electronics exposure. Avoid stimulants here. Mood stabilizers or alpha-agonists can be helpful, though. Consider EMDR, DBT, or biofeedback.

Environmental Issues

What to Look For

Chaotic household, missed appointments, lots of screen time, overwhelmed mom, low parental involvement (often single parent), poor diet, conflicted divorce, violent video game exposure, poor communication, irregular sleep, and lack of follow through with school.

What to Do

Parental support, decrease electronics, remove TV from bedroom, high-protein breakfast, create structure and routine, improve diet, Nurtured Heart Approach, family therapy, or lots of parental education. Avoid medication and supplement with inositol or L-theanine.

Apathy and Learning Issues

What to Look For

Struggle or delay with reading, dislike of school or reading, passive-avoidant style, apathy, right-brained thinker, artistic, slow disengagement from school, movement to marginalized subgroups in junior high or high school (e.g., skaters, punks, goths), dyslexia, and low-grade depression.

What to Do

Consider smaller school, schedule hands-on classes as per preference, exercise, and increased time outside to play. Supplement with EPA/DHA, DMAE, B complex, folic acid, bacopa, or SAMe. Find passions and gifts, explore art and music, and rule out serious depression. Explore for metabolic issues (e.g., methylation, low cholesterol) and check vitamin D levels as well as ferritin levels. High-protein diet can be helpful. Stimulants often fade in value over time; avoid high-dose stimulants as they typically rob this kind of kid of passion and motivation.

Commonsense Adjustments

After assessing subtype, the first step in ADHD treatment is to think about what simple commonsense adjustments you can make to the child's ecosystem:

1. School: Are the school and teacher a good fit? Will a change make a significant difference?
2. Sleep: Is the kid getting adequate sleep? Is there any concern over sleep apnea or sleep-disordered breathing?
3. Overstimulation: Is this child overstimulated?
4. Outdoor activities: Does the child spend too much time in front of a screen? Does he or she spend time outside? Is he or she active enough? Getting enough sunlight and exercise?
5. Other: What else in the child's ecosystem seems out of balance and easy to correct?

Think about these options before moving to the treatment phase. (I wouldn't even consider these treatments per se, just slight tweaks and adjustments to the child's ecosystem.) Making simple adjustments to these realms of a child's life, according to William Pelham's work in the MTA and other studies, can reduce the need for other treatments and will often significantly decrease the medication dose required (MTA Cooperative Group, 1999).

Treating ADHD

Let's begin thinking about ADHD treatment by breaking down the various types of treatments you might employ. There are five main categories of care:

1. Nutrition and diet
2. Natural supplements
3. Neurofeedback and cognitive therapies
4. Parenting and behavioral interventions
5. Medications

I'll move through each of these five categories in turn, explaining the different treatment tools within each category and the ways in which they might be applied in clinical practice.

Nutrition and Diet

Nutrition and diet interventions primarily target three main sources of ADHD symptoms: metabolic poisons and toxins, low-quality diet, and food allergies.

We know that hydrogenated oils are a metabolic poison and that they impair the production of EPA and DHA from the omega-3 precursors in the diet. (Impaired EPA and DHA production results from impairment of the enzyme delta 5 and delta 6 dehydrogenase. High glycemic load in the diet also affects this crucial enzyme.) What we didn't know until recently was that EPA and DHA are central building blocks of a normal nervous system and brain and may be helpful in treating a number of mental health issues including ADHD. That's why many researchers now believe there's a close connection between the rise of the standard American diet—high in metabolic poisons like hydrogenated oils—and the exponential rise we've seen in attentional issues.

Similarly, a number of studies have found a link between pesticide levels and ADHD. In a study of 1,139 kids, researchers measured the levels of organophosphate pesticides (which act via impairment of acteylcholinesterase in the nervous system) and found that 94% of the children had detectable levels. As it turns out, those with higher levels had a 10-fold increased risk of ADHD (Bouchard, Bellinger, Wright, & Weisskopf, 2010). Another study assessed the population effects of exposure to three environmental toxins. The author, D. C. Bellinger of Harvard's School of Public Health, calculated the loss of full-scale IQ points according to exposure. The results, broken down according to poison: lead, 23,000,000 points; methylmercury, 285,000 points; and organophosphate pesticides, 17,000,000 points (Bellinger, 2012). Most people are aware of lead as an environmental toxin, but organophosphate pesticides are a more recent finding. Luckily, we have tools like diet change to limit the burden of exposure. In fact, the switch to an organic diet has been demonstrated to eliminate the excretion of pesticide residue within 6 weeks. Also, remember the clean 15 and the dirty dozen (the list of highly contaminated or predominantly pristine

foods), and avoid highly sprayed fruits and veggies (http://www.ewg
.org/foodnews/).

Regardless of toxin exposure, a high-quality diet can act as a buffer
against mental health issues like ADHD. For kids, a high-protein breakfast is especially important on school days. But also make sure to improve
the overall food quality with a movement to more organic veggies and
fruits, more nuts, lots of protein (grass-fed meat and fish for omega-3),
and the elimination of soda, junk food, hydrogenated oils, fast food, caffeine, processed foods, dyes, colorings, and additives likes high-fructose
corn syrup (HFCS).

In fact, HFCS, found widely in sodas, sweetened juices, and other processed foods, appears to be a significant factor in learning and school
performance issues. Researchers at the UCLA Brain Injury Research
Center in Los Angeles published findings that document the negative effects of a high-fructose diet on learning and school performance. In this
study, a diet high in fructose or deficient in DHA caused insulin receptor
signaling problems in the hippocampus, which impaired learning and
performance (Agrawal & Gomez-Pinilla, 2012). DHA supplementation
actually protected from some of the negative effects of fructose. Sadly,
the average American now consumes 37.8 pounds of HFCS a year. And
research increasingly points to its association with obesity and metabolic
syndrome. It's simple: Too many kids eat too much sugar in this country.

The connection between food allergies and ADHD has been around
since 1975, when Dr. Ben Feingold first published a study demonstrating
the association between artificial food coloring and flavors and hyperactivity. His findings created a quiet controversy, and a slew of widely conflicting data—most of them low quality—emerged in the following years.
However, two large studies support Feingold's conclusions. Collectively,
2,170 kids were followed in the two studies, and both found that colors
and additives such as sodium benzoate create a significant negative effect on a child's ability to focus while also increasing hyperactivity (Mc-
Cann et al., 2007; Bateman et al., 2004). The INCA study, published in
the *Lancet* in 2011, pretty well sums up the link between food allergies
and ADHD. In this Dutch study, 100 children with ADHD were placed on
a restrictive hypoallergenic diet for 5 weeks and showed significant improvement in ADHD symptoms ($P = 0.0001$) (Pelsser et al., 2011). These
kids were then rechallenged with the allergenic responsive food, and
63% responded with a significant increase in ADHD symptoms. (Inter-

estingly, IgE test levels were not predictive. Elimination diet is the most useful way of weeding out food allergies.)

With Feingold and others' data in mind, multiple studies have shown excellent effectiveness in the treatment of ADHD with an oligoantigenic diet. This is a low-allergy diet that eliminates most of the major food offenders: dairy, gluten, soy, corn, eggs, nuts, and artificial colors and flavors. In one study, 62 of 76 children placed on this diet obtained significant benefit (Egger, Carter, & Graham, 1985).

Natural Supplements

A wide range of supplements can be useful in treating the symptoms of ADHD. Here's a list of the (evidence-based) supplements I commonly employ:

- PS omega-3: This combination of omega-3 EFAs and phosphatidylserine creates an enriched molecule with higher central nervous system (CNS) penetration. Try 1–2 capsules a day of Vayarin. (Krill oil may be a cheaper substitute.)
- Bacopa monnieri: Ayurvedic herb used to improve focus and cognition.
- Ginkgo biloba: This herb is most useful for the classic ADHD kid or inattentive child. Try 60–120 mg twice daily. But because of its stimulating effect, it is not very useful in the anxious or agitated ADHD child.
- Centella asiatica (also known as gotu kola): This is a traditional Ayurvedic herb that shows improved outcomes in ADHD kids (Katz, Levine, Kol-Degani, & Kav-Venaki, 2010).
- DMAE: Previously a prescription agent, this supplement has a range of studies showing benefit in learning and attention issues. Try at 100–400 mg a day.
- Fish oil: I put almost every ADHD child on fish oil. A meta-analysis found benefit for fish oil in ADHD with a moderate effect size (0.4) (Bloch & Qawasmi, 2011).
- Chromium: Useful if there are blood sugar issues contributing to inattention or impulsiveness. Use at 400–800 mcg a day.
- Inositol: Excellent for anxiety, stress, or agitation. I use this frequently. The dose is 2–6 g two to three times a day. Use the powder instead of the capsules. It's cheaper and easier to dose for kids.

- L-Theanine: Reduces anxiety, improves focus, and alters EEG in beneficial ways. I use 100–300 mg twice daily.
- Magnesium: Most useful if the child presents with labile mood, explosive temper, agitation, insomnia, or constipation. I use 100–300 mg of magnesium glycinate twice daily.
- Pycnogenol: A powerful antioxidant extract from French maritime pines with good results in ADHD kids. Dose at 50–200 mg a day.
- Phosphatidylserine: Over 25 RCTs document value for memory, learning, cognitive function, mood, and stress.
- Krill oil: High in EFAs and phospholipids. Has a more powerful antioxidant effect than fish oil. More expensive, but comes in a smaller capsule.
- L-Carnitine: An essential nutrient. It is crucial for fatty acid metabolism and mitochondrial energy production. Use 1–2 g daily.
- Iron chelate (aspartate or gluconate): Useful if ferritin levels are low (under 40 ng/ml). Much better tolerated and absorbed than ferrous sulfate. Use 5–20 mg per day.
- Zinc: Crucial in EFA metabolism. Also acts as cofactor for 100 enzymes. Dose at 5–20 mg per day.
- Homeopathy: Individualized remedy selection.
- Chelation therapy: Makes sense only with documented excessive heavy metal burden (lead or mercury).
- Multivitamin: A wide range of population studies show positive cognitive effects.

Neurofeedback and Cognitive Therapy

ADHD looks to be at least in part related to neurodevelopmental delay. The National Institute of Mental Health, in fact, found a pattern of delayed brain development, especially in the frontal lobes, in their study of kids with ADHD. Luckily, we now have treatments that can help these kids catch up on their lost neurodevelopmental time.

Neurofeedback is a type of biofeedback that alters the EEG pattern and retrains the brain. To begin the treatment, the child's brain is mapped with an EEG. This map is then compared to standards and a treatment model is created to guide the child's brain into a more mainstream or mature EEG pattern. This typically takes anywhere from 20 to 40 sessions of neurofeedback to complete. During these sessions, the child tries to increase beta frequency (16–20 Hz) while suppressing the theta frequency (4–8 Hz). This is usually done with some kind of visual and auditory interface: a movie or music video that reacts to beta and theta frequencies. The child learns to control these frequencies through the interface and, in the process, carves out new neural pathways.

Currently, 14 randomized trials of neurofeedback have been published evaluating its effectiveness in ADHD. The majority of the studies are positive, with an average affect size of 0.69 (Lofthouse, Arnold, Hersch, Hurt, & Debeus, 2012). Newer studies are now exploring more sophisticated techniques such as QEEG mapping, which creates a much more individualized EEG pattern. A neurofeedback study employing this technique demonstrated an effect size of 1.78 for attention issues and 1.22 for hyperactivity (Arns, Drinkenburg, & Leon Kenemans, 2012). Continuing improvements in technology will most likely advance the power and effectiveness of neurofeedback even more. The downsides of neurofeedback are cost, availability, and time. That said, in my clinic neurofeedback remains our primary intervention for ADHD.

Children with ADHD typically have deficits in executive functioning, notably working memory. A number of studies document the effectiveness of cognitive training programs to improve working memory (Hurst, Lofthouse, & Arnold, 2010). These studies demonstrate a range of positive cognitive effects, not just on verbal working memory but also on visual-spatial working memory and short-term memory. Given the broad value of working memory and other executive functioning skills, this type of training makes sense, especially for young (4- to 8-year-olds) and at-risk populations. Other training programs such as interactive metronome and attention training offer promise but little convincing data. The important thing is to find one that fits the kid you're working with.

Parenting and Behavioral Interventions

The research on ADHD is clear: The most efficacious treatment in the short to medium term is a combination of behavioral management and stimulant medication. Yet in clinical practice this is very rarely done. The vast majority of children with ADHD are treated solely with stimulant medication. Only a minority of these kids receives counseling or play therapy. Few receive any instruction on behavioral management. So why the disconnect?

Frankly, it is just too simple to prescribe medication. It has an immediate impact and requires little investment of time or effort. Also, parents may resist the implication that they parent poorly, need instruction on behavioral management, or carry any level of blame in the problem at all. And most pediatric mental health clinicians tend to drift more toward conventional one-on-one counseling—mainly because it is simpler and easier.

It's my belief that some form of behavioral management in combination with parental training (BMPT) should be the core of treatment for all ADHD kids. BMPT, with or without stimulant medication, provides a child with the best chance of a sustained positive benefit from treatment. In fact, according to the largest, best-designed, and most important study of ADHD, the MTA study, a combination of BMPT and stimulant therapy provided the best ADHD treatment outcome (MTA Cooperative Group, 1999). A variety of other studies support this conclusion. The American Academy of Pediatric Clinical Practice Guidelines recommends a chronic disease management approach that collaborates with school personnel and uses both stimulant medication and behavioral therapy. The American Psychological Association recommends psychological interventions like BMPT first, as they are safer and have better long-term efficacy.

Part of behavioral management's long-term efficacy for ADHD is related to social outcomes for kids. Researchers have long documented that negative outcomes in childhood ADHD are most closely related to negative peer and social relationships. Over one-half of ADHD children are peer rejected compared to 10–15% of normal youths (Hoza et al., 2005). Youths with poor peer relationships struggle more as adults with dissatisfaction and poor functioning (Hoza, 2007). Thus, if we can improve a child's social functioning at a young age through behavioral management, it might also offer long-term palliative effects for ADHD.

Another part of this long-term efficacy is related to family issues. A range of studies document that ADHD is associated with problematic family functioning, greater stress in the family, higher rates of parental psychopathology, and conflicted parent-child relationships (Deault, 2010). Also, given some of the genetic linkages found in ADHD symptoms between parent and child—maternal ADHD symptoms strongly predict posttreatment behavior problems in the child—it just makes sense to educate the whole family (Chronis-Tuscano et al., 2011). That all goes to show that if we can impact a child at the family level through education, parenting skills, and behavioral management, there's a good chance we can insure that child against ADHD-related suffering.

Social skills, family issues, and ADHD are all connected in their expression, so it only makes sense that they might be connected in their treatment. And it might all come down to parenting skills. In fact, the MTA study looked at just that and found some interesting results. It looked at negative or ineffective discipline by parents as compared to positive involvement. Positive involvement of parents did not relate to improved peer functioning; only a reduction in negative or ineffective discipline improved peer functioning at school. Interestingly, this did not occur in the medication-only group or in the behavior-only group—just in the combination group (Hinshaw et al., 2000).

This makes sense: Medications can set the stage for success but skills must also be taught. The child with ADHD symptoms typically has a deficit of social skills, which are learned through role modeling and instruction, not drugs. Parental training, then, helps to reduce or eliminate the negative role modeling in the home and provides more effective guidance. Remember, skills do not come in pills.

In some ways, it all comes down to core philosophy: Do you target short-term efficacy with medications or the long-term efficacy of BMPT, which builds skills, corrects negative parenting, improves social skills, enhances parental satisfaction, and improves family harmony? According to William Pelham, one of the authors of the MTA study, parental training makes sense for four reasons: Parents of ADHD kids have more stress; they have more psychopathology; parenting style of ADHD parents contributes to long-term negative outcomes; and parents mediate most negative outcomes for ADHD kids (Pelham, 2008).

So how do we apply this in practice?

First off, behavioral management and parental training make sense in almost every case. The primary focus should be on parenting skills and developing the family relationship. This means that there must be rules in the home—best written and posted somewhere clear. It's also important that the parents learn to ignore mild behaviors and praise appropriate ones (pick your battles). Help the family create charts for school and home. This will help instill a sense of discipline and duty in the child, and will keep the parents consistent in reward and punishment. Make rewards like screen time contingent on homework completion. Maybe use a point system that rewards target behaviors (homework completion and cooperation) and creates a known consequence for negative behaviors (not responding to requests and directions). Schedule a homework hour—typically best right before or right after dinner.

The specifics of such systems obviously vary, but the important thing is that the system is built around mutual respect. It's important the parents avoid "power plays" where the child and parent struggle over control of a situation, and the parent puts his foot down just for the sake of maintaining control. Parents with an ADHD kid have to learn to avoid emotional responses to behavior and work on improving communication with their child. Teach parents the importance of addressing the child by name and making eye contact; the child needs to feel respected and noticed if she is going to change her behavior for the better. Parents should make requests that are specific, direct, and simple and match the cognitive age of the child. When parents make demands, they must be reasonable. Sometimes it's good to offer the child an either-or choice: "Do you want to clean your room now or after dinner?" This allows the child to feel some control over the situation.

A similar program should be instituted in the school. Daily report cards that tie into the at-home reward system are the best way to do this. For this to work, though, parents and teachers need to be on the same page and maintain consistent contact. The at-school program should target classroom behavior, academic performance, and social interactions. (I have come to love a BMPT program called the Nurtured Heart Approach that integrates all of these facets. I talk about it more in Chapter 11.)

All together, BMPT offers parents and children the skills that are most likely to be palliative and useful in the long run—skills that empower and set the stage for continual health and happiness. BMPT provides the child with ADHD and the parents with the ADHD child the tool set to create a successful ecosystem.

Medication Safety Issues

Over 300 studies have been completed on the efficacy of stimulant medication. Most indicate a robust reduction in the symptoms of ADHD, though these effects seem to last only a few years and then fade. In fact, stimulant medications offer no sustained benefit to the functional im-

pairments of ADHD within 3 years. The benefits appear to be mainly focused on behavioral changes, not academic gains. Nevertheless, the use
of stimulant medication continues to rise. Today, about 5% of American
children between the ages of 5 and 8 are on regular amphetamine prescriptions, according to one study (Zuvekas & Vitello, 2012). This number has been slowly but steadily increasing since 1996.

Stimulant medications carry significant health risks including elevated blood pressure, cardiac risk, risk of psychosis, weight loss, loss of
sleep, loss of ultimate height, tics, psychotic episodes, and the risk of
triggering manic cycling. In my experience, emotional blunting as well as
depression with explosive temper are the most common side effects. Interestingly, the Raine study documented an enduring elevation of diastolic blood pressure of 7 to 10 points (Smith et al., 2010). If that kind of
elevation continues into adulthood, it means a 30% higher risk of cardio-
vascular disease. Canada banned sustained-release Adderall in 2005
over concerns with sudden cardiac death but reversed it a few months
later. The FDA committee on drug safety voted 8 to 7 to recommend a
black box warning (the strongest warning possible short of banning the
agent) for all stimulants relative to cardiac risk, but the general pediatric
committee overruled it in March 2006 (reasons unclear). Nevertheless,
the use of sustained-release agents continues to increase, as does the
average dosing level. And so should our concern.

More recent studies diminish the concern over sudden cardiac death.
However, the continued rise in average stimulant dose and the increased
use of sustained-release agents will make this an ongoing concern. Tics,
it appears, can be both worsened by stimulants and effectively treated
by them. A large review, however, concluded, "There is no significant
increase in tics when psychostimulants are used in patients with tics
compared with controls" (Erenberg, 2005). But stimulant use is linked
to a modest decrease in adult height and a more significant slowing in
height and weight gain over the growth period (Spencer et al., 2006).
More concerning still, according to an FDA panel that evaluated stimulant medications: 2–5% of children experience hallucinations (Harris,
2006). These are all relevant and potentially decisive concerns that parents should be made aware of during any discussion of use.

These are only the more obvious concerns typical of amphetamine
use, however. There are other, more alarming, less well-known concerns, including the risk of future psychotic illness, brain change, per-

sonality change, and impact on learning. Many doctors and researchers, myself included, are now worried that stimulant use in childhood increases the risk of psychosis and bipolar disorder later in life. A number of reports chronicle acute psychosis in patients on stimulant medications (Greiner, Enss, & Haen, 2009; Kraemer, Uekermann, Wiltfang, & Kis, 2010; Surles, May, & Garry, 2002). The biochemistry makes sense: Stimulant medications raise the level of dopamine in the brain, and excessive dopamine levels are linked to psychotic states. One Canadian study found that as many as 9 out of 98 children treated with stimulants over a 5-year period developed psychotic symptoms (Cherland & Fitzpatrick, 1999). It's probably not a coincidence that the explosion of pediatric bipolar disorder and psychotic symptoms in children over the last 20 years has moved in lockstep with the rapid escalation of stimulant medication use in children (see Chapter 13). These reports are a real cause for alarm, or at the very least apprehension for the prescribing doctor.

Stimulant medications have profound effects on the neurochemical environment in the brain, effects similar to those of cocaine, MDMA, or methamphetamine use. These controlled substances share a structure and neurotransmitter action similar to that of stimulants like methylphenidate, which increases dopamine and norepinephrine levels in the brain through the reuptake inhibition of the respective monoamine transporters. Interestingly, neuroscientists have now documented persistent changes in animal forebrains after exposure to methylphenidate, with long-term behavioral changes that include decreased sensitivity to reward systems (Marco et al., 2011). After even moderate dosing, the brains of adolescents showed significant alterations in neurotransmitter function, systems involved with motivated behaviors, cognition, and stress. Newer studies are showing that the structured anatomy of the prefrontal cortex and hippocampus go through significant changes after exposure to stimulants, with long-term reduction in dopamine receptor density in the striatum that persists throughout adulthood (Moll, Hause, Ruther, Rothenberger, & Huether, 2001). Despite these discoveries, our understanding of stimulants is still far too limited. One excellent review article on this subject concluded, "We know much less than we should . . . about the biological and cognitive effects of more protracted courses of therapeutic stimulants on adult brains and adult behavior" (Berman, Kuczenski, McCracken, & London, 2009).

And we know even less about the effects on children. We know that stimulant medications change the brain rather dramatically; what we do not know is if these changes have good, bad, or mixed long-term consequences. "A growing body of literature suggests that the consequences of modifying neural plasticity with amphetamines vary greatly with both individual and developmental factors," says one group of prominent researchers (Berman et al., 2009). This is enough to warrant caution. Let us harbor no assumption that artificial changes in a complex ecological system like the brain are uniformly positive. We are not that smart.

Personality change is part and parcel of our target outcome in stimulant treatment. But if the personality change is for the worse, there needs to be some consideration of the child's experience and quality of life. Kids on stimulants often become more muted, inhibited, and even robotic. Excessive dosing can create a zombie-like effect where the child is emotionally withdrawn, flat, stiff, and mechanical. This does, however, make their behavior much more manageable. But most kids hate this feeling. In my experience, this negative response is dose related and attenuates with lower doses. But it's still important to ask the child about his or her experience and feeling on the drug: Do you notice a difference in your personality on your medicine? Do you like it? As child mental health professionals, we need to listen to our little patients and advocate as indicated.

Learning and Stimulants

One of the biggest questions surrounding stimulant medication is what dosing works best to enhance learning. The recent trend is toward escalation of dosing and sustained-release medication. I have no doubt that high-dose stimulant medication offers the greatest enhancement of behavior control and maximal reduction of the core symptoms of ADHD. However, questions remain over whether that necessarily equates to maximal support of learning.

The zone of proximal development (ZPD), a concept developed by Russian developmental psychologist Lev Vygotsky, offers some guidance. The ZPD is the difference between what a learner can do without help and what he or she can do with help. In this model, external support can aid in learning through the encouragement of engagement, problem solving, and internalization of new skills. If a teacher merely solves the math question for a child, no real learning takes place. However, if the teacher asks questions, encourages, and provides some corrective guidance, the child can work through the problem with success and true learning. The point is that there should be some gap or difficulty in learning so that the task can be internalized and processed by the child. In this sense, the dosage that most effectively reduces the gap between what a child can and cannot do without teacher assistance, while not closing it totally, is the most effective dosage.

But a question still remains: What dosage best accomplishes this? Most of the dosage studies are not much help as they target behavioral end points. These studies show a linear dose-response curve in which higher doses create more inhibition and control. But this does not seem to be the case with learning assistance. The few studies that do target learning as an end point offer a very different story. A variety of studies show that the biggest change in learning and task completion occurs between placebo and 10 mg of methylphenidate (Brown, Slimmer, & Wynne, 1984; Evans et al., 2001; Peeke, Halliday, Callaway, Prael, & Reus, 1984; Rapport, Quinn, DuPaul, Quinn, & Kelly, 1989). One dosage-response study concluded, "The rate of acquisition and accuracy in learning paired associations were significantly, but differentially, affected by MPH dose and the degree of learning mastery" (Rapport et al., 1989). Some studies have found benefit with higher doses, but most have not. High doses of stimulant medication effectively eliminate the ZPD for many of the crucial compensatory tasks in learning. Perhaps this is the reason that gains typically fade over time—there is no internalization of the learned skills. No challenge; no imprinting. The take-away here is to use low doses and resist the urge to achieve maximal behavioral control. This is not the real target for most kids. Remember, you want to use just enough stimulant medication to give children a little boost in their ability to learn on their own. Learning is a process you do, not a process done to you.

How to Prioritize Treatment Modalities

After assessing a child's ADHD subtype, making commonsense adjustments to their ecosystem, and surveying the various available treatment

Stimulant Cheat Sheet

1. Start with low dose (5 mg) short-acting methylphenidate once, then twice daily.
2. Avoid or use great caution prescribing stimulants to kids with the anxious and overfocused and angry and oppositional subtypes, as they tend to be less responsive.
3. Kids with inattention, developmental delays, or classic subtype will respond best.
4. If the dose escalates to 36 mg or more of Concerta (or equivalent), reexamine to see what subtype or comorbidity issues you might have missed.
5. Consider atomoxetine for anxious and overfocused subtype. Start with low doses (18–25 mg once per day).
6. Consider guanfacine for mood/explosive subtype.
7. Think of medication as the scaffolding, not the building. The goal is learning and growth, not behavioral control.

List of Common Stimulant Medications

- Ritalin (methylphenidate)
- Concerta (methylphenidate)
- Metadate (methylphenidate)
- Daytrana (methylphenidate)
- Adderall (mixed amphetamine salts)
- Focalin (dexmethylphenidate)
- Dexedrine (dextroamphetamine)
- Vyvanse (lisdexamfetamine)

options, you'll need to prioritize one treatment option above the others. Sometimes, this can be a very difficult decision. One way you might come to this decision is to weigh long-term efficacy against long-term risk. Accordingly, treatments would fall into one of these four categories:

1. Evidence-based treatments that correct or heal underlying deficits, improve long-term health, and carry little risk (nutrition and diet,

natural supplements such as probiotics and glutamine to heal the gut, neurofeedback and cognitive therapies, and parenting and behavior interventions).

2. Evidence-based treatments that correct or heal underlying deficiencies and carry some risk (natural supplements such as ferritin and vitamin D to treat deficiencies).

3. Evidence-based treatments that reduce symptoms only and carry little to no risk (natural supplements such as inositol, DMAE, and bacopa to treat anxious ADHD).

4. Evidence-based treatments that reduce symptoms only and carry some risk (medications).

Think about where on this list the treatment options you're thinking about might fall. Discuss it with the patient and the parents and explain the pros and cons of that category according to its long-term efficacy and long-term safety. Ask for input about what style of treatment they're most comfortable with and what fits their current needs and worldview. Going through this process will give you a more informed sense of what treatment styles should be prioritized above the others. Then, according to your informed conclusions, make a list of treatment options for your child in descending order of priority: (1) nutrition and diet, (2) neurofeedback and cognitive therapy, (3) natural supplements, and so on. This way, if the first option fails or the family becomes uncomfortable with it, you'll waste no time and know what to move on to next.

Treatment Plan: Step by Step

1. Comprehensive evaluation of child's six realms (see Chapter 6) and common presenting issues (see Chapter 7).

2. Identify barriers, deficiencies, strengths, and gifts.

3. Examine the child for diet issues, food quality, food allergies, or gut issues. Refer to a nutritionist or naturopath as needed.

4. Mandatory: Survey at least three teachers with standardized form such as Connors or Vanderbilt. I also recommend an open-ended form to gather more information from the teacher (see Figure 6.1). Speak with school counselor as needed.

5. Examine for family conflict, depression or overwhelmed parents, op-

positional behavior, marital stress, poor communication, behavioral issues (home or school, or both), and social skills. Think about BMPT program such as Nurtured Heart, if needed.

6. If the child is depressed, anxious, or traumatized, refer for individual therapy.

7. Lab testing: Check TSH, vitamin D (25 OH), ferritin, serum zinc, lipid profile (low cholesterol), and HS CRP (High Sensitivity C Reactive Protein). Treat abnormalities as they appear. Also think about a sleep study if the child is suffering from insomnia or apnea.

8. Assess for learning issues. If present, consider the 504 Plan (see glossary), IEP for special education (see glossary), tutoring, school change, curriculum change, classroom adjustments, or supplements for focus and learning such bacopa, DMAE, and DHA/EPA.

9. If there are no significant issues in steps 1–7, apply commonsense adjustments and allow 6–12 weeks to see if problem persists.

10. If there are significant issues in steps 1–7, assess further for subtype and comorbidities, and treat accordingly.

11. If there are no gains after treating steps 1–9 or if the family is in crisis, consider medication use (low dose) in tandem with other interventions. Focus on learning, not behavioral management.

12. Continue to reassess, adjust, support, and educate the child and family.

Jack

Jack was a 9-year-old who came in with his mom, Jennifer. She described ADHD symptoms beginning at the age of 5, as well as anxiety and obsessive behaviors that began soon after his stimulant medication dose was increased for the second time. The little boy had long-standing issues with proper growth and was currently underweight. He also had a poor appetite and showed the classic signs of dietary concerns: Dark circles sagged under his eyes and he was pale, with dry scaly skin. Jack also had bright red ears, often indicative of food allergies. The boy acted a bit scattered in my first contact with him, and it was clear he had trouble focusing. When I asked Jennifer about his early history, he had a long run of near-constant ear infections, antibiotics, and tube surgery at age 3. He had some abdominal pain but was more bothered by chronic constipation.

As a first step, I tapered back his stimulant medication (Concerta, 36 mg) to assess baseline. His presenting symptoms—poor focus and inattention—worsened significantly. I then began him on several nutritional supplements: inositol (3 g tid), L-theanine (200 mg bid), vitamin D (vitamin D_3 3,000 iu/day; blood level 18), and fish oils (750 mg of EPA).

I referred Jack to Mary Rondeau, ND, in my clinic to address food allergies, low appetite, and poor diet. Upon further analysis of diet, we learned his overall caloric intake was too low to maintain weight. In addition, his diet consisted mostly of highly processed foods, large amounts of refined sugars, and little protein, healthy fats, fruits, or vegetables. One of the first steps was to remove dairy from his diet as a possible allergen. Other dietary suggestions included at least 15 to 25 g of protein for breakfast, only high-protein snacks, and, because he had a history of constipation, at least 10 oz more water a day (replace soda). Stool testing supported our concern about dysbiosis, so probiotics were added.

Two months after dietary changes and supplementation, his mom reported significant improvements with overall mood and ability to concentrate. As we reduced his stimulant, the anxiety, sleep issues, and appetite improved markedly. Positive school reports started coming in indicating Jack was working in groups better. Diet changes were well tolerated and his appetite increased significantly. Mom noticed a definite correlation with the addition of high-protein breakfast foods and his behavior throughout the day. She said that the increased protein in combination with cereal made Jack calmer and better focused and leveled his mood. Moreover, he tolerated a progressive medication taper without aggravation.

Six months later, we were able to completely eliminate his stimulant medication, and currently he is doing better in school. At least as important, he now seems healthier, looks much better, and has much less anxiety. Jack was a primary food allergy and gut imbalance kid with some secondary anxiety, mainly driven by his stimulant medication. Address the underlying issues and children can recover wholeness without the need for medication.

CHAPTER TEN

Depression

Depression is a common, varied, and potentially devastating illness. It is characterized as a mood disorder with a pervasive negative impact on mood, affect, concentration, motivation, sleep, sexuality, and vitality. There are few illnesses with such a predictable deterioration of quality of life. The negative economic impact of depression has been documented at over $83 billion a year in the United States, not to mention the emotional toll it exacts on the sufferer and his or her community. Depressed people are also more physically ill and contribute less to society. Nearly two-thirds of those diagnosed with depression also suffer from one of the following: hypertension, arthritis, coronary artery disease, diabetes, GI disorders, chronic back pain, pulmonary disease, or angina. Sadly, for almost half of people with depression, the depression first reared its ugly head in childhood.

Pediatric depression carries a significantly greater risk of substance abuse, suicide, poor psychosocial outcome, poor academic performance, and other psychiatric illness. Right now in the United States, about 3% of kids under 13 and about 6–8% of teens experience depression in any given year (Costello, Erkanli, & Angold, 2006; Kessler & Walters, 1998). About 70% of these kids will experience a recurrence and 50% will go on to have chronic mood issues as adults. Most distressing, depression is now the number one cause of disability for people aged 15 to 44 in the United States. These numbers show no sign of going down.

As recently as 30 years ago, the existence of childhood (under the age of 12) major depression was debated in academic child psychiatry. Recently, David Fassler, a child psychiatrist from the University of Vermont and a pediatric depression expert, announced that one-quarter of all children in the United States today will experience serious, significant depression by the age of 18 (1997). Surveys of high school children reveal an incredible prevalence of depression and suicidality. One 2012 study in North Carolina indicated that over 25% of middle school students feel hopeless at times and commonly think of suicide (McNeill, 2012).

And these numbers are starting to sneak into younger age brackets. It's long been known that the age of onset is a consistent predictor of long-term risk and morbidity. And as this epidemic continues to creep into younger and younger populations, it forecasts gloomier and gloomier conclusions for the mental health of our whole population. With earlier onset ages, we're looking at elevated risk levels for the entire population. This phenomenon has consequences for the severity of the disease as well. The younger a child or teen develops a significant depressive illness, the more severe the long-term consequences. For example, preadult age of onset has been documented to be a predictor for risk of suicide and severity of suicidal ideation in long-term adult illness (Williams et al., 2012).

The falling age of onset tells us that the environmental and epigenetic triggers of this illness are changing. And if we're going to effectively prevent pediatric depression and get a handle on this epidemic, we need to first get our hands around these triggers and alter them for the better. What's perhaps most scary is that only about 30–35% of children with major depression find treatment of any kind—much less successful treatment. Also, a prodromal period of as little as 7 days of depressed mood in a child accurately predicts later development of major depressive disorder (MDD; Kovacs & Lopez-Duran, 2010). We need to get these kids better help, faster. Prevention must be a core part of the approach, as even minor symptoms in childhood can herald a lifetime of suffering.

I say this because depression is more than mere illness: It is a response to the stresses of life that becomes habitual, limiting, painful, and destructive. Chronic depressed mood represents a cross-stitched pattern of behavior, physiology, and affect in which many kids become trapped. But neither the brain nor genetics are solely to blame: Depression is neither a chemical imbalance of neurotransmitters nor the production of bad humors. Genetics convey risk—but not fate.

For us to understand—and break—the causal chain that traps kids in depressive symptoms, we must aggressively work to detect early expression, treat triggers, and heal the ecology of the child. The power of wholeness to repair and recover will course through the child naturally once we remove barriers and add supports. As mental health professionals, it is incumbent upon us to demand a focus on prevention, early identification, and treatment. We can't merely struggle to treat the symptoms while more and more children face a lifetime trapped in a state of depression.

The Wholeness Model of treating depression looks for likely triggers and addresses them aggressively, while also enhancing supports to overcome the illness. Given the long-term risk of this illness, mere symptomatic relief carries very little weight and benefit. In fact, even current prevention models have significantly failed to reduce the burden of depression in children (Kovacs & Lopez-Duran, 2010). The wholeness approach aggressively tackles risk factors and strengthens the building blocks of health that may be altered with an eye toward prevention.

Cause

Depression is not well understood. Its cause has been called neurological, biochemical, genetic, environmental, emotional, psychological, and spiritual. And each of these theories, at some level, is right, or at least has some evidence to back it up. Beyond the cause of the disease, there is even less clarity on the most effective treatment. Various researchers have statistically demonstrated the effectiveness of treatments affecting serotonin (fluoxetine et al.), norepinephrine (bupropion), and mixed neurotransmitters (imipramine, duloxetine). Truth be told, no one really knows how conventional antidepressants work, and why some work better than others on certain patients. Other treatments such as electroconvulsive therapy, which uses electrical current to cause a seizure, are also quite effective in treating serious depression. Psychotherapy, such as the cognitive behavioral approach, has been documented as effective in treating depression as well. Also, bright light therapy has been shown to be effective in treating depression. St. John's wort (SJW) has also been shown to effectively treat depression. SAMe works as well as any prescription antidepressant, and it works by enhancing methylation presynaptically. Acupuncture has been shown to effectively treat major depression, perhaps by moving chi. EFAs such as EPA show efficacy, and may work via an anti-inflammatory mechanism (Rabkin, McElhiney, Rabkin, McGrath, & Ferrando, 2006). What's more, the placebo response rates in depression trials are enormous, often 50–90% of the medication response. Yet as we explored earlier, the placebo effect is not simply psychological. In fact, it induces physical brain changes in this process, so you might say it effectively treats depression.

What do we do with all this? How can we sort through it and decide on an effective, or most effective, treatment? We don't need to. What's interesting about this list of effective treatments is that each works via a different mechanism, yet they all have been shown to work. What does this mean? It means depression is a wide-ranging human phenomenon that appears to possess many different paths of causation, as one might expect in an ecological model. And with many paths of causation, there are many paths of cessation. There are many different tools to treat it and many unexplored alternatives as well.

What we can say, then, is that depression is a common expression of dis-ease. It is so wide-ranging and common that this term may have lost its value in describing a specific disorder. Major depressive disorder with clear vegetative signs is a more specific disorder, but only a small percentage of patients fit strict criteria for major depression (13–20% by one estimate for adults, and this is probably much lower in teens and kids).

Rather than a specific disorder, depression might be better seen as a nonspecific response to an imbalance in the body, mind, or spirit. I call it the final common pathway theory. In this framework, imbalance at any level (or levels) can create a depressive response via a final common pathway of expression. This theory holds that the depressive response does not specify an exact cause or treatment. A person might be depressed because of strong genetic loading, interpersonal conflict, or spiritual malaise. Depressive symptoms are simply the final common pathway of that imbalance's expression. As such, in my experience, when there are significant unresolved psychological (mental) or spiritual (existential or attitudinal) issues, biochemical treatments offer only limited and temporary relief.

The final common pathway theory helps to explain why there exist such a wide variety of effective treatment options (e.g., serotonin, norepinephrine, monoamine, exercise, psychotherapy, light, St. John's wort). The logical conclusion is that there are many different expressions of the depression, each requiring a unique treatment plan. The final common pathway theory embraces a more holistic range of both triggers and treatments for depression. It also puts the onus on the practitioner to assess each individual more carefully in order to find out what lies beneath this common presentation of depression.

Cause: Five Common Factors

There are five factors that contribute to the dis-ease of most young sufferers of depression:

1. Hypothalamic-pituitary-adrenal (HPA) axis issues
2. Other physiological ills
3. Inflammation
4. Predisposition
5. Mood repair

I will move through each of these five common factors in turn, explaining the ways in which they contribute to the expression of depression in kids.

HPA Axis Issues

The HPA axis, which plays a key role in stress modulation, reflects the underlying health and vitality of the body's neuroendocrine system. But it may also play a role in the modulation of depressive symptoms. A recent meta-analysis revealed a significant relationship between neuroendocrine dysregulation (such as higher baseline cortisol) and pediatric depression (Lopez-Duran, Kovacs, & George, 2009). Could one source of our current epidemic of childhood depression be an escalation of chronic stress and its impact on the HPA axis? That's what these data suggest. And on a basic level, it makes sense. Kids live in a stressful world, and that stress has an effect on their mood. In fact, evidence suggests that endocrine dysregulation, like stress, precedes the onset of pediatric MDD (Lopez-Duran et al., 2009). This connection does, however, need to be more fully fleshed out.

Other Physiological Ills

Beyond HPA functioning, cardiac vagal control (CVC) and brain hemispheric asymmetry also seem to play strong roles in the development of pediatric depression. These three interlinked and intelligent systems exert a wide range of control on a young human body, so it's no wonder their dysfunction might cause malaise. For many years, these systems have been implicated in the experience, expression, and regulation of affective states (Fox & Davidson, 1988; Korte, 2001; Porges, 1997; Zeman, Cassano, Perry-Parrish, & Stegall, 2006).

Cardiac vagal control is a measure of the activity of the vagus nerve and autonomic nervous system. (Low CVC implies a less relaxed, more aroused sympathetic state.) Depressed adult patients show lower CVC than controls. Recently, CVC levels have been found to be an accurate measure of emotional regulation in children (Vasilev, Crowell, Beauchaine, Mead, & Gatzke-Kopp, 2009). Not surprisingly, these studies show that children of depressed moms have abnormal patterns (reduced CVC) and elevated levels of depression (Ashman, Dawson, & Panagiotides, 2008). And vagal nerve stimulators are now being used in treatment-resistant depression. The exact mechanism at work here is unclear, but it may be related to environmental conditioning and genetic predisposition. More research is needed.

Research on brain hemispheric asymmetry has exploded in the last 10 years. This area of study looks at EEG recordings of children to understand hemispheric differences and how they are related to moods and affective states. A substantial body of these findings has shown that the left and right frontal brain regions are associated with various affects and behavior tendencies. According to these studies, depressed individuals have right frontal asymmetry (relatively greater right than left frontal activation) compared to nondepressed peers (Thibodeau, Jorgensen, & Kim, 2006). Not surprisingly, infants with a currently depressed mother display greater right frontal asymmetry than do infants of nondepressed mothers (Jones, Field, & Almeida, 2009). As these at-risk children get older, the results of their right frontal asymmetry appear to persist. Interestingly, resting right frontal asymmetry correlates with a mother's concurrent and increasing depressive symptoms (Forbes et al., 2006). Other patterns are being identified and evaluated as well.

Inflammation

Inflammation is now commonly recognized as a component of depression. The relationship between depression and inflammation appears to be bidirectional: negative moods activate immune and inflammatory mediators throughout the body, and systemic inflammation triggers a negative mood response. Further, refinement also finds a bidirectional relationship between proinflammatory cytokines and negative mood. One proinflammatory cytokine, interferon, used in cancer treatment, triggers depression in 23–45% of patients. Additionally, an elevation of CRP (a blood test for cardiac-related inflammation) has been shown to be a de novo risk factor for the appearance of MDD in adult women (Pasco et al., 2010). Conversely, some studies show that symptoms of depression occur prior to signs of increased inflammation (Stewart, Rand, Muldoon, & Kamarck, 2009). However, the consensus is clear: Inflammation and depression are closely linked. These studies have not yet begun to explore pediatrics, but the explosion of interest means that it is just a matter of time before we have a greater understanding of the link between pediatric depression and inflammation. Given the vast array of chronic illnesses that have their foundation in inflammation, some attention to this issue makes sense for health care and prevention, especially in at-risk or symptomatic populations.

Predisposition

Family history is a well-known risk factor for depression in children. But what exactly does this mean? Many people interpret this to mean that if you have a clear family history, you will become depressed. But this is simply not the case. Risk is elevated, but ecological factors such as nutrition and emotional state tend to outweigh predisposition. In fact, in adoption studies of twins, very little evidence can be found for a genetic influence on depressive symptoms in childhood depression (Rice, Harold, & Thapar, 2002). A more recent review indicated that specific genetic variations, such as SNPs, make only a very small contribution to MDD (Wray et al., 2012). The clear-cut genetic link we once hoped for just doesn't seem to be there.

Certainly, family history plays an intregral role in the expression of depression, but it may be that environmental factors found in family style or role modeling convey some of the morbidity. This means that while family history sets up a clear risk factor that may triple a child's risk of depressive illness, the complexities of the genetic risk factors preclude us from any simple pharmacological rescues. Instead, we must focus our energy on bringing more preventive strategies to bear on these predisposed kids.

Mood Repair

Mood repair implies the ability of a child to work through negative mood states and move back to a place of balance. Current evidence points to abnormalities of affect development in children of at-risk families as early as the toddler years (Kovacs & Lopez-Duran, 2010). One salient characteristic is the diminished expression of positive affect. In typical children, the displays of positive affect (e.g., smiling, laughing, playing, joking) increase consistently in appearance over the first 8 or 10 years of childhood, while displays of negative affect decrease over the same time frame (Olino et al., 2009). Activation of positive affect is central to the development of normal affective regulation. It also downregulates the negative physiological consequences of negative affect (i.e., the HPA axis). Impaired attentional skills also deplete the ability to activate positive affect. Children with impaired activation of positive affect will increasingly struggle with the typical emotional challenges of childhood. They will be at higher risk for serious mood disorders and for physiological imbalance.

The development of positive affect arises mainly from a complex interaction with caregivers. Low positive affect usually occurs in infants when there is a caregiver (typically the mother) with a recent history of depressive disorder. According to one study, low positive affect in 3- and 4-year-olds was consistently related to maternal (but not paternal) depression, particularly severe or early onset forms (Durbin, Klein, Hayden, Buckley, & Moerk, 2005). Low positive affect may also set a kid up for later depression by attenuating reactivity to external reinforcers or rewarding experiences. (I also view oppositionality as one indicator of systemically low positive affect.) Low positive affect robs a child of the typically positive emotional bias of a healthy youth. Instead, the default mode of the child is neutral to negative. A healthy child needs high positive affect to navigate childhood well.

Any effective treatment must recognize and reflect these five factors. It might look something like this:

1. Stress reduction training through biofeedback, yoga, mindfulness, and DBT (these treatments impact factors 1 and 2).
2. Anti-inflammatory diet, including fish oil supplementation, exercise, sunlight, and vitamin D monitoring.

3. Aggressive family intervention. This would proactively identify depressed and subsyndromal depressed moms and dads. They would be given training in parenting and behavioral management (e.g., Nurtured Heart Approach), positive affective expression (role modeling), HPA treatment (stress reduction like yoga), heart rate variability, biofeedback, and possibly even consideration of neurofeedback to address EEG imbalances (these treatment options reflect factors 4 and 5).

This understanding of causation and treatment builds on existing research, emphasizes prevention, and gets to the core of the issues affecting depressive symptoms. It also tells us that the increasing incidence and prevalence of depression is at least partly due to the growing allostatic load of stress. Stress impacts the HPA axis and the autonomic nervous system, making the body more vulnerable to debilitating outside influences (Wilkinson & Goodyer, 2011). Treatment with an SSRI or individual cognitive psychotherapy does nothing to mitigate this impact and in that way seems superficial and limited, with no acknowledgment of the core issues. Kids deserve something better, something that will get them whole.

Do Antidepressants Work?

It is tough to know whether antidepressants really work. In fact, it seems that the more we unearth about them, the less clear the answer becomes. Erick Turner published a landmark article in the *New England Journal of Medicine* in 2008 documenting a dramatic publication bias in antidepressant trials. Via the Freedom of Information Act, he gained access to all of the antidepressant trials ever submitted to the FDA. What he found was startling: Almost all of the positive trials were published (36 out of 37), but the vast majority of the negative trials were never published. All in all, 74 trials were conducted and 36 had negative results. More than that, Turner found that compared to the FDA analysis of the data, big pharmaceutical companies consistently distorted the statistics to make their products appear more effective. He found that the effect size was inflated by an average of 32% (range 11–69%). It's hard to know what's even evidence-based anymore.

Most of the positive data in these studies were reserved for severely depressed patients. Jay Fournier (2010) and his colleagues at the University of Pennsylvania aggregated individual patient data from six high-quality clinical trials and found that the superiority of antidepressants over placebo becomes clinically significant only for patients who are very severely depressed. This article replicates four other similar reviews in the last few years. Unfortunately for big pharmaceuticals, the majority of patients are not severely depressed. Most are only mildly depressed. If antidepressants only work on the severely depressed, it begs a basic question: How do they work?

Irving Kirsch (2009), one of the world's leading experts on the placebo effect and head of the Harvard Program in Placebo Studies, thinks that antidepressants function as active placebos in which the side effects convince people something is happening, which heightens their expectation and positive belief. For example, in clinical trials the correlation between side effects and improvement with fluoxetine is 0.96 (an almost perfect correlation). Kirsch points out that antidepressants fare much more poorly against active comparators than against placebos. In fact, in 78% of all clinical trials, antidepressants failed to separate from active placebo. He also found that the placebo effect created the majority of clinical effect and was at least twice as powerful as the benefit of the medication alone. In the severe depression group, the most significant treatment effect came not from the increasing value of the medication but from the deteriorating placebo effect. Kirsch also documented that antidepressant medication has no clinical value for anyone with mild to moderate depression (about 83% of patients).

These data, of course, are all for adults. But the research in pediatrics is equally weak. We know that only about 30% of children reach remission of depression with 8 to 10 weeks of treatment via an antidepressant. A review of medication trials for children published in the *British Medical Journal* came to this conclusion: "Antidepressants of all types showed limited efficacy in juvenile depression" (Tsapakis, Soldani, Tondo, & Baldessarini, 2008). The authors agreed that fluoxetine had the best data to support its use.

Efficacy aside, my greatest concern with the status quo in pediatric depression treatment lies with the safety of antidepressant medication. In 2004, the FDA mandated black box warnings for the use of any antidepressant in a pediatric population because of elevations of suicidal ideation. In 2007, that warning was extended up to the age of 24. At that time, 12 of the 15 clinical trials submitted to the FDA had failed in this population. The Cochrane Group took a look at medications in the treatment of adolescent depression in 2007. Their review surveyed the 12 highest-quality studies. The findings are startling. They found that a teen is more likely to experience suicidal ideation (RR 1.80) than to respond (RR 1.28) to treatment (Hetrick, Merry, McKenzie, Sindahl, & Proctor, 2007). This review found that only fluoxetine passed muster as an effective treatment. And yet other antidepressant medications with minimal empirical support are still being prescribed to children in high numbers (Kopas, 2010; Page et al., 2009).

For a more holistic picture of antidepressant efficacy, let's explore the data from the Treatment of Adolescent Depression Study (TADS), probably the largest and most important evaluation ever done on teen depression. The results of this study were first published in 2004 in *JAMA* (March et al., 2004). In it, 439 adolescents (aged 12 to 17) were divided up into four arms: CBT, fluoxetine, combination of CBT and fluoxetine, and placebo. They were followed over 36 weeks at 13 different sites. The medication and placebo groups were blinded for 12 weeks and then open-labeled. The CBT group was, of course, not blinded. At week 12, the response rates were: 73% combination, 62% fluoxetine, 48% CBT. At week 18, the response rates were: 85% combination, 69% fluoxetine, 65% CBT. At week 36, the response rates were: 86% combination, 81% fluoxetine, 81% CBT. When TADS was initially published, the results were widely hailed as support for the use of medications in the treatment of adolescent depression. But, as we all know, the devil is in the details.

A 2007 publication revealed that suicidal events were more common in patients receiving fluoxetine therapy (14.7%) than combination therapy (8.4%) or CBT (6.3%) (March et al., 2007). The article also noted that CBT appeared to "enhance the safety of fluoxetine." The authors speculated that CBT skills enabled teens to better manage the SSRI effects. They went on to summarily downplay the safety risks, noting that not one adolescent committed suicide. However, it was not until the publication of Vitiello's article in 2009 that we were able to actually assess the suicidal events data. Vitiello's report revealed that March et al. summarized the data in such a way that it was impossible to discern which teens from the placebo group and which teens from the CBT groups were placed on medication. Thus, it was impossible to parse out who attempted suicide and on what experimental agent. It was even-

tually learned, however, that at the end of 36 weeks there were 18 suicide attempts, 17 on fluoxetine. At the end of 36 weeks there were also
26 events of suicidal ideation, 19 of those in the drug group.

The TORDIA study looked at a variety of medications in treatment-
resistant teens and found a link between suicidal events and substance
abuse, family conflict, and more severe suicidal ideation. It also identified a link between elevated suicidal events and both benzodiazepines
and venlafaxine. In my mind, the risk raised by SSRI medications makes
it hard to rationalize them as a primary treatment intervention—not to
mention the very limited differentiation from placebo or other treatments. SSRIs convey a very real risk for a very limited reward.

The bottom line is clear. Fluoxetine appears to be among the best—if
not the best—antidepressant medication, though it works only weakly in
teens and probably not at all in children under 13. The value of other
medications—weighted against nasty side effects and the inherent
risks—is not yet totally clear. This much, however, is abundantly clear:
Caution and close monitoring are advised.

General Assessment and Questions

Based on the findings of current research, my approach to treating childhood depression has changed over the years. For long-term benefit, I
place less stock in the value of medications. And increasingly, I have
come to place more emphasis on ecological or family and physiological
interventions.

The wholeness approach to depression requires a comprehensive assessment and appreciation of the individual child. We must acknowledge
that the kids we see are unique, sensitive, and wounded beings of wide-
ranging potential. Only by broadening the scope of our impressions can
we possibly hold a broad enough therapeutic palette to treat appropriately. Depression, perhaps more than any other illness, is a nonspecific
response of the individual to pain, loss, sadness, disappointment, distress, rejection, and isolation on a variety of levels. It is clear that our
culture is becoming less supportive of our emotional, mental, and spiritual health. The epidemic of pediatric depression signals our need for
change on many levels.

Before you meet a young person, center yourself and drop your personal agenda. The personal practice of a meditative technique seems to

enhance the ability to do this effectively and repeatedly. Allow yourself to sense the varied impressions that come to you from this person, including the mental and emotional atmosphere that emerges. The less forceful you are with your format and presence, the more the individual can fill the space with himself or herself. A calm, comforting, and accepting demeanor seems to be less threatening and more helpful.

Ask yourself general questions such as, What is the patient's level of vitality? Does she or he look energetic, fit, overweight, or weary? Does he or she seem comfortable in the body or ill at ease? Many of these observation skills are taught in traditional psychotherapy. However, holistic assessment emphasizes the deeper impressions and intuitions that we all have. The goal is not to form impressions quickly, but to allow impression to form, to "take it all in," as it were. Later, this will empower the intuitive process as you work with someone. The more quiet and accepting you can be, the better this information can be collected. On the other hand, if you are stiff, distant, or intimidating, the young person will be guarded. The key is to create a warm, welcoming space. Start by allowing the person to tell his or her story while you take in as much as you can.

When you are with the patient, try to go beyond words. Try to appreciate that person's presence. Is it vital, joyful, and alive? How is the expression of positive affect? Does he or she open to you and your inquiry? What are his or her passions in life? What are the major burdens? Is there balance, range, or self-awareness? Is there motivation for change? Where do you encounter resistance?

Environment

In assessing the child's environment, you should ask yourself questions like, Is the school healthy, supportive, and nurturing? How is the fit? Are there significant toxins, allergens, or pollutants that affect health? Does this child connect with the earth, plants, and beauty? Is his or her free time crowded with screen time? Is the lack of sunlight a problem? Is the child overscheduled by a well-intentioned parent?

Physical Indicators

Reviewing family history (genetics) is very important. A review of past history (prior episodes) to look at triggers, developmental issues, or traumas is also quite important. Begin to review current medications (prescription, over-the-counter, herbal) in order to assess whether medications may be having an effect (positive or negative) on the child's depression. Stimulant or antipsychotic medication can dull emotions and the ability to generate positive affect. Obesity, lack of exercise, and poor nutrition are huge factors in mood and well-being.

Next, move on to a laboratory workup. Look for thyroid function, adrenal function (DHEA-sulfate, in physical illness or chronic depressive pattern), 25 OH Vitamin D, CBC, lipids (low cholesterol), MTHFR, iron status, and CRP. Also, given the accumulating data, I frequently order an adrenal cortisol stress index with four salivary samples through the day to examine the HPA axis.

Mental Indicators

In the mental arena, assess for patterns that are negative, pessimistic, passive, self-defeating, or those with an external focus of control, which is the opposite of resilience. Assess for the general level of challenge and stimulation in the child's life (too high or too low). Look broadly at addictions (not just substance abuse). Does the child have a profound sense of helplessness or hopelessness? How do creativity, play, and humor come into his or her life?

Emotional Indicators

What is this child's range of emotion? Does he laugh, cry, and emote with vitality? Does she carry baggage from earlier losses and trauma? Can the child generate positive affect and repair negative mood? Do parents step in to repair mood and rescue the child?

Social

Review the number, depth, and variety of friendships. This factor contributes significantly to physical health and well-being. Loneliness and social disconnection are huge risk factors if they exist. Discuss the quality of the primary relationship with each parent, including connection, intimacy, conflict, support, and communication. Spend a bit of time on any romantic relationship, no matter how elementary, as it may give hints about larger patterns. Family life has a tremendous impact on depression for everyone, but especially for a little kid. So look at how well he or she relates to and gets along with the entire family, including all siblings. How are the parents? How strong is their agenda and bias (positive or negative)? How does the child seem to fit in the family and with each parent individually? Is Mom or Dad depressed or on autopilot? Does the person connect or relate to animals? What is the community connection? Do nonparental adults play a role in the young person's life?

Spiritual

Does the family have a spiritual path? Do they have purpose, value, and meaning in life? Do they center or meditate regularly? Are they hopeful about their life? Is love a regular part of each day? Is this person connected to soul or spirit?

Diet and Other Factors

Diet can be an important factor. With kids suffering from depressive symptoms, reducing sugar as well as refined, overly processed foods should be a preliminary step. Next, encourage kids to explore their diet and how they react to it. Many kids find that mood issues benefit from a higher-protein diet, which may improve energy, especially if they have some issues with weight and obesity. A family history of alcoholism will also point you in the direction of a higher-protein diet as well.

If there are any indicators of food intolerance or a significant allergic history, then explore specific items in the diet via a rotation elimination challenge, whereby a common offending food allergen (e.g., corn, dairy, citrus, wheat, soy, eggs, chocolate) is removed for 10 to 14 days and then reintroduced. Two large studies add weight to a nutritionally oriented approach. In a large population-based study of over 1,000 women, adherence to a traditional diet of fruit, vegetables, meat, fish, and whole grains was shown to be associated with a lower incidence of depression and anxiety (Jacka et al., 2010). Also, a very large prospective study of over 10,000 young adults from Spain demonstrated that adherence to a Mediterranean diet protected against the development of depression over the course of 4 years (Sanchez-Villegas et al., 2009).

If fatigue or sleep is a factor, consider the elimination of caffeine, especially coffee. Actually, I recommend that all depressed patients, with their potential for HPA dysfunction, eliminate caffeine as it elevates cortisol and strains the HPA axis. Taper gradually over 2 to 4 weeks. Replace it with herbal teas or grain-based coffee substitutes. Energy drinks are an abomination: They offer no nourishment and create dependence on an external agent for energy. The caffeine dose is excessive and can generate a variety of anxiety, sleep, and cardiac issues.

Treating Depression

The following sections outline various treatment tools, including biochemical approaches, hormonal interventions, and nonpharmacological options, and how they may be implemented safely and effectively in children.

Biochemical Approaches

Several biochemical interventions have sound research backing their use in children:

1. SAMe: I use SAMe frequently, mainly in slowed or retarded depression characterized by fatigue or apathy. In one study, SAMe (1,600 mg orally or 400 mg IM) was compared to 150 mg of imipramine. SAMe was as beneficial and much better tolerated. A large meta-analysis (24 studies) performed by the Agency for Healthcare Research and Quality in 2004 showed that SAMe was safe and as effective as conventional antidepressants. (Interestingly, homocysteine appears to be a better correlate of depression than B_{12} levels.) Additionally, SAMe can be used to help wean someone off antidepressant medication. But be wary; SAMe has a real biochemical impact, so caution and supervision are needed.
2. Folic acid: Folate, like SAMe, works via enhancing methylation. Recently, a prescription form of activated folate was made available with an FDA indication for depression (Deplin, 7.5 mg and 15 mg). Although stand-alone results have been reported, folate is typically used to augment conventional antidepressants. Some people have the genetic variant of the MTHFR enzyme that makes folate turn into the

active form. (A significant family history of mood or anxiety disorders or treatment resistance should prompt this lab test.) These individuals are at higher risk for depression, and supplementation seems to support them.

3. St. John's wort: SJW is as effective as antidepressants in treating major depression, according to a meta-analysis published in 2008 by the Cochrane Group (Linde, Berner, & Kriston, 2008). SJW is a reasonable alternative to conventional antidepressants in treating major depression. It does have herb-drug interactions, and this must be monitored. I find that the side effects and tolerability are much better than with prescription agents. Other studies demonstrated that SJW was an effective treatment in a 1-year follow-up for mild to moderate depression (Brattstrom, 2009; Kasper, Volz, Moller, Dienel, & Kieser, 2008). Another study found SJW to be as effective as paroxetine in preventing relapse of major depression (Anghelescu, Kohnen, Szegedi, Klement, & Kieser, 2006). For patients with chronic depression, SJW presents a reasonable alternative for long-term prevention. For depression with agitation or insomnia, SJW can be an especially excellent choice. I have seen untoward reactions in some highly anxious patients who did not tolerate SSRIs either. Three small studies of SJW in children are positive and point to a need for aggressive dosing (900 mg for age 7 and up) (Simeon, Nixon, Milin, Jovanovic, & Walker, 2005; Findling et al., 2003; Hubner & Kirste, 2001).

4. Ginkgo biloba: Ginkgo appears to work synergistically with SJW for slowed or fatigue-ridden depression (80 to 160 mg BID).

5. Omega-3: Fish oil continues to show increasing value in psychiatric illness across a wide range of issues (Sinn, Milte, & Howe, 2010). For kids and teens with depressive symptoms, target 1,000 mg of this form daily with meals. (EPA is the preferred form in mood disorders.) The increase in hydrogenated oils, the excess of omega-6 oils, and the decrease in magnesium in our diets make omega-3 EFA deficiency a common problem. Perhaps this contributes to the increasing numbers of depressed and suicidal children, and even the skyrocketing incidence of childhood bipolar disorder.

6. Vitamin B: B_6 is a necessary cofactor in serotonin synthesis. In general, I recommend 50 mg per day for any teen dealing with depression. Commonly, I use a B complex at 50 mg with folic acid for all depressed

patients over 12. I also sometimes use a liquid multivitamin for younger kids with at least 5 or 10 mg of B$_6$ and folic acid.

7. Chromium: Although less is known about the role of chromium in mammalian brains, there is research linking it to mood. In one RCT of atypical depression, the investigators reported that 7 of 10 patients taking chromium for 8 weeks responded positively to the chromium treatment, with a significant reduction in depression scores, compared to no response in the placebo group. Chromium supports insulin effectiveness and makes sense in any circumstance of altered carbohydrate metabolism.

8. Vitamin D: One review found a significant association between low 25(OH)-vitamin D levels and mood disorders in women (Murphy & Wagner, 2008). In another study from Norway, investigators followed 441 subjects over 1 year and found that overweight individuals with a 25(OH)-vitamin D level below 40 were at significantly higher risk of depression (Jorde, Sneve, Figenschau, Svartberg, & Waterloo, 2008). One researcher found that fibromyalgia patients with a reduced vitamin D level were much more likely to experience depression (Armstrong et al., 2007). Interestingly enough, obesity in children may reduce vitamin D levels, as the sunlight must travel through the fat to activate the vitamin. Recent studies and clinical experience direct you to test and supplement 25(OH)-vitamin D levels in all mood disorder patients to 40 ng/ml or perhaps 50 ng/ml.

9. Magnesium: As we gain more information about magnesium, we realize that it has a profound influence on many issues including mood disorders. In one rat study, in fact, induced magnesium deficiency created depression-like behavior. The researchers noted that a combination of B$_6$ and magnesium worked best to palliate this behavior (Spasov, Iezhitsa, Kharitonova, & Kravchenko, 2008). In a series of case studies, magnesium supplementation (125–300 mg of glycinate or taurinate TID) was found to be effective in treating major depression (Eby & Eby, 2006). In a large community-based study of over 5,000 individuals, investigators found a clear association between deficient magnesium intake and the likelihood of depressive illness (Jacka et al., 2009). This association was not found with anxiety, however. I often recommend calcium and magnesium supplementation to mood disorder patients. Irritability, headache, muscle pain, insomnia, and constipation are signals that more magnesium could be useful.

Hormones

1. Thyroid: We know that major depression alters the neuroendocrine axis (witness the dexamethasone suppression test). Clinically, we observe a huge overlap between depression and thyroid issues. Thyroid hormone supplementation can be an effective antidepressant, even in people without thyroid abnormalities. Artificial thyroid agents (such as Cytomel/T3 or Synthroid/T4) have been used for decades by psychiatrists as an augmenting agent. Many holistic physicians use low-dose natural thyroid hormone (desiccated thyroid), which contains both T3 and T4. The mental health benefits seem to be better than with either T3 or T4 alone. Often, there is a positive family history of thyroid disease. When used as a first-line treatment, this approach can be rapidly effective for mild depression. Interestingly, elevated TSH (over 2) appears to be connected to gluten sensitivity. The autoimmune thyroiditis underlying most elevations in TSH may relate to immunological sensitization by gluten; if you see this, consider a gluten-free trial.
2. DHEA: Available over the counter, this hormone strengthens the body (as opposed to the catabolic effects of cortisol). Low DHEA levels are a common problem in any chronic debilitating illness or in severe chronic stress. Before initiating supplementation, baseline blood levels are recommended. And blood levels should be continuously monitored in those taking DHEA supplementation. Supplement to average level for a young adult of the same sex as reported in normograms. Doses are typically 10 to 25 mg for teen girls and 25 to 100 mg for teen guys. I think of this intervention in anyone with chronic disease or physical illness with fatigue. I save this intervention for ages 12 and up.

Nonpharmacological Options

1. Bright light: Bright light therapy continues to shine as an effective treatment for a variety of psychiatric maladies. It has been demonstrated to help premenstrual dysphoric disorder and pregnant mothers, and to augment conventional antidepressants. Researchers are finding that bright light therapy improves temperature regulation as well as mood. Side effects for bright light therapy are few: There are rare reports of manic activation in bipolar patients and autonomic arousal.

2. Cranial stimulators and melatonin: Most depressed kids sleep poorly, and the Western response is often a sedative hypnotic. This dangerous trend needs to stop. I am inclined to offer safe sleep aids, such as melatonin (0.5 to 1.0 mg), but only in the short run. Focus should be brought to sleep hygiene, exercise, stress, and stimulation reduction. Cranial electrical stimulators have also been shown to help sleep and improve mood. They look to be low risk, with over 30 years of intensive use. The device is easy to use, costs about $400 to $700, and should be used about 20 minutes before bed.

3. Talk therapies: CBT remains a gold standard for treating depression. For depression, I also like to use DBT, as it builds awareness and skills in emotional regulation. Furthermore, we now have neuroimaging studies that show the positive ways in which DBT and psychotherapies alter the brain.

4. Experiential therapies: Most of the body-oriented therapies such as Hakomi or Somatic Experiencing fall under this category. These are good options for sensitive kids who want to go deeper and build new levels of awareness. Expressive therapies such as art, music, and dance make good sense to me as an adjunct for kids who are out of touch with their emotions. One RCT found music therapy effective in treating depression (Erkkila et al., 2011).

5. Acupuncture: A review of acupuncture for MDD in adults concludes that it is an effective and well-tolerated treatment as a monotherapy for MDD (Wu, Yeung, Schnyer, Wang, & Mischoulon, 2012). As of right now, we have no studies to guide us in the use of acupuncture in children, but acupuncture has been documented to be safe in childhood. In fact, I have practiced acupuncture for almost 20 years, and I find teenagers to be interested in and to benefit from this treatment quite often. It makes good sense for anyone with autonomic or HPA abnormalities. Generally, I use it as a complement to a range of interventions.

6. Meditation: Practicing meditation complements psychotherapy by teaching individuals to be more present and aware. One meta-analysis found that mindful physical exercises such as tai chi improve depression as a stand-alone intervention (Tsang, Chan, & Cheung, 2008). According to another study, mindfulness-based cognitive therapy is effective at preventing depressive relapses—as effective as antidepressants—and also effective for reducing residual

symptoms in patients with major depression (Chiesa & Serretti, 2011).

7. Biofeedback: Given the increasing data about HPA dysregulation in mood disorders in children, biofeedback makes good sense as a tool to support autonomic balance. I think of it especially when anxiety and depression are comorbid, as they often are. Neurofeedback, a type of biofeedback that focuses on brainwave patterns, has developed quite an evidence base in recent years, especially in the treatment of mood disorders and ADHD. The documentation of EEG frontal asymmetry in mood disorders lends further credence to the use of this tool. In all, we now have somewhere around 21 articles and six studies on neurofeedback, and they all show positive results (Dias & van Deusen, 2011).

8. Massage: Massage can be valuable in helping kids recover and feel connected. This may be particularly helpful for any child who has suffered physical or sexual abuse. Really, any form of healing that involves gentle physical contact may be helpful in depression, where kids commonly feel unloved and isolated.

9. Socialization: Depressed patients are commonly isolated. I generally find that socialization and friendship can both be major factors to improve mood and activity. Recreation, group activities, and even a phone call to a friend can be useful. We know from good research that the strength of an individual's social network correlates to protective effects against depression (Ornish, 1999).

10. Spirituality: The more chronic the depression, the more spiritual issues come into play. A strong sense of purpose can contribute to recovery from depression or the prevention of it. I commonly recommend that older kids spend some time in spiritual inquiry and explore a spiritual path. Prayer, meditation, retreat, and worship can begin to open this realm up for someone suffering with depression. Service in the community can heal and lift spirits for kids of all ages. Simple volunteer work for those in greater need does wonders for the soul. A gratitude journal may be one of the simpler and more powerful tools to help anyone regain a positive attitude toward life. Simply have children write down a few things once or twice daily that they are thankful for. All of the truly spiritual—and healthy—beings I have encountered in my life radiate gratitude.

Treatment Plan: Step by Step

1. Comprehensive evaluation of child's six realms (see Chapter 6) and common presenting issues (see Chapter 7).
2. Identify barriers, deficiencies, strengths, and gifts.
3. Examine the child for diet issues, food quality, food allergies, or gut issues. Refer to a nutritionist or naturopath as needed.
4. Examine for family conflict, depressed or overwhelmed parents, oppositional behavior, marital stress, poor communication, behavioral issues (home or school, or both?), and social skills. Think about family therapy if needed.
5. If the child is depressed, refer for individual therapy. If previously or already in therapy, contact prior or current therapist for background and collaboration.
6. Lab testing: Check TSH, vitamin D (25 OH), ferritin/CBC, lipid profile (low cholesterol), homocysteine, and HS CRP. Treat abnormalities as they appear. Consider DHEA-sulfate or MTHFR screen if chronic illness. Also think about a sleep study if the child is suffering from insomnia or apnea.
7. Add B-complex 50 mg with 1 mg of folate, 500 to 1,000 mg of EPA, and 500 to 1,000 mg of vitamin C.
8. If chronic depression or fatigue, explore adrenal health (DHEA-sulfate and salivary cortisols) and consider adaptogens such as rhodiola or ashwaganda.
9. Make sure sleep, exercise, and sunlight are at appropriate levels and limit electronics as needed.
10. If emotional regulation is an issue, think of DBT.
11. Look at adding needed supplements to support mood and energy.
12. Select SJW, SAMe, or fluoxetine as appropriate.
13. Address social concerns as relevant.

Jordan

Jordan came to me in severe pain. For more than a year she'd been plagued by bad headaches. At my clinic, her folks doted on her in the waiting room, finding a quiet alcove and moving some chairs so that she could lie flat. When she walked into my office she immediately slumped down onto the couch and curled up into a ball. She was stocky with long brown hair, and looked much older than her 15 years. When I asked her how she was doing, she spoke in a smoky whisper, and it was hard for me to make out anything more than a murmur.

Jordan grew up in a tight-knit, religious family that did lots together: played games, camped, attended service, and enjoyed the same TV shows. Dad worked in computers and Mom devoted herself to her kids in the home full time. Both parents were devoted to their child and were desperate to assuage her suffering.

The headaches had started a few years earlier. At first, they were only intermittent and pretty mild, but as the months rolled on they had increased in frequency and intensity—so much so, in fact, that by the time I saw her she was no longer attending school and was seeing a home-bound teacher. Her effort, according to the therapist, was inconsistent and meager. This struck me as odd. Jordan was sharp as a whip and had been a straight A student since early elementary school. It wasn't like her to go halfway on anything.

As you might expect, Jordan was upset about many things, not just her headaches. Her eyes could barely contain the coiled anger behind them. With her folks out of the room, she acknowledged the hopeless-ness of her situation and blamed herself for it, using some pretty harsh words to describe herself and her efforts. Tears came intermittently as she talked, but she fought them back, each time regaining composure and stiffening her back. Jordan had lofty goals for her life. But frustra-tion with herself and her headaches was beginning to eat away at them.

The amount and variety of treatments Jordan had been through was impressive. She had tried acupuncture, homeopathy, various diets, tons of supplements, and massage, as well as the gamut of conventional care options: numerous pain medications and even opiates. Nothing seemed to help for long, though. Nothing slowed her steady decline in function-ing and activity. She had no friends, no social contact with peers, and now couldn't even do schoolwork. She rarely left the couch, much less the house.

Her parents had been remarkable agents for Jordan. She had been to Denver's Children's Hospital and another local hospital for pain workups. Initially, her parents were hesitant to share the reports, but after some consideration they handed them over. I wasn't surprised by what they found. Both institutions felt that family dynamics and personality factors contributed to the pain problem, and they recommended therapy. The parents said they felt violated by the insinuation that nonbiological factors were to blame and rejected it out of hand. They believed that with enough exploration the biological cure would be just around the corner, and they were determined to find it. Really, they only came to see me because Jordan had been started on two psychiatric medications (an antidepressant and a sleep aid), and her primary care doctor told them they needed to find a psychiatrist to manage them.

After I reviewed everything and talked at length to all three of them, I shared my view. I said that I thought Jordan was a bright, highly ambitious young woman who had developed a severe physical condition that reflected her intensity and drive. The pain was real and needed treatment. But there were software issues that needed to be addressed alongside the hardware. Most importantly, I said that we needed to design a rehabilitation program to get her back to school and studies and connected with her peers.

I made some slight adjustments to her supplement intake, mostly trimming back the unneeded items and boosting support for her mood (B vitamins, fish oil, and inositol). I recommended DBT training, individual psychotherapy, and perhaps a few family sessions once she was ready. I also recommended biofeedback to help her learn how to control her imbalanced autonomic nervous system. I outlined an exercise and activity plan to gradually move her back to some level of fitness and bodily control.

As I somewhat expected, Jordan and her folks just went through the motions for a few therapy sessions, which Jordan hated and soon refused to attend. She did not want to talk about herself or any "problems" she had. After a time, her parents decided that Jordan's issue was not emotional or psychological at all but was in fact related to chronic Lyme disease. She began a year-long program for treatment, which included some harsh antibiotics and a bagful of new supplements. During the treatment, they saw me only a few times a year, mostly for medication management.

After some initial progress with the new treatment, Jordan had a relapse. Now, a year and half later, she goes to two classes at school but must return home immediately afterward to rest on the couch. Headaches still limit her on an almost daily basis. We have seen little progress in activity or social connectedness. Jordan denies being depressed but refuses to stop her antidepressant medication. "It does help somehow," she told me. She hopes to go to college someday, perhaps after the Lyme treatment finally finishes. I continue to reflect my earlier recommendations, but money is tight and Jordan is too overwhelmed with school to consider a new therapist. So I work to support rehabilitation as best I can.

Jordan's case reflects a few truths in our business: Not everyone gets better, at least right away, and not everyone will follow advice. Many families and patients just get stuck in a biological mind-set—seduced by the idea of fast-acting scientific solutions—and balk at the idea that anything psychological might be part of the problem. We can nudge people in the right direction and make recommendations, but they don't always stick. It's tough to swallow, but as practitioners we don't always have what it takes to reach patients and motivate them to help themselves.

It pains me to see Jordan and know how much she is suffering.

CHAPTER ELEVEN

Behavioral Issues

Childhood is that period of time in which a child, uninitiated into the patterns and customs of family and social life, learns to behave in an appropriate manner. Some children manage this learning curve better than others. Sometimes, children's struggles during this period can reach such a point that we slap them with a specific label to describe their difficulties. These labels, like attention-deficit/hyperactivity disorder (ADHD), oppositional defiant disorder (ODD), and conduct disorder (CD), are the bane of schools, law enforcement, and overwhelmed parents. And they share a few common traits: They can be diagnosed at a distance by a clinician, the child typically has no concern or sense of the problem, and it causes considerable stress and turmoil for those managing the child.

ADHD, ODD, and CD make up the category of externalizing disorders (EDs) first proposed by Achenbach in 1978. According to Achenbach (1978), the common traits connecting these disorders are a lack of emotional control, interpersonal aggressiveness, and lack of adherence to social norms. The latter of these two disorders are called "disruptive behavior disorders" and entail a persistent pattern of behavior that may include defiance of authority figures, aggression, blaming others for one's own mistakes, hostility, irritability, lying, angry outbursts (e.g., temper tantrums), intentionally annoying others, arguing with adults, and refusing to comply with requests. Externalizing disorders are tied to a number of negative long-term outcomes including low academic competence, juvenile delinquency, adult smoking, and adult crime, as well as a vulnerability and persistence of substance abuse.

These issues represent massive public health concerns and common challenges in pediatric mental health. According to a survey, 13.8% of children met criteria for ED at school entry (compared to 11.1% for internalizing disorder) (Carter et al., 2010). Interestingly, about 60% of these children had both an externalizing and an internalizing disorder in this large survey. The authors also noted that risk for boys is the same as girls, until age 4. From then on, boys strongly predominate.

It should come as no surprise that genetic factors play a role in these patterns. An extremely violent, aggressive dad and an impulsive, substance-abusing mom will, probably, end up passing a number of high-risk traits on to their children. Unfortunately, beyond risk assessment, this knowledge is almost totally useless to us. It hasn't led us to any preventative measures or, really, any reliable biochemical intervention. On the other hand, new research data tell us that specific environmental factors contribute to the development of EDs and can be readily modified. More than that, a range of useful parenting and systemic interventions can effectively treat or even prevent these problems. Let's explore the relevant research.

Risk Factors: Parental Psychopathology

We know that a variety of adverse parenting events are highly predictive of ED (Rothbaum & Weisz, 1994). For example, behaviors such as less parental involvement, hostility, and limited monitoring are correlated strongly with ED symptoms. How these behaviors are passed on, however, is a little more of a difficult question. Stoolmiller, for one, suggested that it is ineffective parental discipline rather than role modeling of aggression that connects these behaviors to ED in kids (Stoolmiller, Patterson, & Snyder, 1997). Conversely, a number of researchers have reported direct links between parental depression and ED (Burcusa, Iacono, & McGue, 2003). In fact, recurrent maternal depression has been identified as a significant risk factor for the development of ED, internalizing disorders, and general behavior problems (Giles, Davies, Whitrow, Warin, & Moore, 2011).

It's simple: If the child's primary emotional caregiver (Mom, 98% of the time) is not functioning at full strength emotionally, the child may begin to express psychiatric issues. Studies on maternal depression, in particular, document that a child's risk of having a psychiatric diagnosis rises fourfold with a depressed mom (Hammen, Shih, Altman, & Brennan, 2003). Interestingly, the issues seen in children are not just depression, as one might logically conclude, but also behavioral, anxiety, and attentional problems. Curiously, having a healthy father in the home offers only partial protection.

If Mom gets help and her problems are addressed, then about 33% of those psychiatrically "ill" kids will recover completely, without any specific treatment. If Mom's issues go unaddressed, then an additional 17% will develop a psychiatric illness. One study followed these kids into adulthood and found that 23 years later, children of depressed moms have more depression, chronic pain, disability, psychiatric medications, avoidance, and fewer friends (Weissman, John, & Merikangas, 1986; Weissman et al., 2006).

In my practice I find that at least half of kids showing out-of-control behavior have a depressed, overwhelmed, anxious, or emotionally unavailable mom. Of course, it varies based on the child's temperament and how that fits with the mom. Some children have easy temperaments, and for them gentle or aloof parenting works well. However, with willful, intense, or traumatized kids, a fierce lioness of a mom is needed to manage the extremes of behavior and to socialize the child early on. If Mom cannot rise to meet these challenges, the child will run amok and take behavioral control through the use of aggression, tantrums, intimidation, and a wild persistence that wears everyone down. And if this behavioral pattern gets imprinted over years, it is very difficult to change. The imperative here seems quite clear: Assess, treat, and support all parents to seek the treatment they need in order to be the emotionally sound parents their children require.

The struggles of moms often go well beyond depression, however, and often include anxiety and interpersonal difficulty, which can negatively affect the child long before the appearance of ED-like behaviors (Harnish, Dodge, & Valente, 1995). For example, one study showed that a caregiver's perception of his or her toddler as unresponsive was a consistent predictor of later ED in the toddler (Olson, Bates, Sandy, & Lanthier, 2000). Other early risks, according to this study, included a perception of the child as difficult to control, as well as a relationship low in warmth and affective enjoyment. More interesting still, the caregiver's environment during infancy can be linked to the development of ED at school entry (Shaw, Owens, Giovannelli, & Winslow, 2001). This is consistent with social learning and attachment models, inasmuch as it shows that a deficit in early caregiving and environment is connected to the later expression of ED.

Whenever I mention maternal depression as a risk factor for anything, I am always asked, "But what about paternal depression?" Good question. For obvious reasons, mothers are usually the principle test subjects in studies of parental psychopathology, so we don't know that much about paternal depression. In fact, of all the studies looking at parental psychopathology, only 1% examined fathers alone. But, from these data, parental depression appears to be much more common than we think. One study looked at over 80,000 mother, father, and infant triads, and the incidence of depression (per 100 person-years) was 3.6 for fathers and 13.9 for mothers (Davé, Petersen, Sherr, & Nazareth, 2010). As an aside, in this study, younger parents (aged 15 to 24 years), parents with a history of depression, and parents from deprived areas were found to be at the highest risk for depression.

Another meta-analysis looked at 43 different studies of postpartum dads, and the overall rate of paternal depression was 10.4% during the first trimester and 1 year postpartum (Paulson & Bazemore, 2010). It is important to note that the highest rates of depression (25.6%) were found during the 3- to 6-month postpartum period. Also, a moderate positive correlation ($r = 0.308$) was found between maternal and paternal depression. So, while paternal depression appears to be less common than maternal depression, it's still fairly common, particularly in young, recent dads living in poor areas. And since paternal depression is linked to more aggressive parenting practices, which, in turn, are linked to the development of ED, we'd be wise to ask about any history of paternal depression in a child with ED symptoms.

It appears to be a burden stretched across both parents, though. A study from Columbia University found that about 18% of parents who bring their child in for evaluation by a psychiatrist meet *DSM* criteria, mainly for internalizing disorders like depression and anxiety (Vidair et al., 2011). Interestingly, in most cases the mom's diagnosis was directly linked to the child's while the dad's diagnosis was not. However, the severity of both parents' symptoms was directly linked to the severity of the child's symptoms. In another study of kids brought in for evaluation, 31% of mothers showed symptoms suggesting current psychiatric diagnosis, while 43% reported subsyndromal symptoms. One researcher assessed 222 mothers who brought their children in for evaluation and found that 61% met *DSM-IV* criteria for an Axis I disorder, most commonly depressive and anxiety disorders (Swartz et al., 2005). And it's not uncommon to see these symptoms in pregnant women, either: A large survey (over 4,000 women) in the Pacific Northwest found that over 15% of pregnant women were depressed at some point and many continuously through the study, as well as before and after pregnancy (Dietz et al., 2007). Since parental psychopathology is so closely linked to development of ED symptoms in kids, it's not unwise to focus some (or a lot) of your attention on the parents—getting them healthy as a way to get and keep the child healthy.

And this phenomenon holds true beyond depressive or anxious symptoms. A mom with a history of abuse as a child or intimate partner violence conveys a high risk of CD to her child (Miranda, de la Osa, Granero, & Ezpeleta, 2011). In fact, maternal PTSD predicts an infant's emotional regulation abnormalities at 6 months and predicts ED, ID, and dysregulated emotions at 13 months. The added risk, in this case, is not driven by maternal depression, however (Bosquet Enlow et al., 2011). The risk stems from the mom's attachment history as an infant (Brook, Zhang, Balka, & Brook, 2012). In fact, according to one three-generational study, a grandmother's relationship with her daughter predicted the development of ED in the grandchild (Brook et al., 2012). Conversely, a secure maternal attachment was protective against the intergenerational transmission of adverse parenting practices.

The risk factors go both ways, of course. A child that is hyper and aggressive early on has higher risks. And when this behavior meets high levels of negative parenting and high levels of family stress—as it often does—it's much more likely to create an ongoing ED (Campbell, Shaw, & Gilliom, 2000). I have no doubt that these kids are challenging temperamentally, and when they're combined with a high-risk mom or high-conflict family, these families very often struggle to break the cycle of mutually deteriorative behavior.

By the time EDs manifest, the child has likely weathered a very stressful early emotional environment. It should come as no surprise, then, that the child has developed indicators of autonomic and neuroendocrine dysfunction (Herpertz et al., 2003). Studies point to abnormal autonomic arousal and electrodermal skin resistance. Cortisol abnormalities are common in ED kids, with a consistent pattern of blunting in adolescence (Ruttle et al., 2011). While the HPA axis may show hyperarousal when these behaviors first display in childhood, long-term exposure may lead to a hypoarousal of the HPA axis, which culminates in a dysregulated diurnal rhythm. This may help to explain the heightened comorbidity with a range of other psychiatric disorders linked to these disruptions of the child's internal ecology. Thus, a dysregulated HPA axis and abnormal autonomic activity may provide a window into the exposure of a child to life stressors or the accumulation of emotional distress over time, and serve as a psychobiological mechanism whereby stressors manifest as a risk for the onset and persistence of mental health problems (van Praag et al., 2004).

This pattern, needless to say, tends to evolve over time into more parent-child conflict and distress. But is this cycle biology or behavior? In a significant study, researchers from the University of Minnesota evaluated parent-child conflict and explored genetic versus environmental factors. They found that parent-child conflict strongly predicted ADHD, ODD, and CD (Burt, Krueger, McGue, & Iacono, 2003). Based on the nature of this link, the authors concluded,

> Parent-child conflict appears to act as a common vulnerability that increases risk for multiple childhood disorders. Furthermore, this association is mediated via common genetic and environmental factors. These findings support the idea that the comorbidity among these disorders partially reflects core psychopathological processes in the family environment that link putatively separate psychiatric disorders. (Burt et al., 2003, p. 609)

We need to appreciate the ecological nature of EDs and not get caught up treating end point symptoms. This does little to alter the underlying imbalances—in both the child and the parents. As we move forward to treat these issues, we have a choice: We can either effectively treat these kids with cost-effective systemic interventions or blame the child, blame the brain, and look toward medication for short-term relief.

Group-based parenting interventions are effective in producing sustained positive change in both the parent's perception and the child's behavior (Barlow & Stewart-Brown, 2000). According to a Cochrane analysis, parent training programs for kids with ADHD aged 5 to 18 look to be positive and also decrease parental stress and improve parental confidence (Zwi, Jones, Thorgaard, York, & Dennis, 2011). In a look at CD, behavioral and cognitive behavioral group-based parenting interventions were effective and cost effective for improving conduct problems, parental mental health, and parenting skills for kids 3 to 12 (Furlong et al., 2012). Research also suggests that these programs improve maternal mental health, a crucial risk factor (Barlow & Coren, 2004). Parental or systemic interventions have been shown to have positive effects in decreasing disruptive behaviors, and the benefit seems to increase over time, unlike cognitive behavioral interventions, which seem to require booster sessions (Bell & McBride, 2010).

Attachment should continue to play a role in treatment, as well. A secure maternal attachment and a positive therapeutic alliance predict positive outcome in very high-risk populations (Guzder, Bond, Rabiau, Zelkowitz, & Rohar, 2011). In fact, a mom's trust in her oldest child predicts how positive the therapeutic alliance will be. A growing research base documents the value of therapeutic alliance in family therapy as a useful predictor of outcome. Famed attachment theorist John Bowlby (1988) described the therapeutic relationship as an attachment relationship crucial for success. The closer we examine and the more we learn, the more we find that it all comes back to relationship: the depth and quality of a parent's relationship with the child and the depth and quality of the parent-therapist relationship. With those two relationships in harmony, it's much easier to get the child healthy and happy again.

Family History and Genetics

For every kid with behavioral issues, I also make sure to ask about the psychiatric family history. When I see a large number of blood relatives with depression, bipolar disorder, substance abuse, or ADHD, I assume there is an impairment in a crucial metabolic pathway. In turn, I begin to think about supplementation and diet. In behaviorally difficult kids (or their parents), my goal typically centers on two basic elements: relationships (parental well-being and parent-child connection) and biology. I look for mood, anxiety, sensory, and gut issues and food allergies and support them via supplements, diet change, or both. The goal in this process is to soften the brittle mood, reduce the extreme anxiety, improve sensory integration, enhance proper absorption, and eliminate allergens. Combining this step with the more relationship-oriented work creates synergetic results, because often the excessive reactivity of the child, as the result of biological problems, magnifies and stresses the parent-child relationship. One needs to work both sides of the biology-relationship divide to soothe the child's mood and get him or her back on the right track with the parents.

Treating Externalizing Disorders

In my experience, EDs are neither a disorder nor an illness, nor best viewed as such. The terms are simply useful common descriptions of behavior patterns, a pattern that needs to be addressed as young as possible, as it's a specific indicator that the child feels powerless, unsuccessful, and angry. ODD, as a pattern of behavior, is a common, primitive response, not an illness. Most 2- and 3-year-olds, for example, display some ODD behavior, just as many 4- to 6-year-olds at some point exhibit some pattern of behavior that might be construed as the result of CD. What's important, then, is to address the problem as soon as possible and in a way that teaches the child to cope with and control these behaviors. That's why the predominant conventional approach to these problems involves the use of behavioral-based parenting interventions such as the setting of clear, firm limits and consistent consequences—basically, training a difficult child to be better behaved. And they do learn, albeit slowly sometimes.

Sadly, there has been a huge trend toward medicating these children, often with powerful and dangerous atypical anti-psychotic medications like risperidone, aripiprazole, and quetiapine. These medications sedate and reduce the level of aggression, but only for a period of time. And just because it works in the short run does not mean it's the right thing to do. This is a common refrain of mine. And just as with ADHD, we need to dig deeper and weed out triggers and predisposing factors, rather than just mask symptoms. This way, we can try to understand what these difficult children really need to get better, what they need to get whole.

I have spent almost 30 years in psychiatry assessing and treating kids like this in a variety of settings. Some common themes emerge that are useful in taking an ecological approach to assessment and treatment. First, most of these children do not seem to have established a secure attachment to one or both of their parents. Second, the parents of these kids are often depressed, anxious, highly stressed, distracted, or embroiled in their own struggles. Third, the family history is often rife with issues such as depression or alcoholism indicative of some genetic or metabolic issues. Fourth, these kids seem to do poorly in school for a number of reasons. Fifth, a pattern of abuse (of any style) or neglect will magnify the problems significantly and often causes aggression as a reactive challenge.

So, based on that, the first step in treatment is to enhance the parent-child relationship. This relationship has typically deteriorated into a policing role intent on identifying infractions and doling out consequences. No matter how loving and supportive, parents become frustrated and resentful when they have to handle kids like this. It's a perfectly natural response. But as a result, the positive connection between parent and child fades. The child, often frustrated with limited attention, finds that this problematic behavior pulls in and engages the parent—negative attention is still attention. For the first time, they feel seen and connected with, even if by hostile and frustrated parents.

This mutually frustrating trap can be transformed, however. The research indicates parent training programs work. Howard Glasser developed one such program, called the Nurtured Heart Approach (NHA), which supports parents to rebuild their bond with their child (Glasser & Easley, 1998). It works by challenging parents to alter their interactions with the child on a regular basis, most importantly, by making neutral comments on behavior. For example, rather than saying, "Good job on that homework assignment," the parent might swing by a bit earlier and say something more innocuous, like, "I noticed that you look up at the ceiling when you are figuring out those math problems" or, "When you are getting ready for school you line up all of the stuff you need to take with you." This removes judgment—positive or negative—and instead generates simple feedback. This way, the child feels seen and understood, and thus connected to, without any hint of judgment. This nourishes the spirit, and gives the child confidence and stability.

Glasser also coaches parents on the ways to downplay reactions to inevitable infractions. Children recognize that they can create a dramatic response by acting out or, as Glasser says, "The parent is the child's favorite toy." If they can connect with their parents deeply, they will; however, if they are hungry for a connection, actions that trigger hot button responses become the next best thing. They want to get a rise out of the parents; they need to see some, any, reaction. Similarly, the NHA uses a variety of parental interventions to build positive behavior. I have worked with Glasser's NHA for many years and have been astounded by how well it works to improve the parent-child relationship and eliminate behavioral issues in children.

The evidence supporting the value of behavioral management and parent training programs (BMTP) is broad and well documented, especially for externalizing disorders such as ADHD or conduct problems (Furlong et al., 2012). One BMTP program, NHA, has fair evidence for safety and effectiveness. In fact, Tolson Elementary of the Tucson United School District implemented the NHA program and, over a 10-year period, students referred for special education dropped from 16% to 1%, and no new children were placed on antipsychotic medication. The ideal situation would be to adopt NHA at home and in the school at the same time. This program gets at the heart of the problem—the spirit of the child that feels hungry and needy. When children feel recognized and closer to the parents (or teachers), they stop fighting for attention. At that point, parents can begin to adjust behaviors much more readily with coaching and support. This work indeed transforms the child's ecology.

School Fit and Learning Style

Many young people suffering from behavioral issues also struggle in school. They may struggle with some mild dyslexia or attend poorly to cognitive tasks. They may be right brained and thrive in a more artistic or creative setting not available to them. Often they are athletic and hands-on learners. Whatever the case, they just don't seem to be part of that 60% or 70% of kids who take school in stride; they struggle to do well and have few successful experiences. Self-esteem and confidence, as a result, suffer. To make things worse, they're usually marginalized in school social settings, plunging them deeper into worry and pain. By junior high they are often failing and ditching class. Failure in school only compounds their frustration and creates a spiral of anger, sadness, and resentment, often leading to substance abuse and dropout.

Finding the best match for learning style and passion is the best way out of this spiral. Researchers have documented a range of learning styles, and kids with behavioral issues typically don't fit the normal pedagogic setting. So evaluate the whole child, identify learning style, and support it with the child's passions and interests. Smaller schools, charter schools, hands-on classes, a focus in the arts, school athletics, vocational practices, or other adaptations can all create opportunities for successful experiences that help turn around behavioral issues. That's why it's so important to look for learning style, passions, and gifts, which are often the best antidotes for failure, anger, and difficult behavior.

Social-emotional education is also a great option. These programs focus on building life skills such as communication, problem solving, conflict management, and self-awareness—traits that support lifelong success. A close friend of mine, Eric Larsen, developed the Discovery Program at a local alternative high school to instill these skills in high-risk youth. As a teacher, Eric knows that these "soft skills" are crucial for transforming high-risk kids into successful students—and adults. Over 6 weeks, the Discovery Program develops a mutually respectful environment where teens are held accountable for their actions in a supportive yet realistic manner. They learn about their behavioral triggers and how to control them, but also about relationships and how to navigate them successfully. By the end, they're able to move beyond their oppositional past and develop healthy habits and relationships. Programs like the Discovery Program should exist in every school to support those children who are not lucky enough to internalize the relational and behavioral skills needed for adult life. School success is just a small part of the gain.

Trauma and Abuse

Any history of trauma or abuse (think emotional abuse and neglect) will magnify the likelihood of behavioral issues. Clearly, we must identify traumatized kids and treat them as such. Traumatized kids are prone to overreact and need a sense of safety and comfort in order to develop healthy behaviors. The treatment plan, therefore, must address relationships, as the trauma will impair their ability to attach and connect with others. It must address the altered HPA axis and autonomic nervous system, which is fried as a result of hyperreactivity. With trauma everything becomes more difficult, so it's important for the parents and practitioner to make every effort to bridge the divide, building a connection that gives the traumatized youth security and care.

Treatment Plan: Step by Step

1. Comprehensive evaluation of child's six realms (see Chapter 6) and common presenting issues (see Chapter 7).
2. Identify barriers, deficiencies, strengths, and gifts.
3. Examine the child for diet issues, food quality, food allergies, or gut issues. Refer to a nutritionist or naturopath as needed.
4. Examine closely for family conflict, depressed or overwhelmed parents, marital stress, poor communication, and social skills. Think about NHA or other BMTP for parents as cornerstone of care.
5. If the child is depressed, anxious, or traumatized, refer for individual therapy. If in therapy, contact prior or current therapist for background and collaboration.
6. Lab testing: Check TSH, vitamin D (25 OH), ferritin, lipid profile (low cholesterol), homocysteine, and HS CRP. Treat abnormalities as they appear. Also think about a sleep study if the child is suffering from insomnia or apnea.
7. Assess for learning issues. Some behavior issues in children come from expressive or receptive language issues.
8. Treat mood dysregulation with such things as magnesium, inositol, or EMPowerplus.
9. If anxious, consider biofeedback or yoga.
10. Coordinate program and interventions with school to echo the same behavior plan and goals.
11. DBT may be of some help for labile moods.
12. Explore the need to severely limit electronics, as this is often one sign of an out-of-control child or teen.

Tyler

Tyler was an active kid, full of life. At 6, he was struggling in first grade with some aggression, some defiance, some inattention, and lots of impulsivity. Thin, tanned, always moving, we just barely sighted his buzz cut as he zoomed around the office. Teachers brought the issue to his mom's attention after repeated conduct violations at his elementary school. A big woman, Donna had the look of a former athlete. Both she and her husband, Tom, were ambitious and career oriented in a large insurance group. Upon inquiry, Donna told me that she had been on Celexa for 6 years, since Tyler's birth. "It helps—I don't do well without it," she said. Tom traveled quite a bit and didn't really do much parenting: Donna did it all, in many ways.

Tyler was robustly healthy but had some anxiety about sleep and Dad leaving. No food or GI issues were found. There was a family history of depression (maternal), and Tyler could be explosive if challenged. Donna told me that when he upped the ante in public and became explosive, she often just gave in to prevent "a scene." Donna admitted that she felt overmatched by his energy and intensity. I told Donna we would do some hardware and software adjustments.

First, the hardware. We added some inositol, some EPA, and some magnesium to reduce Tyler's volatility. His labs looked good, so there was nothing more to do. Now, the challenging part: the software. I told Donna that we needed to give her lots more support to deal with a challenging kid like Tyler. We needed to get her and Tom on the same page and get him more involved. I referred her to Anca Niculae, a marriage and family therapist with whom I had worked closely for a decade.

In the initial session, with both parents present, the therapist addressed the importance of giving attention to wanted behaviors, while giving minimal attention to the unwanted behaviors. Therapy also focused on increasing the bond between father and son, as Tom typically used harsh phrases such as "man up" or "boys don't cry" when his 6-year-old son became upset. A month later, a follow-up session was done with Donna alone, due to travel issues for Tom, with more specific lessons on reinforcing rules and consequences. By Donna's report, the relationships in the household had already improved significantly and the dynamics in the family felt much more fluid and warm.

Donna and her therapist explored ways to further energize positive behaviors and limit the opportunities for acting out. On the third and final session, Donna shared great admiration for the Nurtured Heart Approach, as all three household members interacted positively on a consistent basis, and Tyler now displayed a lot of empathy and cooperation both at home and in the school setting.

No medications were needed, and Tyler was now much more success-ful in school and with peers. Donna felt much more confident and better supported by Tom, who stepped up with more direct parenting and more time with the kids. There is no "cure," but Tyler is now making consis-tent gains and exploring his potential for wholeness. The crucial thing is that he is learning, thanks to an environment that holds him accountable and provides the structure he needs.

CHAPTER TWELVE

Anxiety and OCD

Americans have by far the highest rates of anxiety in the world, with a lifetime risk of 31%, according to a World Health Organization study (Kessler et al., 2009). New Zealand, Colombia, and France come in a distant second, third, and fourth, trailing us by a large margin. In fact, most countries have one-half to one-fifth of the anxiety we do, even though many of them are poor, rural, and isolated, conditions we might assume to be more anxiety inducing than those of the typical American life. But it's just not the case. Most Americans now experience and, indeed, endorse a rapidly increasing rate of anxiety.

This trend has now worked its way into our children. Studies show that students feel increasingly overwhelmed, anxious, and depressed entering college—what's supposed to be a bright and buoyant chapter in a kid's life. The Higher Education Research Institute, based at UCLA, has surveyed students entering American 4-year colleges since 1966, and according to their 2011 survey of 201,818 full-time students, anxiety has reached an all-time high (Pryor, DeAngelo, Palucki Blake, Hurtado, & Tran, 2011). (According to the study, young women experience two times the anxiety of young men.) And these are our best, brightest, most successful, and most affluent students.

Part of the reason for Americans' recent descent into anxiety may have to do with a shift in locus of control. Over the past 50 years, Americans have moved from a society of internal locus—we believe that we have control over our lives—to a culture of external locus—we blame external forces for life's trajectory. According to one study surveying over 18,000 college students, the average undergraduate in 2002 had a more external locus of control than 80% of college students in the early 1960s (Twenge, Zhang, & Im, 2004). The implications of this study are almost uniformly negative, as externality is correlated with poor school achievement, helplessness, ineffective stress management, decreased self-control, depression, and anxiety.

Anxiety disorders represent a wide range of related problems in a pediatric population, including but not limited to separation anxiety disorder, simple phobia, generalized anxiety, panic disorder, PTSD, OCD, acute stress disorder, agoraphobia, social phobia, and anxiety disorder NOS (not otherwise specified). The incidence and prevalence varies by specific diagnosis, but in general, anxiety disorders are among the most common impairing conditions of childhood and adolescence. Rates fluctuate from study to study, but the best estimate is that between 5.7% and 12.8% of kids suffer from some kind of anxiety-related disorder (Ramsawh, Chavira, & Stein, 2010).

In teens the numbers are even higher. The National Comorbidity Survey–Adolescent Supplement (NCS-A), a nationally representative face-to-face survey of 10,123 adolescents aged 13 to 18 years in the United States, reports that anxiety disorders are the most common condition in teens, coming in at about 32%. (In fact, 8.3% of teens suffer from a severe impairment from an anxiety disorder.) Rates among specific disorders ranged from 2.2% for generalized anxiety disorder to 19.3% for specific phobias. All anxiety disorder subtypes are more frequent in females (the greatest sex difference appears to be in PTSD). More distressing still, anxiety appears at the youngest age of any psychiatric disorder: The median age of onset for an anxiety disorder is 6 (Merikangas et al., 2010).

What makes things worse is that these kids usually also suffer from other issues. Rates of comorbidity among kids with an anxiety disorder are quite elevated, with significant overlap with ADHD, major depression, and dysthymia. And if these issues go untreated, they tend to have a chronic and unremitting course (Ramsawh et al., 2010). Longitudinal studies that follow children into adulthood suggest that most chronic mood and anxiety disorders in adulthood begin with high levels of anxiety in childhood. In fact, childhood anxiety predicts adult depression as well as it predicts adult anxiety. And since anxiety disorders are more common among children than either mood disorders or ADHD—those disorders most often associated with children's mental health—it means that we have a huge, unrecognized pediatric health crisis on our hands.

Well, if the problem is so pervasive, chronic, and laced with comorbidities, then why are anxiety disorders so often missed in children? The problem is twofold. One, anxiety disorders are internalizing conditions with little external reflection of the issue. And two, kids with anxiety disorders often try to please adults by minimizing or hiding their distress. So while an impairing anxiety disorder may account for up to 10% of children and teens, only a fraction of that is diagnosed. Symptoms of anxiety in childhood often go unnoticed or unreported because they revolve around sleep or other more personal, physical complaints. In fact, in a sample of kids with anxiety disorders, 88% had a sleep-related problem and 55% had three or more (Alfano, Ginsburg, & Kingery, 2007). That's why I often ask questions about sleep onset to test for the presence of anxiety in kids.

The presence of somatic complaints like sleep onset are associated with more anxiety severity, more functional impairment, greater school refusal, and poor school performance (Hughes, Lourea-Waddell, & Kendall, 2008; Ginsburg, Riddle, & Davies, 2006). In one look at kids with anxiety, 41% met criteria for a functional GI disorder versus 6% of controls (Waters, Schilpzand, Bell, Walker, & Baber, 2012). Recurrent abdominal pain is classic in this category. The prevalence of an anxiety disorder in kids with RAP is around 42–79%, with rates of depression only slightly lower (Campo et al., 2004). I immediately think of anxiety disorders when I encounter vague somatic issues or chronic physical distress.

The link between anxiety disorders and chronic medical conditions like migraine, gastrointestinal disorders, and particularly atopic disorders may indeed be a bidirectional link, in which one condition increases the likelihood of the other (Egger, Costello, Erkanli, & Angold, 1999; Spady, Schopflocher, Svenson, & Thompson, 2005). These chronic health problems share some similar ecological triggers with anxiety (childhood adversity, low socioeconomic status, and parental smoking), and according to at least one study, about half of anxious children have a chronic medical condition (Roy-Byrne et al., 2008; Chavira, Garland, Daley, & Hough, 2008), which is double the rate of the typical population. Asthma and allergies (atopic illnesses) are the most common conditions. There may be a shared pathway to both atopy and anxiety that explains the link, but it hasn't been completely fleshed out yet. In my experience, children with anxiety often have gut pathology and nutritional issues that may underlie both problems. A whole child evaluation and treatment model can identify and address this commonality.

Risk Factors

Though the more obvious risk factors of genetics, temperament, and parent psychopathology (e.g., depression and anxiety) seem to play a role in the development of anxiety, they don't appear to be either necessary or sufficient (Epkins & Heckler, 2011). For example, there's some research that leads us to believe that something as seemingly innocuous as having parents who don't listen is in fact a risk factor for teen anxiety (Dumont & Olson, 2012). And regardless of whether it appears abusive, early life stress, such as harsh physical punishment and trauma, is probably the most damaging risk factor (Nugent, Tyrka, Carpenter, & Price, 2011).

Child abuse is pretty clearly linked to later anxiety and PTSD. It is most likely mediated by the HPA axis and autonomic nervous system (McCrory, De Brito, & Viding, 2012). Neuroendocrine studies indicate an association between early adversity and atypical development of the HPA axis stress response, which may predispose the child to psychiatric vulnerability in adulthood. Brain imaging research in children and adults provides evidence for several structural and functional brain differences associated with early adversity. Structural differences have been reported in the corpus callosum, cerebellum, and prefrontal cortex. Functional differences have been reported in regions implicated in emotional and behavioral regulation, including the amygdala and anterior cingulate cortex. These differences at the neurobiological level may represent adaptations to early experiences of heightened stress that lead to an increased risk of psychopathology through life.

Identification

Primary care docs and therapists are usually pretty good at identifying disruptive and mood problems, but they often miss most anxiety disorders other than frank OCD. That's why, as a childhood mental health practitioner, my antennae are constantly on the lookout for signs and symptoms of anxiety. The challenge is to understand the developmental context of anxiety and know when bedtime rituals or preoccupation with a fear is part of normal growth and development and when it is a cause for concern. The important factor here is severity and chronicity. Does the little kid worry about bedtime excessively, with rituals to stave off that fear? Often, with older kids, looking back on temperament and early childhood patterns can give us a road map to current problems and their origins. This can, in turn, inform care. Were they overly sensitive as kids, with excessive stranger anxiety? Did they always have some sleep issues that accelerated over time?

In the patient history, ask about sleep issues, worry, and rituals as well as somatic complaints like abdominal pain, headaches, or other chronic pain. The interview may be the most critical element to treating the child well. Meet with the child alone and ask if the child worries a lot or has fears about things. Watch how the child separates from the parents in the time with you. Does he or she seem reluctant or scared to be without them? Ask parents about the need for reassurance. Ask about family history, especially anxiety in either parent or a history of trauma.

Shyness may be a useful indicator, but it's not uniform. In the large NCS-A study, over 10,000 kids aged 13 to 18 were surveyed, and while about half of the kids self-identified themselves as shy, only 12% of those shy kids met the criteria for social phobia (Merikangas et al., 2010). The kids with social phobia displayed significantly greater role impairment and were more likely to experience a multitude of psychiatric disorders, including disorders of anxiety, mood, behavior, and substance use. However, those adolescents were no more likely than their peers to be taking prescribed medications (Burstein, Ameli-Grillon, & Merikangas, 2011). These kids look more impaired, suffer significantly, and possess greater risk.

The best way to identify these kids is to provide a universal screen that only takes a few minutes. The SCARED (Screen for Child Anxiety Related Emotional Disorder) screen is a great assessment tool and comes in both a parent and child version. It's only five questions and has been shown to be useful in clinical populations (Chavira, Stein, Bailey, & Stein, 2004). A free version (for children 8 and older as well as the parents' form) can be found at the University of Pittsburgh Web site (http://www.psychiatry.pitt.edu/research/tools-research/assessment-instruments).

Treating Anxiety and OCD

Anxiety patients are often the kindest and most sensitive kids I see in a given week. They're usually much more cooperative and motivated than most. And their motivation usually pays off, as all types of interventions, both conventional and alternative, seem to work well for these kids.

Cognitive behavioral therapy (CBT) is very effective: A Cochrane metareview found that anxiety-based CBT worked well for children and adolescents, with no difference between individual, group, or parental or family-based interventions (James, Soler, & Weatherall, 2005), though it is often hard to locate psychotherapists who practice formal CBT and not a diluted variation. One answer may lie in online services. A recent RCT examined online CBT versus in-person CBT versus wait-list controls for adolescent anxiety, and it found that online CBT was as effective in reducing anxiety as the face-to-face version (Spence et al., 2011). For many kids, this may be the best way to get high-quality focused CBT.

One novel variation of cognitive therapy that is gaining traction is attention bias modification treatment. This approach recognizes that anxious folks scan their environment (internal and external) for indicators of threat and pay more attention to it than do controls. In one RCT of 186 anxious children, attention bias modification significantly reduced anxiety levels compared to two control interventions (Eldar et al., 2012). This intervention appeals to me as it tries to alter that underlying "threat" mechanism that may drive the anxiety.

I am a big fan of biofeedback, particularly heart rate variability, as an effective intervention for pediatric anxiety. A wide range of studies supports its use in children, especially with somatic issues like headaches and recurrent abdominal pain (Konichezky & Gothelf, 2011) (see Chapter 16).

In terms of drug treatment, SSRIs seem to work much better for childhood anxiety than they do for depression (Bridge et al., 2007). Kids with OCD almost always have an intermediate response, but typically it's not as sustained and beneficial as it is for kids with general anxiety. There are some downsides, however. SSRIs remain somewhat unpredictable in children, with notable side effects, including activation, nausea, and impaired concentration, in a significant minority.

Combining drug treatment with CBT appears to get the best results. The Child/Adolescent Anxiety Multimodal Study explored the use of CBT, placebo, sertraline, and combination (CBT plus sertraline) for pediatric anxiety in 488 kids (ages 7 to 17) (Compton et al., 2010). The 6-year, six-site study tried to assess the best practice for treating three common forms of pediatric anxiety (social phobia, generalized anxiety, and separation anxiety). The results were as expected: The combination group exhibited the best response (81%), while the CBT (60%) and sertraline groups (55%) were better than placebo (24%). The sertraline group, however, experienced more side effects—insomnia, fatigue, sedation, and restlessness—than the CBT group. (It should be noted that the CBT and combination group were, of course, not blinded.) The evaluation of combination therapy is particularly important because approximately 40–50% of children with these disorders do not have a response to short-term treatment with either individual therapy (James et al., 2005).

The body of literature for alternative medicine and pediatric anxiety is still quite small, but some approaches have shown some promise. Massage therapy, for instance, was found to be effective in reducing the anxiety of children with asthma, according to one study (Ghazavi et al., 2010). Similarly, according to another study, massage was effective for reducing anxiety in children on a burn unit (Parlak Gurol, Polat, & Akcay, 2010). One review of pediatric massage found anxiety reduction to be the most consistent effect (Beider, Mahrer, & Gold, 2007). And yet another review of RCTs found pediatric massage effectively reduced anxiety (Beider & Moyer, 2007). It is really no wonder that massage helps soothe the anxious child, given its calming, body-wide impact. The only challenge here is to make the delivery methods and client selection appropriate.

Beyond massage, other alternative tools such as mindfulness-based stress reduction and acupuncture make solid sense, but are not yet widely studied. In general, the number of pediatric studies—conventional treatment methods or otherwise—in anxiety disorders is still quite small. A review that covered the material in detail showed that the data are still sparse and mainly extrapolated from adults (Feucht & Patel, 2011; van der Watt, Laugharne, & Janca, 2008).

Many supplements show good success in treating pediatric anxiety. A few deserve special mention.

Inositol

Inositol is a sugar alcohol that works as a second messenger within the cell. This means that it is involved in relaying messages from the outside (e.g., hormones, neurotransmitters) to the cell nucleus so that changes can occur in the cell's machinery and thus gene expression. It has been shown in some studies to effectively treat anxiety, panic, bulimia, and agoraphobia, as well as unipolar and bipolar depression in adults (Brown & Gerbarg, 2001; Taylor, Wilder, Bhagwagar, & Geddes, 2004; Palatnik, Frolov, Fux, & Benjamin, 2001; Fux, Benjamin, & Belmaker, 1999). It also improves insulin resistance and has been helpful in polycystic ovarian disease (Fux et al., 1999).

In little kids, inositol is primarily good for anxiety, stress, agitation, and OCD. Inositol is found in our food and is extraordinarily safe. I really like to use it in kids because it comes as a sweet powder that looks and tastes like powdered sugar. I have 2- and 3-year-olds in my practice taking it. The dosing is simple: about 1 gram per 25 to 30 pounds per dose, two or three times daily. There can be mild stomach upset or loose stools, but it's fairly rare. Give it after food. Use the powder, not the capsules, as it is much cheaper and goes down easier for the kids.

L-Theanine

L-theanine is a natural supplement found in green tea (*Camellia sinensis*) and may work as an antidote to caffeine. A nonprotein amino acid, L-theanine naturally increases alpha brainwave activity and focused relaxation. It beneficially increases BDNF (associated with learning and new neuronal growth) and DHEA-sulfate (associated with reduced stress and improved adrenal health) (Miodownik et al., 2011). I find it particularly useful in the child who has both anxiety and impaired school performance (or ADHD). I use doses of 200 mg twice daily to 400 mg three times daily depending on age. It is very safe.

Kava Kava (*Piper methysticum*)

Kava kava is a root, harvested traditionally from a shrub in Oceania, and has been shown to be the most effective natural supplement for treating significant anxiety. It easily clears the Cochrane Review's standards for effectiveness in the treatment of anxiety, and other reviews concur (Pittler & Ernst, 2002; Sarris, LaPorte, & Schweitzer, 2011). Over the last few years, reports of hepatotoxicity and death have occurred, however. And in spite of intensive research, no clear cause has been identified. Various theories about aflatoxins or nonrhizome components continue to be the focus of speculation.

Herbalists traditionally focus on the medicinal use of an aqueous extract derived from peeled rhizomes and roots of a nonmoldy noble kava cultivar, limited to a maximum of 250 mg kavalactones daily for acute or intermittent use with routine testing of liver function (Teschke, Sarris, & Lebot, 2012). The most cautious stance would be to withhold treatment with kava completely until this argument is settled.

Lemon Balm (*Melissa officinalis*) and Valerian (*Valeriana officinalis*)

Two herbal remedies, lemon balm and valerian, have a long tradition of use for anxiety in children. They both appear to act on the GABA neurotransmitter system via different mechanisms (Awad et al., 2007). One large open-label study in children 12 and younger found good effectiveness, tolerability, and safety for anxiety and sleep issues (Muller & Klement, 2006). These botanicals are quite safe and can be used in traditional dosing ranges for children.

Dietary intolerances such as celiac disease play a much larger role in anxiety than previously thought. In fact, celiac disease may provide some instruction about how diet alters psychiatric signs and symptoms in general. Celiac presents most commonly with GI distress and digestive issues, but can also manifest as "silent" celiac disease (i.e., few or no symptoms), which can only really be detected through testing. This may account for the long delays in making a proper diagnosis and the recent "explosion" of kids symptomatic with non-GI issues. Surveys confirm the high and growing rates of silent celiac in school-aged populations (Cilleruelo Pascual et al., 2002). The clinical spectrum is extremely wide, however, from low-end sensitivity all the way up to frank intolerance (Bottaro, Cataldo, Rotolo, Spina, & Corazza, 1999). In children, iron deficiency anemia, apthous stomatitis (canker sores), severe insomnia, or short stature may be the first clues to a problem. Check for elevated TSH, low ferritin, and any history of autoimmune disease (e.g., thyroiditis), as they are also useful clues to a gluten intolerance.

According to a wide array of literature, the presenting symptoms in celiac disease may also be neurological or psychiatric (Zelnik, Pacht, Obeid, & Lerner, 2004; Bushara, 2005; Vaknin, Eliakim, Ackerman, & Steiner, 2004). This theory was parsed out from the observation that children with celiac disease often suffer from a common pattern of neurological and psychological disorders, including headaches, ADHD, learning and tic disorders, hypotonia, developmental delay, cerebellar ataxia, depression, and anxiety (Lionetti et al., 2009; Pynnönen et al., 2004, 2005; Niederhofer & Pittschieler, 2006). The cause of this pathology, however, is poorly understood. Some have hypothesized the role of deficient folic acid, vitamin E, and biopterin (which is well documented in these patients), whereas other studies have identified cross-reacting antibodies, immune complex disease, and direct toxicity as possible key players (Addolorato et al., 2008). More recently, additional factors have been suggested, including brain perfusion abnormalities, which have been found in the superior and anterior areas of the frontal cortex and anterior cingulate cortex in patients with celiac disease (Abenavoli, 2010). An alteration of perfusion in the same brain areas has also been reported in patients with neurological and psychiatric disorders, including depression and anxiety, thus providing a possible explanation for the association between the two conditions (Versino et al., 2009).

Treatment obviously makes a big difference here. One study reported that ADHD-like symptoms were markedly overrepresented among untreated celiac patients (age range 3–57), and that a gluten-free diet improved the symptoms within a short period of time (Niederhofer & Pittschieler, 2006). In another group, anxiety fell significantly after 1 year of a gluten-free diet (Addolorato et al., 2001). All told, what we can take from these studies and associations is that dietary issues are much more closely related to psychiatric issues like anxiety in kids, and that we need to actively test for them, particularly celiac disease, if we're to get ailing kids healthy again. The most reliable test for food allergy or intolerance is an elimination diet.

Other specific food intolerances beyond gluten appear to affect anxiety and can be ameliorated by dietary intervention alone (in the discussion of OCD I include a case report that echoes this finding). To weed out the specific food intolerance, try an elimination diet starting with one or more of the most common offenders (e.g., dairy, gluten, corn), and perhaps consult a nutritionist or naturopath. Once again, the theme here is the interconnection of body and mind, with the implication that we have to look for these problems in symptomatic children and not just jump to symptom management with external modifiers like psychiatric medication.

Unlike gluten, which has a range of sensitivity, no child should be exposed to caffeine, especially if experiencing significant anxiety. Studies have found that adults with anxiety respond in a significantly worse manner to caffeine administration, with a strong subset likely to experience panic attacks at higher doses. Now, considering that this reaction is within a well-developed, well-controlled brain, we can well imagine the havoc caffeine wreaks on a still-developing, immature nervous system and brain. Researchers have found that caffeine induced threat-related midbrain-periaqueductal gray activation (Smith, Lawrence, Diukova, Wise, & Rogers, 2011). Effects of caffeine on the extent of threat-related amygdala activation correlated negatively with levels of dietary caffeine intake. In concurrence with these changes in threat-related brain activation, caffeine increased self-rated anxiety and diastolic blood pressure. These results demonstrate potential neural correlates of the anxiogenic effect of caffeine, and they implicate the amygdala as a key site for caffeine tolerance in regular users. Caffeine increases the perceived sense of stress and cortisol markers of HPA activation, even in regular users. It's just not a good idea for anxious children—ever.

In sum, CBT endures as the best treatment for pediatric anxiety. It's safe and we have evidence that the skill building at the core of the therapy lasts up to 7.4 years for kids (Kendall, Safford, Flannery-Schroeder, & Webb, 2004), which might be enough time to break the cycle of anxiety and reinforce new, better coping skills. As a result, CBT should be the first approach to treating chronic anxiety in children. It's also important to make a strong push to improve the environment (i.e., change of school or family dynamics), address the diet and gut as needed, and support with safe nutritional agents like inositol or L-theanine. I also encourage a modality that will reset the autonomic nervous system and HPA axis such as yoga, biofeedback, or even meditation. CBT can be done in person or online. If 8 weeks of CBT plus nutritional support, diet, and ecological interventions fail to provide adequate relief, then SSRIs can be considered.

Treatment Plan: Step by Step (for General Anxiety)

1. Comprehensive evaluation of child's six realms (see Chapter 6) and common presenting issues (see Chapter 7).
2. Identify barriers, deficiencies, strengths, and gifts.

3. Examine the child for diet issues, food quality, food allergies, or gut issues. Refer to a nutritionist or naturopath as needed.

4. Examine for family conflict, depressed or overwhelmed parents, oppositional behavior, marital stress, and poor communication. Family therapy as needed.

5. If the child is anxious, refer for individual therapy with CBT. Address social isolation or social skills as needed. Identify underlying trauma. If previously in therapy, contact prior or current therapist for background and collaboration.

6. Lab testing: Check TSH, vitamin D (25 OH), ferritin, lipid profile (low cholesterol), and HS CRP. Treat abnormalities as they appear.

7. Most anxious kids sleep poorly. Consider melatonin and/or magnesium. Also think about a sleep study if the child is suffering from significant signs of apnea or snores loudly.

8. Treat with appropriate natural supplements such as inositol, L-theanine, kava (if comfortable with risk), or herbals such as California poppy, lemon balm, valerian, and so on.

9. Consider yoga, biofeedback, and/or meditation to reduce autonomic overactivity and provide lifelong skills.

10. Education: Anxious patients become less anxious when they are educated about their concerns.

PANDAS

Sydenham chorea, a neurological side effect of acute rheumatic fever characterized by unpredictable jerky movements of the limbs and face, is thought to be an autoimmune-mediated response to group A β-hemolytic streptococcus (GABHS) infection. In this well-accepted effect of the common strep infection, up to 70% of those affected also show OCD symptoms (Swedo, 1994). In 1998, Susan Swedo suggested that the side effects of a GABHS infection to the central nervous system may not be restricted to Sydenham chorea but may also include a spectrum of neurobehavioral disturbances, which they termed pediatric autoimmune neuropsychiatric disorders (PANDAS for short) (1998). Swedo hypothesized that GABHS infection can lead both to the onset of PANDAS and to clinical exacerbations over time. She and her colleagues proposed five diagnostic criteria:

1. The presence of OCD or a tic disorder or both
2. Pediatric onset
3. Episodic course of symptom severity with abrupt onset or dramatic symptom exacerbations
4. Temporal association with GABHS infection
5. Association with neurological abnormalities during symptom exacerbations

Despite growing support for an association between GABHS and OCD, and the causal relationship between GABHS infection and OCD, its pathophysiology and its possible clinical implications remain controversial. The details of this ongoing debate are extremely complicated, and both camps have solid evidence to back up their stance. (A review of the evidence for both sides and their corresponding arguments is worth the time to parse out this thorny issue: see Moretti, Pasquini, Mandarelli, Tarsitani, & Biondi 2008). We may not know for some time the outcome of this dialogue.

Regardless, it can inform our treatment decision making. We know that kids with PANDAS respond to conventional interventions such as CBT and SSRIs (Swedo & Grant, 2005). We also know that a subset of children resistant to these interventions responds to a PANDAS-oriented treatment including antibiotics and immunologically oriented therapies such as intravenous immunoglobulin. In one study, these interventions were more effective than placebo for a PANDAS OCD group, and the results were sustained at 1-year follow-up (Perlmutter et al., 1999).

But how do we identify PANDAS-type children with OCD or other neuropsychiatric symptoms? Studies examining the presentation of PANDAS and non-PANDAS children reveal significant differences. PANDAS children were significantly more likely to present with separation anxiety, urinary urgency, hyperactivity, impulsivity, deterioration in handwriting, and decline in school performance during their initial episode of neuropsychiatric illness compared with children with OCD (Bernstein, Victor, Pipal, & Williams, 2010). These PANDAS-related issues look to be related to basal ganglia function, which is perhaps why total tics and vocal tics are more severe in PANDAS children.

Treating Obsessive-Compulsive Disorder

About one-third of adults plagued with OCD (a subtype of anxiety) note onset of the problem in childhood. In fact, the mean age of onset for OCD is 10 (Mataix-Cols, Nakatani, Micali, & Heyman, 2008). Juvenile OCD is, however, a little different from adult OCD, with higher rates of tics (20% lifetime), ADHD, and other disruptive disorders. And up to one-half will have concurrent anxiety disorders (Mancebo et al., 2008). Like many syndromes first encountered in childhood, the diathesis looks to be more severe with greater genetic loading (Nestadt et al., 2000). This connection of severity can be found in the fact that up to 70% of childhood-onset cases of OCD have a continuous course (Mancebo et al., 2008). In younger samples, males are overrepresented, but by adulthood the sex distribution evens out.

The four most common presentations of pediatric OCD are (1) symmetry, (2) forbidden thoughts, (3) cleaning and contamination, and (4) hoarding. The hoarding subtype is more common among kids and is a particularly difficult version to deal with. It is associated with slowness, increased sense of responsibility, indecision, and pathological doubt. This subtype is linked to poor treatment response for both CBT and medications. In this and other subtypes of OCD, the rates of depression are significant (Storch et al., 2012).

It's often difficult to identify children with OCD because they often minimize their symptoms. These kids recognize and indeed are ashamed by the illogical nature of their actions, so they hide them or else say they're not a problem. Thus, statistically, parents and children often disagree on the severity of symptoms (Canavera, Wilkins, Pincus, & Ehrenreich-May, 2009). I find the use of an objective scale such as the Yale-Brown Obsessive Compulsive Scale (YBOCS) to be almost mandatory to properly evaluate these kids.

There are a number of predictors of treatment response. The three best, beyond symptom severity, are insight, depression, and family accommodation (Storch, Larson, et al., 2010). Comorbidity and cognitive deficits also limit the response to CBT (Storch, Bjorgvinsson, et al., 2010). Levels of family accommodation, which refers to ways in which the family members take part in the performance of rituals, avoidance of anxiety-provoking situations, or modification of daily routines to assist a relative with OCD, are negatively associated with treatment outcomes for both behavioral and pharmacological treatment. In the same way, significant improvement of OCD symptoms with treatment is associated with reductions in family accommodation. Accommodation is also strongly and consistently associated with symptom severity as well as rates of parental anxiety and OCD (Lebowitz, Panza, Su, & Bloch, 2012). Family-based CBT may make more sense for the child with significant indicators of increased accommodation.

In terms of treatment tools, exposure response prevention (ERP), a behavioral variation of CBT for OCD, seems to work well in kids, with response rates typically higher (though not always statistically) than SSRI alone (Pediatric OCD Treatment Study Team, 2004; Franklin et al., 2011). Unlike medication, it does require a significant investment, however, as the typical treatment time is in the range of 10 to 14 sessions.

General CBT can also be effective. We know from the POTS study that CBT and sertraline are more effective than placebo, and that the combination works best for OCD (Pediatric OCD Treatment Study Team, 2004). Based on this and the follow-up study, recommendations are that children with OCD should receive either CBT alone or CBT plus sertraline.

In terms of isolated medication interventions, the efficacy of SSRIs for pediatric OCD has been established for clomipramine, fluvoxamine, sertraline, and fluoxetine. The pediatric literature is consistent with the adult literature in revealing a 30–40% reduction in OCD symptoms with pharmacotherapy, which leaves the great majority of patients who respond to medication management alone with clinically significant residual symptoms (Pediatric OCD Treatment Study Team, 2004).

In addition to CBT and medication, preliminary support for pediatric anxiety has been found for mindfulness meditation, electroacupuncture (the use of low voltage, low amperage current with acupuncture points), and kundalini yoga. The nutrient glycine, milk thistle, and borage also show positive results in kids. N-acetylcysteine is effective in trichotillomania. In general, anything that positively affects the serotonergic or glutamatergic pathways appears to be helpful (Camfield, Sarris, & Berk, 2011). Counterintuitively, we have two small RCT studies showing effective augmentation with 30 mg of dextroamphetamine and one showing beneficial augmentation with 300 mg of caffeine (Koran, Aboujaoude, & Gamel, 2009). Some studies suggest that inositol has value, but it appears limited. St. John's wort, EPA, and meridian tapping appear to be ineffective in treating pediatric OCD (Sarris, Camfield, & Berk, 2012).

Beyond these treatments, I typically look at food allergies and intolerances and see if there is anything negatively impacting the child's well-being. Given the well-documented connection between gluten sensitivity and anxiety, it's very likely that OCD might be connected to some kind of food allergies as well.

Treatment Plan: Step by Step (for OCD)

1. Comprehensive evaluation of child's six realms (see Chapter 6) and common presenting issues (see Chapter 7).
2. Identify barriers, deficiencies, strengths, and gifts.
3. Examine the child for diet issues, food quality, food allergies, or gut issues. Consider a gluten-free trial. Refer to a nutritionist or naturopath as needed.
4. Examine for family conflict, depressed or overwhelmed parents, oppositional behavior, marital stress, or poor communication. Family therapy may help. Often a traumatized family may need help with parenting support.
5. Monitor and educate about family accommodation. Address it as needed.
6. Make sure the young person is referred to a therapist trained in ERP. If no one is local, consider online options. Consider ERP workbooks for parents and kids. If already in therapy, contact prior or current therapist for background and collaboration.
7. Lab testing: Check TSH, vitamin D (25 OH), ferritin, lipid profile (low cholesterol), homocysteine, and HS CRP. Treat abnormalities as they appear.
8. Kids with OCD often sleep poorly. Rule out sleep apnea. Consider melatonin and/or other agents to support sleep.

9. Consider inositol, 5-HTP, L-theanine, and/or herbals to reduce ambient anxiety.
10. Consider N-acetylcysteine.
11. If signs or symptoms consistent with PANDAS, order appropriate screening tests.
12. Consider medication (fluoxetine or sertraline) if 8-week trial of above interventions fails to make progress or if family wants to do this concurrently.
13. Monitor progress with YBOCS.

Cliff

Cliff was a sweet 12-year-old boy who came in to see me a few years ago with his mom, Cathy. Cliff was burdened with notable signs of OCD that had been present for about 2 years and were progressively increasing. He had fears about dirt, contamination, and germs. He was locked for hours each day in slow rituals, cleaning and washing his clothes. His YBOCS score was 27, indicating severe OCD.

As I was taking his history, a few things jumped out at me. He had loose stools and a lot of gas. His early history was notable for colic and moderate reflux as an infant, as well as chronic ear infections. I also noted stunted growth: Cliff was quite small for his age. But my ears really perked up when his mom said, "Cliff's aunt has celiac disease, but we don't think Cliff does as he does not have abdominal pain like she did as a kid." I told Cathy that Cliff needed to go on a 4-week gluten-free trial while I obtained some labs and surveyed his school.

Cathy came back a few weeks later with a smile on her face. "Cliff is so much better. His OCD is almost gone." I retested him, and his YBOC score was 8, the low end of mild (probably about what mine would be). He was basically, almost miraculously cured. I placed him on some low-dose inositol for a few months to help further break the behavioral pattern and talked to them about the crucial importance of remaining on the diet. I had a few more follow-ups over the next year, but, really, Cliff no longer had OCD. He also felt much better overall and no longer had gut issues.

CHAPTER THIRTEEN
Bipolar Disorder

Pediatric bipolar disorder (PBD) is perhaps the most difficult, dangerous, and confusing challenge a clinician faces today. Even something as simple as measuring the incidence rate proves to be a tricky task with PBD. In fact, most of what we know today about PBD comes right out of the adult numbers. Currently, full-blown bipolar disorder (BD) affects about 1% of adults, though an expansion of diagnostic criteria to include subsyndromal disorders may enlarge the affected population to around 4–7% of adults. The actual incidence rate in adults is probably somewhere between these two figures, something like 2–4%. This gives us some sense of where the childhood numbers might fall, and adolescent studies confirm these estimates (Goldstein & Birmaher, 2012).

This sense is strengthened by the fact that having one parent affected by bipolar disorder conveys a risk of 15–30% for a child. If both parents are ill, the risk jumps up to somewhere around 50% or 75%. The connection between childhood and adult bipolar incidence is even further strengthened by the fact that most adults with BD report the onset of their illness before the age of 18, suggesting a potential continuity between the numbers. About 30% of those affected by BPD noted very early onset (age 13 or younger), while 40% cite early onset (age 14 to 18) (Perlis et al., 2004). But as it turns out, the question of childhood incidence is much more complicated than heredity and continuity. In fact, those clues might be a red herring.

Part of the reason why PBD incidence is so difficult to measure is that the diagnostic criteria are splintered and at odds with those of adult BD. Right now, PBD can be divided into two rough subgroups: broad phenotype (irritability and generalized unstable mood; does not fit *DSM* criteria) and narrow phenotype (fits adult criteria, with true mania and mood cycling). Strangely, the vast majority of our current PBD patients fall into the broad phenotype (Pavuluri, Birmaher, & Naylor, 2005), and thus look different from the typical adult patient with BD. What's more, the vast majority of PBD patients are male (66%), whereas the vast majority of adult BD patients are female (67%) (Moreno et al., 2007). This makes it very difficult to track the incidence rate in children according to adult numbers. Some short-term studies in adolescence point toward continuity, but the question remains unanswered. In fact, at this time, we can't say with any certainty that PBD patients become adult BD patients, which means either there's something askew with our categorization and understanding of these disorders or something magical occurs at age 18.

This issue becomes even more confusing as we consider recent trends. Prior to the 1990s, PBD was rarely diagnosed and treated. PBD patients made up less than 10% of both child and adolescent inpatient discharges in 1996. But by 2004, the rate had shot up to 34% for children and 26% for teens (Blader & Carlson, 2007). According to the National Ambulatory Medical Care Survey, the rate of PBD in outpatient settings rose 40-fold between 1994 and 2003. And yet, the rates for adult illness did not even double over the same time (Moreno et al., 2007). If PBD were simply the prepubertal manifestation of BD, we might reasonably expect some continuity to these numbers. But it's just not the case. It looks like PBD is something entirely different than adult BD.

In fact, there's some reason to think PBD may be a geographically specific illness. When child psychiatrists in Australia and New Zealand were surveyed recently, the vast majority reported that they had not diagnosed prepubertal PBD. Most participants in this survey were of the opinion that bipolar disorder in prepubertal children was either "very rare (less than 0.01%)" or "rare (less than 0.1%)" (Parry & Allison, 2008; Parry, Furbe, & Allison, 2009). On the other side of the globe in Germany, only 7.8% of child and adolescent psychiatrists had ever diagnosed PBD (Meyer, Koßmann-Böhm, & Schlottke, 2004). And this trend holds true for most European countries. But it's the exact opposite of the trend in the United States, where each year we see more and more PBD cases. In fact, today PBD kids make up a significant proportion of the caseload for every American child psychiatrist.

The skyrocketing rates of PBD in recent years and the huge disparity in the rate of diagnosis from country to country tells us that something unique is occurring in the United States with PBD, something more complicated than increased awareness, better diagnostics, or differences in cultural standards. Remember, these kids are not subtle or easy to miss.

This is not a quiet, internalizing disorder like anxiety or depression. These kids throw chairs and chase their parents with knives. It doesn't matter where that happens or in what time period—it's cause for alarm. And it's highly unlikely that prior to 1990 we were simply unaware of this symptom pattern or else were misdiagnosing it.

Maybe we're just catching these kids at the wrong time. In my experience, a change of venue or in supervising adults can lead to a remarkable shift in behavior for many of the children with these symptoms. For example, a surprising number of these kids will rage and show symptoms of PBD while at home, but never do so while at school, in spite of 5 years of consistent in-home symptoms. If this were true PBD, we would see some continuity in symptoms. The noted pediatric bipolar researcher Gabrielle Carlson observed that once hospitalized, fully one-half of pediatric bipolar patients fail to display any of the remarkable rages and manic behaviors that led to hospitalization (Carlson, Potegal, Margulies, Gutkovich, & Basile, 2009). According to Carlson's study, "One third of children with rages had been given a bipolar diagnosis prior to admission. However, only 9% of children with rages were given that diagnosis after careful observation." What accounts for this change in behavior? It's hard to know exactly, but what it does suggest is that environmental or parent-child fit issues may be masquerading as PBD or perhaps exacerbating its symptoms in certain settings. If nothing else, it certainly leads us away from thinking PBD is a clear-cut biological issue or can be easily diagnosed.

Bipolarity is characterized by extremely high comorbidity—perhaps more so than any other illness in pediatric psychiatry—which further clouds the already muddied diagnostic waters. Among children with PBD, the overlap with ADHD has been reported at 91%, 98%, and 57% (Carlson, 1999; Wozniak et al., 1995; West, McElroy, Strakowski, Keck, & McConville, 1995). Joseph Biederman (2005) of Harvard once quipped, "The children with PBD meet more criteria for ADHD than the kids with ADHD do." The comorbidity goes beyond ADHD. One study found that 98% of PBD cases also met criteria for another illness (Tillman et al., 2003). Those illnesses most highly represented included ODD (46–75%), conduct disorder (5–37%), anxiety (12–77%), and substance abuse (40%). The presence of this comorbidity complicates treatment and often indicates an increased likelihood of family conflict, further exacerbating the child's pain (Esposito-Smythers et al., 2006). At a basic level, this pattern of comorbidity reflects a group of underlying issues common to all sufferers of PBD and needs to be fleshed out more fully.

The combination of diagnostic uncertainty, regional pattern of incidence, confusion about continuity into adulthood, and the massive comorbidity lead me to believe that the dramatic increase in PBD diagnosis over the last two decades is something other than an increase in neurochemical disorder. But what could be going on? As I mentioned earlier, the increase in PBD is mainly due to a rise in the number of kids diagnosed with the broad phenotype subtype. A growing body of evidence suggests that children with the broad phenotype (those who do not meet *DSM* criteria, as well as those with BP NOS or severe mood dysregulation) look quite different from those afflicted with narrow phenotype symptoms (those who meet *DSM* criteria)—so much so, in fact, that it may be a totally different disorder. As it turns out, these groups differ in EEG patterns of arousal and frustration, as well as family genetics (positive for narrow; negative for broad) and attention to emotional stimuli (Rich et al., 2010, 2011; Brotman et al., 2007). Children with the broad phenotype have much more severe impairments in executive functioning and attention, and are also much more strongly associated with ODD symptom severity (Rich et al., 2007). Increasingly, research shows us that these two phenotypes represent two very different illnesses. What we're calling broad phenotype just might be an outdated name for a new, modern disorder, something totally different from bipolar disorder.

How has psychiatry dealt with this new phenomenon? Well, as you might imagine, psychiatrists began by creating a new diagnosis to fit the broad phenotype. First called severe temper dysregulation disorder but more recently changed to disruptive mood dysregulation disorder (DMDD), this new diagnostic proposal for the *DSM-V* would be applied to those children with explosive temper, rages, and extreme irritability. Actually, this new diagnostic category has more in common with ODD than with adult BD. In fact, almost all of the kids in this category would fit criteria for ODD, and about 15% of kids with ODD would fit into the DMDD category. This new disorder would be placed in the mood disorder category, not under behavior disorder as ODD is. As a result, these kids would be more eligible for treatment with antipsychotics and mood stabilizers, while much less likely to encounter behavior therapy or parenting support. The rationale of the *DSM* work group is well outlined on their Web site: "The data differentiating the TDD/SMD phenotype from

BD in terms of longitudinal outcome is reasonably strong, and the family history, demographic, and pathophysiologic data are suggestive. On the other hand, TDD/SMD cannot be differentiated from ODD. Indeed, the TDD phenotype can be conceptualized as the most severely irritable of patients with ODD." This is a half victory. One the one hand, the committee appears to understands that the broad phenotype is not a subtype of BD, but on the other, it seems compelled to lump it in with another vague and ambiguous disorder.

This new proposal has generated a firestorm of controversy. New diagnostic entities have been created before. Perhaps no psychiatrist is in a better place to comment on this process than Allen Frances, professor emeritus and former chair of psychiatry at Duke University, and chair of the *DSM-IV* Task Force:

> Everyone must have known that DMDD is a made up and unstudied diagnosis with no real scientific support. The review group probably bought the child group's argument that DMDD is a lesser evil replacement for childhood bipolar disorder. But their proposed fix is a disaster in the making that will most likely make an already bad situation much worse. DMDD will capture a wildly heterogeneous and diagnostically meaningless grab bag of difficult to handle kids. (Frances, 2011)

In a later article Frances (2012a) continued his dissent: "Why introduce Disruptive Mood Dysregulation Disorder when it has been studied by only one research team for only six years and risks further encouraging the inappropriate use of antipsychotic drugs for kids with temper tantrums?" He could only draw shady conclusions:

> The general lesson to be learned is clear—never have the fox guard the henhouse. The DSM-5 experts who are suggesting untested psychiatric diagnoses are too close to their pet proposals to be objective about them. The scientific review group is too close to the DSM-5 leadership and the APA institutional goals to provide anything resembling the needed independent review. (Frances, 2012a)

An independent review, as Frances suggests, would be the best way to corner this illness (if it even is one). According to what we've parsed so far, a review would tell us two things for certain. First, no one is sure what this problem is exactly (illness, disorder?), how to diagnose it (according to new or old criteria?), how to prevent it, or how we can treat it.

Second, highly risky antipsychotic medication can often reduce symptoms in the short run, much in the same way they make ODD kids less oppositional in the short run, but there are no good data linking medication to long-term remission. If we look a little deeper into the expression of this mercurial problem, however, some answers about prevention and treatment crop up.

Expression and Prevention

Here is a short list of underlying factors that may contribute to the expression of BD symptoms in our children:

1. Nutrient deficiency: Falling intake of omega-3 EFAs, vitamins, and minerals—especially magnesium—may be related to increased PBD symptomatology. These crucial nutrients relate to mood control and affective regulation. The decline of the American diet has moved in lockstep with the increase in PBD. Furthermore, the progressive rise in the intake of hydrogenated oils and glycemic load may also be to blame. Both of these factors impair delta-5 and -6 dehydrogenase—a crucial enzyme in the production of EPA/DHA and anti-inflammatory eicosinoids from dietary precursors. Kids also show a low decline in executive control and mood regulation when exposed to additives and dyes.

2. Overstimulation: Lack of sleep, excessive video games, violence, and sexuality. In a nutshell, lack of downtime. This phenomenon of the modern era increases autonomic arousal and CNS imbalance and decreases self-regulation. Social rhythms therapy is built upon the theory that mood disorder patients, particularly bipolar-spectrum patients, have disrupted biological rhythms. Having a consistent sleep and wake time keeps a child well balanced and healthy. Research supports that mood disorder patients have less social rhythm regularity and that social rhythm disruptions, such as meal interruptions, contribute to affective symptoms (Malkoff-Schwartz et al., 1998). This builds upon the concept that social zeitgebers, any external trigger that synchronizes an organism's internal time-keeping system, drive the functioning of our hypothalamus, and this has critical interplay with neuroendocrine regulation (Grandin, Alloy, & Abramson, 2006). The application of this

idea, mainly regulation of these social rhythms with more structure and predictability, has shown value in preventing manic episodes in adults (Frank et al., 2005). While it has not yet been tested in children, it makes perfect sense that better structure and regulation in a bipolar child's life would be beneficial, hopefully breaking the cycle of dysregulation that's plagued the child. Sure, the triggers are multifactorial here, but the value of correctional structure makes sense.

3. Inflammation: The idea that bipolar disorder could be a multisystem inflammatory disease has become a hot topic lately, and the research base has exploded over the last few years. The general conclusion is that bipolar disorder represents a manifestation of multisystemic inflammation (Leboyer et al., 2012). This makes sense given the rates of comorbidity. And the fact that several key studies showed success in treating BD with omega-3 EFAs and N-acetylcysteine (NAC), which are anti-inflammatories, also lends support to this theory. NAC is the precursor to glutathione, the primary antioxidant in the human body. Its anti-inflammatory effects also help dopamine and glutamate pathways in the CNS. In one large, well-designed RCT of 76 adult BD patients treated with NAC, a 6-month trial period resulted in significant improvements in a wide range of clinical measures (Berk et al., 2008). (This topic is covered in more depth in Chapter 10.)

4. Inadequate behavioral control: Depressed moms, conflicted homes, and overwhelmed parents—these three ecological disasters can make any child go out of control. When a mom is depressed, for example, the child may not have adequate behavioral containment, and may develop severe behavioral symptoms. In fact, when a mom is depressed, a child has a four-fold risk of developing mental illness. These numbers reflect both mood and behavioral issues. And be aware, depressed moms are not a small group: They represent somewhere around 15% of moms. As mentioned previously, when depressed moms are treated, the behavioral and mood issues in the children improve dramatically. When mom's issues are not treated, children become more symptomatic. In challenging children—those who need the most behavioral management—the presence of maternal depression or overreactivity caused ODD and externalizing symptoms in the mother's children (Harvey, Metcalfe, Herbert, & Fanton, 2011). Kids from depressed moms are less controlled, more oppositional, and more aggressive. In my experience, maternal depression is a major factor in the rapid rise of this phenomenon.

Other factors come to mind, but you get the drift. These four triggers—combined or in isolation—are the most likely culprits of the faux bipolar epidemic sweeping the nation today. They also help us understand the tight link between PBD and ADHD, as well as Biederman's earlier observation that PBD patients have more symptoms of ADHD than ADHD kids do. The foundation of both problems may arise from similar pathophysiology, only with more severe expression of mood dysregulation and ODD in PBD. Also, this helps to explain the overlapping epidemic rise in these two syndromes over the last three decades, as well as PBD's high rates of comorbidity with other disorders. All speculation aside, this list does address—and provide solutions to—the growing recognition that psychiatry's traditional focus on genetics and pharmacology cannot resolve the suffering of kids with PBD.

Treating Pediatric Bipolar Disorder

The Wholeness Model of treatment for PBD can indeed resolve the suffering of kids with PBD. The model is predicated on reducing triggers, eliminating barriers, and enhancing support of the child's wholeness. The following pages outline the basic model of treatment and are divided according to eight principal treatment methods: nutrients, diet, mineral and supplement support, contraindications, environmental adjustments, light and dark, psychosocial, and medications. When necessary, each treatment subsection includes a short segment titled What to Do, which covers recommended dosages and styles of treatment.

Nutrients

In the past 50 years, the American diet has steadily deteriorated. Among other things, this deterioration has reduced levels of crucial micronutrients such as magnesium and EFAs in the average American's diet. EFAs, in particular, are crucial, as they create flexible, responsive neurons. And omega-3 deficiency alters dopamine transmission in brain control systems, contributing to emotional and cognitive dysregulation. Chronic dietary deficits of omega-3 EFAs produce an imbalance of two crucial circuits, in which the mesocortical system becomes inhibited and the mesolimbic system grows hyperactive. In effect, this cascade of deficiencies creates an emotionally labile and undercontrolled brain in a child, a series of symptoms similar to those of PBD (Chalon, Vancassel, Zimmer, Guilloteau, & Durand, 2001). A consistent stream of publications has linked omega-3 levels to neurotransmission efficiency and behavior, as well as mood regulation. It's not surprising, then, that omega-3 supplementation has been demonstrated to improve outcomes in bipolar disorder, for both children and adults. What's more, according to newer research, omega-3 deficiency is a putative risk factor for the development of BD (McNamara, Nandagopal, Strakowski, & DelBello, 2010). More fascinating still, evidence now supports the predictive value of a lipid profile (which characterizes serum EFA ratios) in assessing suicide risk in PBD (Evans et al., 2012). Most importantly, omega-3 EFAs have demonstrated clinical efficacy in treating PBD (Wozniak et al., 2007).

In fact, one study found that adding 9.6 g per day of omega-3 fatty acids to standard medications led to longer periods of remission (Stoll, Locke, & Marangell, 1999). Interestingly enough, although flaxseed oil is rich in omega-3 precursors, it has not been shown to improve mood in PBD (Gracious et al., 2010). A small subset responded to flaxseed oil, according to one study, but these kids had elevated levels of eicosapentaenoic acid (EPA, one of the crucial end points of omega-3 metabolism, and a primary building block of brain development), indicating a differential response based on metabolism or absorption. Research has indicated SNPs of this metabolic pathway might make a significant portion of symptomatic kids unresponsive to precursors. That's why I prefer using fish oil over flaxseed oil in any patient with mood disorder symptoms. For vegetarians, I recommend a docosahexaenoic acid (DHA, another crucial omega-3 building block for brain health) preparation from algae.

EPA looks to be more clinically useful in treating mood disorders than DHA. The physiology makes perfect sense; the safety margin is incredibly high, and benefits accrue for preventing other illnesses. Needless to say, omega-3 supplements form a core element of my treatment recommendations for any young person presenting with symptoms of PBD.

What to Do

I recommend 1 gram-plus of EPA for any child 8 years or older. I use 500–750 mg for younger kids. Typically, I use liquid preparations for younger kids. I like the microemulsified formulas, which are easier to mix into smoothies or juice. The new molecularly distilled products have little negative taste. For extremely sensitive kids, the capsules can be frozen or taken at the beginning of a meal. Generally, the fish used here are small, so mercury is not an issue. You can also recommend eating fish or eggs high in EPA/DHA (a label on the box will advertise their presence), as well as plants high in the omega-3 oils (flaxseeds, walnuts, pumpkin seeds, and many green leafy vegetables) that the body can actively convert to EPA and DHA.

Diet

In general, a whole-foods diet that balances complex carbohydrates, protein, and fats is best. Avoid simple sugars, fatty foods, and especially caffeine. The challenge here is that many children and teens with PBD crave sweets and carbohydrates (e.g., bread, pasta, cereal, baked goods). As a matter of fact, in one study, bipolar disorder was associated with a higher glycemic load (more sugar), lower-quality food, and more processed items (Jacka, Pasco, et al., 2011). That's why it's so important to wean kids off these unhealthy and addictive substances and move them toward a healthier diet.

Mineral and Supplement Support

Lithium, the mainstay of bipolar treatment for the last 60 years, is actually a naturally occurring mineral. For PBD, I strongly support the use of minerals, as well as vitamins and a few supplements. (For an excellent overview of the physiology and theory behind mineral supplementation, consult Kaplan et al., 2007.) Besides the clinical form of lithium carbonate, an over-the-counter amino acid chelate is also available: lithium orotate. It comes in much, much lower doses than the prescription form, and the legend is that it is much better absorbed— and safer. However, a recent PubMed search pulled up six hits for the substance, and not one documented any evidence of efficacy in mood disorders, or showed any advantage in safety over lithium carbonate. Lithium orotate looks to be more poorly excreted with no difference in absorption. That's why I do not recommend it very often.

Another mineral that helps stabilize mood, particularly manic cycling, is magnesium (Heiden et al., 1999; Giannini, Nakoneczie, Melemis, Ventresco, & Condon, 2000). Many researchers have noted how the overall effect of magnesium in the CNS is very similar to that of lithium. Actually, I would say that lithium has an effect similar to that of magnesium, as our nervous system evolved with significant amounts of magnesium, not lithium. This is one reason for its calming effect on the CNS, and why in a variety of population studies it has been shown to correlate with mood symptoms. In various studies, magnesium has been shown to suppress hippocampal kindling, dampen protein kinase C-related transmission, regulate NMDA receptors, and alter glutamate activity (Murck, 2002; Swek, 2005). Unfortunately, most Americans are deficient in magnesium.

What to Do

I use magnesium alone or in combination with calcium for milder mood complaints like irritability. In these cases, I use a combined calcium and magnesium supplement, as magnesium is a laxative and calcium is constipating, so together they tend to create less problems. I use magnesium alone if constipation is an issue. I prefer minerals bound to citrate or aspartate. The daily dose of each mineral by age is as follows: 150–200 mg for children under 6 years, 300–400 mg for kids 7 to 11, and 400–600 mg for kids 12 and older. Dose to bowel tolerance or response. Giving the supplement at bedtime may also improve sleep.

However, when signs and symptoms of a severe unstable mood disorder such as PBD present, I almost always recommend a vitamin-mineral combination called EMPowerplus (EMP). It contains 36 different vitamins and minerals. As of this year, 19 peer-reviewed journal articles have shown success with the product (Rucklidge, Gately, & Kaplan, 2010; Frazier, Fristad, & Arnold, 2009). A publication from researchers at Ohio State University's Department of Psychiatry found effectiveness in using EMP to treat PBD (Frazier, Fristad, & Arnold, 2012).

Perhaps the oddest part of using this product is that you can't just add it to psychiatric medications. It is not complementary; it is not an add-on, like omega-3 EFAs. This has taught me quite a bit about bipolar disorder and about psychiatric medications. Over the last decade of clinical trials in my practice, I have watched psychiatric medications, pain medications, and over-the-counter agents impair the ability of EMP to effectively stabilize BD. In the most severe cases, even mild agents (Benadryl, caffeine, antibiotics) can yank a BD patient out of stability and back into crisis. Certain medications (aripiprazole, benzodiazepines, quetiapine, SSRIs, narcotics) throw the balance of the CNS off to such a degree that they are not compatible at all with EMP. In general, one needs to taper all psychiatric medications (simultaneously) while increasing the dose of EMP in what can be a challenging cross-taper over 6 or so weeks. Many of the people I treat have never been on psychiatric agents, so this is a piece of cake: Simply ramp up the EMP over a week or two to the full loading dose of five capsules three times daily (given with meals, of course). Most kids respond within a few weeks. Explosive anger and irritability are often the first symptoms to fall away. Occasionally, it takes 6 weeks or more for response, but this is usually for kids with a long psychiatric medication history. It also comes in a powder form for the very young or difficult. I have engaged it effectively with 3- or 4-year-olds.

A few other interesting pearls: The more psychotic features the individual has, the better the response to EMP. About 90% of the people I start on EMP stay with it. Their comments are almost always positive: "I feel like myself again"; "I don't have any side effects"; "I have lost all of the weight I gained from meds"; "I can think again"; "I will never go back." About 80% of those that stay with it become fully stable on EMP alone and require no psychiatric medications. About 20% require a very small amount of one psychiatric medication to find balance (usually kids with a long medication history). In these circumstances, you can add a very small dose of a compatible medication (often a mood stabilizer like lamotrigine or atomoxetine for ADHD issues, if severe). The trick here is that the dose must be very small—I mean, *very small*. Often, it is one-fifth or even one-tenth or less of standard dosing. The EMP appears to magnify both target effects and side effects of psychiatric medications. The other difference is that once patients respond to EMP, they remain stable and do not require any "medication adjustments" unless they ingest a contraindicated substance.

Patients with poor EMP response are of four types usually: mitochondrial patients with odd energy production issues (often significant developmental issues); gut patients with severe dysbiosis or yeast overgrowth (much more common in kids with long-term antipsychotic use, obesity, and appetite stimulation); oppositional kids with significant family conflict; and kids with a long history of psychiatric medication use. With this last group, just remember: It takes a long time for the CNS to find a state of balance again. So be patient and taper carefully. We often see medication withdrawal effects as far down the road as 6 months or more. Psychiatric medications are often lipophilic and store in fat tissues with accelerated release in weight loss, hard exercise, or heat. Most of these issues tend to be quite treatable, but can give the appearance of nonresponse at first glance. But the power of wholeness works wonders if we can remove the barriers and be patient.

The more I work with EMP, the more respect I hold for the ability of the CNS to find balance when the needed building blocks are present. EMP appears to deliver crucial ingredients to an overstressed, imbalanced, and probably deficient CNS. It is a new frontier for working with severe mental illness. This is indeed a strange new world for psychiatrists used to the old paradigm of constantly remedicating a moving target.

The other component of my treatment protocol for PBD is inositol, a unique natural agent that stabilizes mood and reduces anxiety with few side effects and a high degree of safety. In the STEP-BD study, one arm examined inositol versus risperidone and lamotrigine in the treatment of bipolar depression in adults, with inositol outperforming risperidone and almost as effective as lamotrigine (Nierenberg et al., 2006).

With inositol, I use the powder form, as it is cheaper and easier to use. As a sugar analogue, it is sweet tasting. I use it for all ages. Under age 7, I start with 2 g two or three times daily and may work up to 3 g three times daily. For ages 7 to 12, I start with 3 g two or three times daily and may work up to 4 or 5 g. For 13 on up, I start with 4 g two or three times daily and will go up to 6 g, three times daily. Inositol is well tolerated; only rarely do I hear of mild GI distress.

Occasionally, I also recommend NAC as an augmenting agent. I do this if there is evidence of inflammation (elevated C-reactive protein, or CRP), cutting, or the child complains of wanting to jump out of his skin. I start with 600 mg once or twice a day for younger patients and will go up to 1,200 mg twice daily for teens. The response time may take up to 9 weeks, but be patient.

Many kids with PBD have mitochondrial issues. The connection between mitochondrial issues and mental health is an exploding field of research right now, and it carries with it massive implications for many psychiatric patients (Nierenberg et al., 2013). Interventions for mitochondrial disorders include CoQ10, EFAs, alpha-lipoic acid, acetyl-L-carnitine, melatonin, and medium-chain triglycerides found in coconut oil. I expect that this arena of research will continue to rapidly change and expand in importance over the next few years.

Contraindications

Here are some supplements and medications that people with BD should not take, or else should take with caution. I discourage people who have a family history of BD from taking 5-HTP, St. John's wort, or SAMe because they may trigger mania or rapid cycling. I'm also cautious with standardized extracts of ginseng (*Panax ginseng*) and *Ginkgo biloba*, as they have an activating effect on the brain, and both have been reported to trigger mania. None of these herbs are stimulants on the order of amphetamine, but extreme caution is in order. In general, anyone with BD should avoid any substance that stimulates or sedates the CNS, even caffeine or nicotine. Stimulants are not a good idea.

Environmental Adjustments

Agitated, irritable kids displaying symptoms of PBD are exquisitely sensitive to their environments. A calm and nurturing home life is important. Soothing music and calming scents such as lavender can be particularly helpful. Predictable schedules (e.g., mealtimes, sleep and wake cycles, study times) help anchor moods. Radically reducing exposure to sexual or violent media will go a long way in soothing the child's psyche.

Loving touch improves self-soothing, so remember to give every child plenty of hugs. Believe it or not, one study found that maternal warmth decreased the likelihood of relapse in children and teens diagnosed with bipolar disorder (Geller et al., 2002). Consistent but gentle parenting skills (and a huge amount of patience by the parents) can mold behavior while preserving self-esteem. You may find that family therapy helps in the development of such skills. Remember, the patient probably already feels badly about his or her lack of control over moods and actions, so be patient and kind.

Light and Dark

A number of studies show light therapy to be helpful in treating BD. In fact, in one study, morning sunlight reduced the duration of stay for patients hospitalized for BD (Benedetti, Colombo, Barbini, Campori, & Smeraldi, 2001). Reports also suggest rapid-cycling BD can be broken with long nights of sleep in darkness and the addition of daytime light therapy (Wirz-Justice, Graw, Roosli, Glauser, & Fleischhauer, 1999). Try installing full-spectrum lightbulbs in the home and, if teachers will permit it, in the classroom as well.

Exposure to darkness at night is also important. During the winter months, I recommend starting low-intensity lighting at 7 P.M. and, as the evening progresses, having fewer and fewer lights on in the home. This will help prepare the child for bed and control his or her intensity level. Installing dimmers on lights can make this easier. Dawn simulators are also helpful in regulating sleep-wake cycles for kids who have difficulty rising.

True light therapy involves using a light box. The timing of the exposure depends upon the child's mood. Bright light exposure helps to shift circadian rhythms in a normalizing direction. During bouts of depression, morning exposure is best. But if mania develops, cut off light therapy immediately. As a general rule, keep the light box 18 inches from the eyes. Obviously, keeping a consistent schedule with little kids is difficult, particularly during the school year, but try to establish a routine of giving the child a dose (30 minutes) of light therapy right before school. Though there is some evidence that light therapy can trigger mania, I find that kids respond to it better and more quickly than medications or supplements.

Psychosocial

One of the techniques that I strongly endorse for anyone with BD or unstable mood swings is dialectical behavior therapy (DBT). This combination of CBT and mindfulness was originally developed by Marsha Linehan in the early 1990s to treat highly suicidal patients with borderline personality disorder. At its core, this therapy works to enhance emotional self-regulation through skill building and increased self-awareness, teaching the patient how to manage his or her moods under pressure. The research base for DBT is still building, but there is good evidence to support its use in kids with PBD. According to a few studies, it can improve manic and depressive symptoms in as few as 15 sessions (Goldstein, Axelson, Birmaher, & Brent, 2007; Feeny, Danielson, Schwartz, Youngstrom, &

Findling, 2006). CBT can also play an important role in the treatment of PBD. Perhaps the most impressive data for CBT come from a long-term study of a family-focused program that was effective in maintaining the management of mood symptoms over 3 years in youths with BD (West, Henry, & Pavuluri, 2007).

I have been less impressed with the value of play therapy for kids exhibiting this kind of behavior. Perhaps most of all, these kids need an ally who will listen, provide emotional support, and educate the whole family about the disorder. That's why CBT seems to be so successful; it provides structure and skills.

A social skills group can help younger kids, who often have extremely impaired social skills. Older children may find comfort and benefit in group therapy and peer-support groups. As in the management of ADHD, family, behavioral, and systemic interventions like CBT make good sense. In fact, if there is a component of oppositional behavior (which is typical in this disorder), I almost always include a family- or parenting-based intervention. The Nurtured Heart Approach is extremely useful for these families. It is a practical application of a variety of parenting and family-based techniques, which gently and effectively guide parents to a new attitude and style in their parenting. It has a smaller research base than other family-based programs, but I swear by it.

Like the Nurtured Heart Approach, family-focused therapy—an approach that builds psychoeducation, communication skills, and problem-solving skills—has been shown to improve both depressive and manic symptoms in PBD (Miklowitz et al., 2004). Other programs like individual family treatment and multifamily psychoeducation groups were designed to provide support, psychoeducation, and communication in families with a mood-disordered child. And they work great. These have been shown to increase the parents' understanding of mood disorders, reduce mood symptoms, and improve family functioning (Fristad, 2006) (see Chapter 11).

What to Do

I almost always recommend family therapy and/or parenting support for a child with an unstable mood disorder. There is typically a component of behavior control and family conflict in the home, and parents love the support and direction. For children under 12, this is much more crucial than individual therapy. But while most reverse this priority, I do not.

This is relevant for most adolescents as well. My preference is the Nurtured Heart Approach developed by Howard Glasser. I will most often recommend individual therapy for teens as well to help with self-esteem, coping skills, and relationships. I also recommend a DBT class or books for teens. This can be enormously helpful in building crucial skills and empowering teens to take control of their emotions and their lives.

Medications

Given the severity of true bipolar disorder and its devastating impact on children and their families, most conventional child psychiatrists and parents opt for drug treatment as the first step. Generally, I recommend nutritional work, psychosocial care, and the use of supplements prior to initiating medications. When medications are indeed needed, I continue to utilize psychosocial approaches, such as DBT, and nutritional care. The use of supplements such as EPA and inositol often allows for lower drug doses.

Used cautiously and in conjunction with other supportive treatments, prescription medications can be a valuable element in the treatment program. But, in general, they are vastly overused today. Mood stabilizers, including lithium, divalproex sodium, carbamazepine, oxcarbazepine, and the like help to level mood, putting a damper on the radical ups and downs. I prefer oxcarbazepine and lamotrigene as they do not require blood levels and have no weight gain or sedation issues. Some research supports their effectiveness; however, most of those studies are geared toward use in adults, so be cautious and dose mildly.

Occasionally, I will use alpha central agonists (a type of older medication originally used to treat blood pressure in the 1970s) such as clonidine or guanfacine to provide some short-term calming effects. These are much safer than mood stabilizers, which is one of my prime goals in working with kids. I avoid the use of antipsychotic medications in most circumstances. I also avoid stimulants and antidepressants in anyone with an unstable mood disorder.

Other Treatments

Acupuncture is, in my experience, very useful in anyone ages 12 and older. It has a calming effect and seems to reset the autonomic nervous system. It also seems to help regulate sleep and wake cycles and to remedy coexisting anxiety, headaches, or gastrointestinal problems. Chinese herbs can augment acupuncture treatments. The exact combination of herbs depends upon the child. Consult a local acupuncturist if you believe one of your patients could benefit.

Body work, including therapeutic touch and massage therapy, can help calm and center agitated children. These approaches are particularly useful if there is a history of abuse.

Osteopathic cranial manipulation and craniosacral therapy can also help calm children with symptoms of PBD. One of my young patients, who was quite agitated, wild, and destructive, became noticeably calmer as the practitioner began the manipulation, and was markedly different in mood and demeanor following the treatment. And the results lasted. I particularly emphasize cranial manipulation if there is a history of a traumatic birth, concussions, head injuries, or chronic headaches.

Scientific evidence has begun to suggest that, in true bipolar disorder, the two halves of the brain, called the cerebral hemispheres, don't communicate well (Pettigrew & Miller, 1998). Such findings have led me to the use of EMDR, which helps synchronize electrical activity between the two hemispheres, in some of my young patients, particularly those who also have a history of trauma.

Another therapy that hones mental steadiness is martial arts. It gives kids a positive outlet for their intense energy and encourages them to develop mental discipline and to work effectively with adults. I routinely witness markedly enhanced executive functioning skills with martial arts training.

Most children diagnosed with bipolar disorder feel a great deal of remorse about the way they have behaved, and also pain about the fact that they have a serious mental illness. They experience turmoil in both their outer and inner environments. The ability to step back and talk about broader spiritual issues with a counselor, pastor, rabbi, or minister can come as a relief. The acceptance, compassion, and forgiveness of such elders can be balm to the soul. And, in receiving these spiritual bounties, children may come to accept and forgive themselves. Also, opening a channel through which guilt and remorse can flow easily may reduce the risk of lapsing into severe depression.

As a rule, parents of a bipolar child are stressed. These children are, from an early age, tough to manage and difficult to live with. The parents will find themselves frustrated, challenged, and in a constant swirl of conflict (with both the child and each other). Because a child with bipolar disorder can be impulsive and exhibit poor judgment, parents are always on the lookout, stressing about the fact that, once again, the child has gotten into trouble or has come into harm's way. Stress reduction skills for the parents such as yoga or meditation can be a useful tool, not only for their own emotional survival but for the environment it creates for the child in the home.

So, in reflection, is PBD a psychiatric epidemic or merely a multifactorial debilitation of our youth? As I've suggested, there is not much evidence for the former, and seeing it that way keeps us locked in a paradigm of care that just doesn't seem to be working. Through an approach based on wholeness, however, we can arrive at safer, more thoughtful preventative treatment options, options that promise to palliate much of the suffering plaguing young people with PBD today.

Treatment Plan: Step by Step

1. Comprehensive evaluation of child's six realms (see Chapter 6) and common presenting issues (see Chapter 7).
2. Identify barriers, deficiencies, strengths, and gifts.
3. Examine the child for diet issues, food quality, food allergies, or gut issues. Refer to a nutritionist or naturopath as needed.
4. Examine for family conflict, depressed or overwhelmed parents, oppositional behavior, marital stress, poor communication, behavioral issues (home or school, or both), and social skills. Think about family therapy if needed.
5. Add Nurtured Heart or other parenting and behavior support program—a crucial component.
6. If the child is depressed, anxious, or traumatized, refer for individual therapy. If already in therapy, contact prior or current therapist for background and collaboration.
7. Lab testing: Check TSH, vitamin D (25 OH), ferritin/CBC, lipid profile (low cholesterol), homocysteine, and HS CRP. Treat abnormalities as they appear. Consider DHEA-sulfate or MTHFR screen if chronic illness. Also think about a sleep study if the child is suffering from insomnia or apnea.

8. Add 500–1,000 mg of EPA and inositol 3–6 g two or three times daily.
9. Make sure sleep, exercise, and sunlight are at appropriate levels and limit electronics as needed—often a serious problem.
10. If emotional regulation is an issue (it most likely is), think of DBT.
11. Avoid St. John's wort, SAMe, ginkgo, ginseng, stimulants, and anti-depressants.
12. Address social concerns as relevant with social skills group.
13. Consider martial arts training for discipline and philosophy.
14. Consider EMPowerplus as central biochemical intervention. If no current psychiatric or contraindicated medications, ramp up to five capsules three times daily after food over a few days. If on psychiatric medications or contraindicated medications, find guidance to undertake cross-taper. The EMPowerplus people have a professionals' guide designed for physicians to understand the complexities of this approach for complicated patients. It is very helpful.
15. If manic issues persist, consider choline bitartrate 300–500 mg two or three times daily.
16. If needed, consider trial of NAC.
17. Consider some self-regulation support for calming skills such as bio-feedback or yoga.

Brittany

Brittany was a tall 15-year-old with auburn hair and long legs. She played volleyball for her high school, and loved to text and talk with her many friends. A decent but not stellar student, over the last few years she'd become more erratic and irritable, mainly at home. There was a family history of depression as both her dad's mom and her mom had been treated in the past with good benefit. There was no history of abuse. Medically, she suffered from migraines with a past history of asthma. Brittany had been sleeping poorly, and it was getting steadily worse over the first semester of school.

The second semester started okay but soon deteriorated into falling grades, more bad moods, and some explosive fights at home with her mom. Jenna, her mom, worked part time in a consulting business and Tom, her dad, had a high-level job with a governmental agency that required lots of travel. Brittany did some cutting and even tried some binging and purging. She struggled with her social group at school and her boyfriend of 3 months.

This all came to a head when she felt so despondent and overwhelmed following a breakup with her boyfriend that she took a handful of Tylenol and ended up treated overnight at the local hospital, followed by a transfer to the freestanding psychiatric hospital, where she spent a week. Discharged on 50 mg of lamotrigine and 100 mg of quetiapine, it was recommended that she find a psychiatrist and therapist. Her diagnosis was bipolar disorder, rule out bulimia.

That's where I came in. Brittany came into my office 5 days after being discharged. She smiled readily and made nice eye contact with me. Her folks, clearly both bright and direct, were quite engaged. I started my session by gathering a more in-depth history. Brittany ate poorly, with a horrific diet characterized by fast food, sweets, carbs, and soda on the fly. She had two or three Diet Cokes each day to keep up with her aggressive curriculum and sports, which ran year round. She stayed up late studying and messing around on her cell phone.

Her family seemed supportive but was clearly ambitious and tense. Dad appeared disconnected, off in his own world. Brittany rarely saw him. Her 18-year-old brother had had some struggles with drugs in midadolescence but seemed on track in his first year of college. Brittany had no interest in drugs or alcohol. There was no history of abuse or neglect.

As I spent more time with Brittany alone, it became abundantly clear that what she struggled with most were her self-esteem and identity. She was insightful for a high schooler: She talked openly about her behavior and made comments about how reactive she was and how much she regretted what she had done. From what she said, the cutting and purging seemed superficial, like she was just trying them on for size. She had mood swings but, overall, her mood was positive and bright—she didn't want to hurt herself. She was excited to see her friends, loved volleyball, and was quite good at it. There was no mania, no hypomania really. Brittany acknowledged being sensitive and slightly anxious about friends and relationships, but she seemed basically in control of her behavior. She had big goals for herself in life and wanted to become an environmental attorney to support the planet. Brittany was easy to like, easy to talk with.

At the end of our session together, I collected my thoughts and reflected back to Brittany how I understood her:

> You are a sensitive, bright, caring, and slightly insecure young woman who is trying to sort out how to succeed in life with friends, romance, school, and sports. Things sometimes move faster and stronger than you are ready for. At times you feel desperate and overwhelmed and, as a result, overrespond. You feel wound up and tense inside with little ability to calm yourself down. You love life, your family, and your friends dearly and do not want to die.

She nodded tearfully and looked at me with appreciation and acknowledgment.

Her parents shared the same view as Brittany and me. "Since we are all in agreement, let's develop a plan to get you to where you need to go," I said. I contacted her school and ordered labs before the treatment planning session. Her labs came back with some notable problems: Her CRP was over 3, indicative of high levels of inflammation. Her cholesterol was low—about 100—which signaled an issue with mood and reactivity, as the body needs cholesterol to make neuronal membranes and hormones. Her MTHFR gene showed a defect known to affect mood. Her vitamin D level was on the low end, hovering around 21 ng/dl, which might have contributed to her depression. Her homocysteine level was about 11 ng/dl, consistent with problems in methylation and probably tied to her MTHFR abnormality.

The school forms from her teachers found her to be motivated, socially focused, and at times overwhelmed with tasks. Overall, her teachers really liked her and made positive comments about her presence in the classroom. There were no notes from her school on issues with behavior or mood.

So, after surveying the landscape, I sat down with Brittany and her folks and we came up with a plan. The basics of the plan were derived from the idea that she needed skills to be successful and the knowledge that she was capable of becoming whole and solid again. I started by addressing four health factors. First of all, she had a miserable diet and was experiencing high levels of inflammation and HPA stimulation. Second, Brittany desperately needed skills to manage her emotions, which were volatile and raw. Third, she needed to learn how to relax and destress.

Fourth, we needed to enhance the family bond, especially between her and her dad.

To begin the process, I made some referrals. I sent her to Dr. Mary Rondeau, a naturopathic physician at the Wholeness Center who mainly works with food and diet. Beyond merely cleaning up her diet and improving glycemic load, Mary removed caffeine and added an anti-inflammatory diet. Given the low cholesterol, Mary also added positive fats and oils.

Next, I hooked her up with Anca Niculae, a psychotherapist at the Wholeness Center who teaches DBT classes for teens. Anca mixed Brittany's individual sessions with a few family sessions to enhance the family ecology. Anca likes to take kids outside and walk on the trails with them near our office to stay active and informal. This intimacy helped Brittany unwind and feel at ease as she discussed her personal life. Between sports, friends, and school, Brittany had a lot going for her, which made Anca's work of empowering her that much easier.

Finally, we connected Brittany with Jen Strating, the Wholeness Center's biofeedback therapist and yoga teacher, who helped her relax and let go of some of her inner tension. Brittany was a physical girl with a good sense of her body and how to control it; she took to these tasks like a natural. A few massages didn't hurt, either, and later Brittany even asked about trying acupuncture.

My work, as it turned out, was the easy part. I told Brittany and her folks that I didn't see any bipolar disorder present, and that, frankly, I didn't see much that needed to be labeled or medicated. But I did start her on a few supplements to help her find balance. I added EPA at 1 g daily, inositol at 4 g twice daily to reduce stress and anxiety (which is often more of a component of mood issues than most recognize); and magnesium glycinate at 250 mg twice daily to help stabilize mood, reduce reactivity, and treat migraines. I also added a B vitamin with activated folate. Over the next month or so we started to taper her off her medications.

As you might expect, Brittany has done well. She's a young woman of incredible strength and resolve, and I'm lucky I get to watch her grow and find wholeness. I know that my tenure with her is short, so I enjoy every minute I get to spend with her. She remains volatile at times, but these episodes are less intense and less frequent than before. She can be insecure with friends still but has learned to navigate relationships without cutting and intense dysphoria.

Brittany's story is a story of success, a story of everything gone right. But not all stories at the Wholeness Center turn out this way. Not all kids return to wholeness so quickly and easily. Some kids are much more challenging than Brittany, and test the basic framework and foundation of our system. However, we always work from a place of optimism.

CHAPTER FOURTEEN

Substance Abuse

As kids grow and mature into teens and young adults, they'll begin to experiment with substances. It's inevitable: They'll party, get wild with their friends, and try new things—sometimes a lot of them. In this developmental window, which starts around age 12 and usually lasts into the mid-20s, kids often binge and abuse substances, trying to work out their relationship and attitude toward various agents. Most of the time, the learning curve is sharp, and kids find a middle, more sustainable road on which to imbibe; they figure out what they like and what they don't. But sometimes, binging and abuse become indiscriminate, habitual, excess-ridden behaviors that seep in and impact other facets of their lives—most of the time negatively.

This kind of behavior, while potentially dangerous, is not the kind of addiction and dependency we so often see in adults. In truth, it's less common to see signs or behaviors of true addiction in teens, even young adults. But that's not to say that unhealthy patterns of excess don't exist. They surely do. It's just that teens and young adults have a different, more rowdy, more up-and-down relationship with substances. That being the case, this chapter explores the particular ways in which teens and young adults abuse substances (e.g., binging) and how those behaviors can be brought back to a healthy medium.

Current Research: What's Trending Now

In the last two decades, there have been some encouraging trends in teen substance use. Cigarette use, that badge of teenage angst, continues to fall among teens. Daily use has dropped to 2.4% in 8th graders and to 10.3% in 12th graders (National Institute on Drug Abuse, 2011). These falling numbers bode well for the public health disaster that is lifelong nicotine dependence and related illnesses. Likewise, binge alcohol use has fallen in all categories to 6.4% of 8th graders and 21.4% of 12th graders. Considering that 29% of all motor vehicle accident–related fatalities for those 15 to 17 years old are alcohol related, this is great news. Fewer grief-stricken families, fewer lives cut short.

On the other hand, there's some bad news. While marijuana use had fallen for a decade or more through the mid-2000s, the medical marijuana movement has reversed the trend. In the last year of the study alone (2010), use increased to 12.5% of 8th graders and 36.4% of 12th graders—which means that pot use is now more common and frequent than cigarette use (22.6% vs. 18.7% reporting past 30-day use), a first for teenage statistics. What's most alarming about these numbers is that about 26% of teen pot users meet criteria for a substance use disorder. So it's not just kids experimenting; it's kids using.

With respect to cannabis use, a powerful study out of New Zealand highlights what many of us have suspected for some time. In a 38-year prospective study of over 1,000 consecutive births in Dundein, researchers showed that adults meeting criteria for cannabis dependence as adolescents and young adults demonstrated a significant drop in IQ from age 13 to 38 (Meier et al., 2012). The more years of dependence, the greater the drop, which averaged 8 points for those who had the longest use. Sadly, cessation of use did not fully restore capacity in adolescent-onset users. Dependence was associated with broad declines on repeat neuropsychological testing even when controlled for education. Cannabis may have more than psychosocial morbidity—it may be neurotoxic.

But the most dangerous trend is that of nonmedical use of prescription drugs (NMUPD). In terms of rate of change, this is our most pressing concern in teenage substance abuse. There has been a significant increase in past-month use among adolescents and young adults (Riggs, 2008). According to numbers collected in 2010, 5.6% of middle and high schoolers acknowledge that they've used a nonmedical prescription within the last month, with a third of them meeting criteria for a substance use disorder (McCabe et al., 2012). In high schoolers, NMUPD is well on its way to becoming the major abuse concern: over 8% have abused Vicodin and over 8% have abused Adderall.

The source of this trend can in fact be directly linked to the prescription habits of American physicians. The prescribed use of stimulant medications and opioid pain killers has exploded in the last decade, making it much easier for kids to use, abuse, and, unfortunately, sell these agents.

Interestingly, according to a survey of pediatric prescriptions from 2002 until 2010, the total number of prescriptions actually fell, while the number of stimulant prescriptions increased 46% (Chai et al., 2012). A similar rise has occurred with the use of sustained-release opioids like Oxycontin. According to the Centers for Disease Control (2011), deaths from NMUPD now exceed those from all illicit drugs in the 15 to 24 age group (and every other age group, for that matter).

A friend or relative supplies most of those teens that abuse prescription medications. This trend is the most prevalent with college students: 62% have been offered a stimulant by a friend; 31% have used; and 74% know someone they can readily access (Garnier-Dykstra, Caldeira, Vincent, O'Grady, & Arria, 2012). A front-page article in the *New York Times* drew attention to the culture of performance and competition at elite high schools around the country and how it feeds into the abuse of prescription stimulants like Adderall, Concerta, and Ritalin (Schwarz, 2012). "Peers estimate that one in three engage in NMUPD" to aid studying and project completion, the author noted. The article also touched on how easy it now is to obtain these agents either by asking a friend or gaming a well-intentioned physician. Like it or not, this is the culture we've created by medicating school performance. For a penetrating look at this issue, I highly recommend Lawrence Diller's (1998) book *Running on Ritalin*.

Though it's not as visible as NMUPD, inhalant abuse is a topic that deserves attention. In my experience directing adolescent day treatment and inpatient substance abuse programs, no category of substance abuse worries me more. I have seen rapid, severe cognitive and neurological changes with inhalant use—changes that look permanent. It's also a severe risk factor for suicide. In one study, 67% of huffers had thought of suicide at one time and 20% had attempted (Howard, Perron, Sacco, et al., 2010). Huffing increases the risk for all categories of illness, but is highly correlated with aggressive and antisocial behaviors (Howard, Perron, Vaughn, Bender, & Garland, 2010). If you come across a young huffer, pull out all the stops to provide care, treatment, and support.

Adolescence is the time to address and change this massive public health concern. We know that adult addictions typically begin with substance use and abuse in adolescence. If we can stop the behavior upstream, we can save a lot of heartache, suffering, and economic fallout.

But the first step is awareness. A massive survey of over 72,000 adolescents aged 12 to 17 showed that the extent of the problem is vast: 37% have used a drug or alcohol in the past year and 8% meet criteria for abuse or dependence (Wu, Woody, Yang, Pan, & Blazer, 2011). In ethnic populations, these numbers are even higher. For example, 32% of Native American youth and 21% of Hispanic youth are in trouble with abuse or dependence. These problems all too quickly become adult addictions and create a lifetime of suffering. Beyond the human toll, the Substance Abuse Policy Research Program has estimated the price tag for addictions in this country at $275 billion per year (McCarty, 2007).

Identification

Let's be honest: We do a poor job of identifying adolescent substance abusers. One large study looked at primary care visits and screened adolescents for substance use and abuse. It found that only 18 out of every 100 teens suffering from a substance problem were identified by their primary care provider. Of the 50 abusing alcohol or drugs, only 10 were identified. Surprisingly, zero of 36 teens with frank alcohol or drug dependence were spotted. Clinical impressions massively underestimate drug use and abuse, and casual interviews do a poor job of identifying these issues in teens (Wilson, Sherritt, Gates, & Knight, 2004). Structured screens and questionnaires looking for risk factors help and make good sense.

Risk Factors

Risk factors can be divided according to family, individual, peer, and media. Family risk factors for teenagers include low parent supervision, poor communication patterns, family conflict, inconsistent or severe parental discipline, and a family history of alcohol or drug abuse. Heredity or any family history can increase a teen's risk fourfold.

Individual risk factors include learning issues (dyslexia or other learning disorder), emotional problems (anxiety or depression), difficulty managing impulses (ADHD), thrill-seeking behaviors, and poor risk assessment, as well as any history of trauma or physical or sexual abuse.

Numerous studies demonstrate that significant stressors or negative events in early childhood, like trauma or abuse, are a strong independent predictor of adult alcohol and drug dependence (Eaves, Prom, & Silberg, 2010). Stress on the HPA axis appears to be the mediating effect here.

Peer risk factors include peer use, peer pressure and approval, and low concern over use. Last but not least, identification with media images has been found to be a significant risk factor (Scull, Kupersmidt, Parker, Elmore, & Benson, 2010). Manufacturers of medications, alcohol, and tobacco spend $25 billion well-considered dollars each year to influence young people—and it works. Results from a number of correlational and longitudinal studies have confirmed that exposure to television and movie smoking is now one of the key factors that prompts teenagers to smoke (Sargent, Gibson, & Heatherton, 2009). According to a meta-analysis, media may account for nearly half of smoking initiation in young teenagers (Dalton, Adachi-Meija, & Longacre, 2006). In fact, exposure to movie smoking may even outweigh parents' smoking status as the key factor in adolescents' initiation of smoking (Sargent et al., 2009).

Conventional wisdom holds that the ecological influence on substance abuse (media, peers) is about equal to that of genetic (individual, family) risk factors (Enoch, 2012). So try not to focus too much attention on one particular risk factor, and instead take a balanced, more holistic approach to mitigating risk factors.

Prevention

In terms of prevention, it all comes back to the family. We know that the peer group that a child associates with can become a risk factor through peer pressure, peer use, and social norms. However, parental variables drive most of the protective factors (Scull et al., 2010). Some family issues can create enhanced risk, such as family drug use and family conflict, and things like family bonding and parental support can reduce it (Denton & Kampfe, 1994; Anderson & Henry, 1994). In terms of alcohol misuse, a Cochrane Review found that family-based programming was most effective in preventing use, and that some school-based programming was effective as well (Foxcroft & Tsertsvadze, 2011).

Treating Substance Abuse

If we can't prevent it, our biggest challenge is to properly identify teen substance abuse and provide some treatment. Sadly, only 1 in 10 young people who meet criteria for abuse or dependence receive any form of treatment (Lord & Marsch, 2011). In a major review of outpatient treatment programs for adolescent substance abuse, family-based programming showed the most consistent improvement (Tanner-Smith, Wilson, & Lipsey, 2012). All types of programming reduced substance use, but family therapy and peer groups provided the greatest benefit. In another major review of psychosocial treatment of adolescent substance abuse, three treatment approaches—multidimensional family therapy, functional family therapy, and group CBT—emerged as the best models for substance abuse treatment (Waldron & Turner, 2008). However, a number of other models are efficacious, and none of the treatment approaches in this study appeared to be clearly superior in terms of efficacy. In my experience, residential treatment programs provide perhaps the greatest benefit, given the intensity and duration of treatment, and ongoing aftercare is crucial to success (Dasinger, Shane, & Martinovich, 2004). Many of the kids in these programs are traumatized youths who have much more severe substance abuse problems and may require more specific, more prolonged treatment (Williams, Smith, An, & Hall, 2008).

Whatever the setting, our modern health care system has a horrible track record in the treatment of chemical dependency, with folks of any age. In fact, in response to this systemic failure, a huge, self-directed network of 12-step programs (e.g., AA, NA, OA, GA) has spread over the world since Bill W. and Bob S. created Alcoholics Anonymous in 1935. Working outside the framework of health care, the success of these 12-step programs seems to flow from two distinctly different facets: group support and spiritual reassessment. While these programs seem to work best for adults, teens can benefit as well, although teens tend to do better with a program built around peer group input and family work.

Prior to founding AA, Bill W. searched in vain for a remedy to his chronic alcoholism. In correspondence, C. G. Jung told him that the only cure for alcoholism was intense spiritual involvement. Bill W. used this input and refined his views about treating alcoholism. He believed that treatment needed to address three aspects of health: the physical, the mental, and the spiritual. In his view, AA provided good treatment for the mental and spiritual, but not the physical. Bill W. never quite figured out how to integrate physical health into AA, and the problem still persists in rehab programs: How can we address the physical disorders found in addictions?

Acupuncture

The two most useful modalities for rebalancing a physical body drained by substance abuse and addiction are nutrition and acupuncture. At Lincoln Hospital in the Bronx, New York, Michael Smith has pioneered the use of auricular (ear-based) acupuncture in the treatment of severe chemical dependency. His protocol has been adapted by the National Acupuncture Detoxification Association and is being implemented in over 700 treatment centers worldwide, representing over 40 countries.

For a number of years, I worked as the medical director of an inpatient substance abuse treatment center. I routinely treated individuals hospitalized against their will with acute withdrawal from heroin, methamphetamines, alcohol, and cocaine. I don't think I have seen anything nearly as magical as the response of these agitated people to acupuncture. A threatening and aggressive man would become tranquil and often fall asleep within 15 minutes of having the needles placed.

Acupuncture soothes the autonomic nervous system and endorphin system, both of which become extremely disrupted and chaotic in the addictive process. Clinical research from the Hazelton Foundation and Hennepin County support the usefulness of acupuncture in treating severe, chronic chemical dependency. The National Acupuncture Detoxification Association (NADA) protocol as well as the data from Hazelton and Hennepin County focus on the use of a simple, identical four- or five-needle program for each patient's ear (Bullock, Culliton, & Olander, 1989). I believe the results would be even stronger with an individualized acupuncture treatment program and the addition of Chinese herbs. When combined, these treatments seem to be most effective for rebuilding the body's reserve and calming the nervous system over the long haul.

The NADA protocol, however, was investigated as a stand-alone treatment for cocaine addiction and found not to be helpful (Margolin, Kleber, & Avants, 2002). And it didn't reduce opiate withdrawal symptoms, either (Ramchand, Griffin, Harris, McCaffrey, & Morral, 2008). This does not refute the earlier work that indicated the protocol as a significant addition to a comprehensive plan for chemical dependency; nobody in the field has ever advocated for acupuncture as a solitary treatment. It needs to be part of a more comprehensive, complementary treatment plan. In fact, a more recent study demonstrated that auricular acupuncture was a useful adjunct to conventional addiction treatment for women (Courbasson, de Sorkin, Dullerud, & Van Wyk, 2007). And in urban Vancouver, acupuncture was found to be an effective tool for recovery in inner-city addicts (Janssen, Demorest, & Whynot, 2005). What's more, auricular acupuncture has been documented to reduce anxiety and alter a wide range of neurotransmitters and neuropeptides. Given the low risk and high potential reward, I support the use of acupuncture (typically full-body treatment, not just ear-based) in any teen with a chemical dependency or usage that goes beyond experimentation or casual use. Also, acupuncture may have more value for the teen with a trauma history or altered HPA axis.

One of the most useful concepts I gleaned from learning acupuncture is the difference between patterns of excess and patterns of deficiency. Western medicine effectively deals with acute illnesses, which are generally patterns of excess. However, nowhere in my medical or psychiatric training did I receive any instruction about supporting the physical body of individuals suffering from chronic disease. This tends to be a pattern of deficiency in which most Western pharmacological approaches actually worsen the problem by further draining the physical resources of the body. The approach to health care in the Orient, on the other hand, recognizes the need to replenish the body, especially with aging or chronic illness. The common use of herbal tonics such as ginseng is one example of this approach. When a young person becomes dependent on a substance such as cocaine, methamphetamine, or stimulants, the body becomes depleted by lack of sleep and poor diet. Helping to correct these imbalances and deficiencies will support wholeness and help in the return to health.

Diet

In addiction the diet suffers. The body is drained and overtaxed, underfed, and unrested. A body that has been strained by addiction and depleted by the addictive cycle needs nourishment and rebalancing. Some basic guidelines would include a diet high in fiber, adequate in protein, and low in saturated and hydrogenated fats. This will help to soup up the body after prolonged bouts of malnourishment and poor eating. Obviously, this diet should also be low in sugar, caffeine, and processed food. Beyond that, a number of practitioners take a symptomatic approach to additional nutritional supplementation and individually target areas of the diet that are suffering (Larson, 1992).

What gets targeted depends on the individual, of course. But one study shows that addicts have low serum levels of iron, as well as vitamins E, C, and A (Hossain, Kamal, Ahsan, & Islam, 2007). These nutrients play an important role in general and psychiatric health, and should be included in any treatment plan (Nazrul Islam, Jahangir Hossain, & Ahsan, 2001). One study found that inclusion of a nutrition-based educational component positively altered addiction treatment outcome (Grant, Haughton, & Sachan, 2004).

I would encourage a nutritional approach for anyone with a true chemical dependency or addiction, as well as any self-destructive, compulsive behavior (especially if there is a family history of alcoholism). There is not, however, one cure-all diet. For some, a high-protein diet seems to work. Others do well on a vegetarian diet or even going vegan. Encourage people to explore options, listen to their own intuition, and heighten their awareness about the impact of food choices upon their body, mind, and spirit. Watch out for the strong tendency of substance abusers to have an abusive relationship with sugar, a close cousin of the alcohol molecule. For more information on this topic, see the wonderful classic, *Body, Mind and Sugar* (Pezet, 1967).

The Ayurvedic approach provides a lot of useful guidance about diet. Similar to the Chinese system, this approach seeks balance by examining the basic constitution (or *dosha*) of the patient and looking for current excesses or deficiencies that need to be addressed. Seek out advice from an Ayurvedic practitioner or manual if you believe this approach could help one of your patients.

Another, less tested approach uses amino acids to address drug withdrawal. I have found free-form amino acids to be extremely useful for drug withdrawal issues. This can be acute withdrawal from cocaine or meth or prolonged withdrawal from Effexor or clonazepam. The research on this topic, however, is meager: Some studies indicate that essential amino acid supplementation reduces liver damage from alcohol abuse and L-tryptophan can reduce oxidative damage in the CNS (Corsetti et al., 2011; Del Angel-Meza et al., 2011). Despite the low evidence base, it's a low-risk treatment that seems to offer some help. I use 3 to 6 capsules three or more times daily on an empty stomach.

Physical Activity

It's often overlooked, but physical exercise can be a wonderful tool for reenergizing and balancing the body. I am occasionally reluctant to recommend it because in our culture it's often done to excess, which effectively duplicates the primary illness: Individuals often become exercise addicts. However, this may be a positive addiction overall, depending upon the individual. Gentle activity such as walking, swimming, or tai chi can be helpful in the recovery process. But it's important to emphasize the need for moderation and to encourage individuals to build awareness about what their bodies want, what they need, and what's too much. An obese, sedentary middle-aged woman will obviously require different guidance than a young male distance runner. Balance and individuation are the key here.

Exercise found some supportive data in Weinstock's (2008) large study. Another study found that even low-intensity exercise of short duration benefited smokers in their recovery from addiction (Taylor, Ussher, & Faulkner, 2007). In fact, yogic breathing and yoga helped cancer patients quit tobacco and improve their immune function as measured by natural killer cell counts (Kochupillai, Kumar, & Singh, 2005). Hatha yoga, the more physical style of yoga primarily practiced in the West, did not improve outcomes for addicts when compared to methadone maintenance (Shaffer, LaSalvia, & Stein, 1997). More and more addiction programs are including physical activity for the support of recovery.

Healthy Mind

One of the qualities in short supply in the addicted individual is peace of mind. Techniques that retrain the mind to open to more peace and serenity can be invaluable. EEG biofeedback, also called neurofeedback, helps get the brain back on healthy neuropathways and has been demonstrated to be an effective treatment for some substance abusers (Scott,

Kaiser, Othmer, & Sideroff, 2005). Mindfulness meditation, an analogue to neurofeedback, has built a strong following in the substance abuse world in the last few years. Both of these approaches rehabilitate an imbalanced, wracked neuroendocrine system. The downside to neurofeedback is that it can be costly, but it may be a better choice than meditation in the short term if there are significant functional physical issues, such as migraine headache or irritable bowel.

If there are significant body image issues or a history of physical or sexual abuse, consider body work (e.g., massage, Rolfing) and referral for a body-oriented psychotherapy such as Hakomi or a trial of cranial osteopathy, which has shown promise in resolving PTSD and addiction.

Creative outlets are important tools as well. Many individuals with addictions have high levels of creative energy, and if this energy is not channeled properly, it may become destructive. If you see this, talk to your patient about what he or she likes to create and try to match up a creative outlet. Also remember that educational and vocational adjustments factor in here. If a teen or young adult does not feel properly challenged or expressive in the school or job setting, it can devolve quickly into substance use and abuse.

For most, addiction carries a sense of isolation. AA and NA as well as other 12-step programs address this lack of intimacy by meeting in a group setting. Beyond this, most people in recovery need to progressively address their lack of (or distorted) social connections, as well as the lack of true intimacy in their lives. Addiction often ends up distancing the addicted person from friends and family because of resentment and tension. Guidance from a mental health professional may be needed to bring them back together, as the individual may lack useful role models or may have had maladaptive early experiences and as a result may struggle to reorient or reconnect. These barriers to intimacy make excellent topics for therapeutic sessions.

Spirituality

The success of AA has opened our eyes to the value of the spirit in treating addictions. But beyond the structure of a 12-step program, many other modalities can be helpful in reenergizing the spirit and soothing the soul. Spiritual healing and therapeutic touch are nonspecific modalities that can be of great aid to the drained, disconnected, and dispirited person dealing with addictions. Supporting a deeper spiritual process through journaling, retreat, and spiritual practice could serve the struggling teen or young adult and strengthen recovery. Meditation is perhaps the most profound spiritual exercise. It acts as a nonspecific tool for opening the door to our human spirituality. It can be learned in many styles free of religious dogma or structure.

Many people, myself included, find great peace and serenity in nature; it's one of the best healers for the troubles of abuse and dependence. I often recommend an experiential outdoor program such as Outward Bound or one of the many therapeutic variations on this theme for teens or young adults. As medical director of one young adult residential program for substance abusers in Boulder, Colorado, I routinely asked each of the young people as they were discharged what they thought helped them most in their recovery. For most of them the path involved a few hospital stays, drug rehab, a wilderness program, and a residential treatment center. Over 90% of them indicated that the wilderness stay— anywhere from 1 to 3 months—was the most valuable component of their recovery. Sometimes, more than anything a young person just needs to get away from a toxic family, toxic culture, and toxic peer group and find an inner quiet.

In sum, substance abuse and dependence in teens represents a significant, highly underidentified, and massively undertreated problem in America. Although genetic risk factors are significant, they only alert us to added risk. The ecological factors in a young person's life such as family environment, parenting, support, peer group, and media represent the other half of risk, one that can be readily managed. Trauma in childhood and adversity also convey added risk that may alter the HPA axis and autonomic balance.

Substance use and abuse, more than dependence or addiction, are the major concerns here, as they can predispose the teen or young adult to a lifelong cycle of addiction. The path out is as simple as Bill W.'s three-pronged approach to body-mind-spirit. If you can remove the barriers in a teen's ecosystem by addressing potential negative input from family, peers, and media while simultaneously enhancing psychological, nutritional, and family supports, then recovery and wholeness become more than possible—they become probable.

Additional Supplementation for Substance Dependence

1. Free-form amino acids (should include L-tryptophan): 3–6 capsules tid on empty stomach (higher end if in acute withdrawal).
2. Glutamine: 1,000 mg tid.
3. Ester C: 1,000 mg bid.
4. B complex: 50 mg bid.
5. Melatonin: 1 mg at bedtime
6. Calcium citrate: 500 mg bid.
7. Magnesium glycinate 300 mg bid.
8. EFA omega-3 (EPA 400 mg) tid.
9. Inositol: 4–6 g tid (powder is better).
10. For severe addiction or malnutrition, consider IV nutritional support in first month.

Treatment Plan: Step by Step

1. Comprehensive evaluation of child's six realms (see Chapter 6) and common presenting issues (see Chapter 7).
2. Identify barriers, deficiencies, strengths, and gifts.
3. Examine the child for diet issues, food quality, food allergies, or gut issues. Refer to a nutritionist or naturopath as needed. Consider higher-protein diet.
4. Examine for family conflict, depressed or overwhelmed parents, oppositional behavior, marital stress, poor communication, behavioral issues (home or school, or both), and social skills. Think about family therapy if needed. These families may be more chaotic than most, and parenting support may be quite useful.
5. Screen carefully for depression, anxiety, or trauma and refer for individual therapy. If previously in therapy, contact prior or current therapist for background and collaboration.
6. Lab testing: Check TSH, vitamin D (25 OH), ferritin/CBC, lipid profile (low cholesterol), homocysteine, and HS CRP. Treat abnormalities as they appear.
7. Add inositol 3–6 g two or three times daily as powder in water.

8. Acupuncture may be quite helpful.

9. Add B-complex 50 mg with 1 mg of folate, 500–1,000 mg of EPA, and 500–1,000 mg of vitamin C. If true dependence, glutamine 1,000 mg or more three times daily and calcium/magnesium (1:1) 250–500 mg twice daily.

10. Add free-form amino acids for the first few months to help with any withdrawal issues with true dependence. Use 3–6 capsules three or five times daily on an empty stomach.

11. If chronic depression or fatigue, explore adrenal health (DHEA-sulfate and salivary cortisols) and consider adaptogens such as rhodiola or ashwaganda.

12. Make sure exercise and sunlight are at appropriate levels. Encourage time in nature and physical activity to help the person fully inhabit his or her body.

13. Sleep is likely to be an issue. Consider melatonin and other natural agents as indicated.

14. If emotional regulation is an issue, think of DBT.

15. Consider a self-regulation technique such as meditation or yoga.

16. Consider school fit and learning style.

17. If highly motivated or chronic, consider neurofeedback training.

18. If severe dependence and impaired nutrition, consider IV nutritional support over the first 2 months of recovery.

CHAPTER FIFTEEN

Autism Spectrum Disorders

Autism alters every aspect of the child's interaction with the surrounding world. It strikes at the very essence of communication, language, and sense of self. This disorder dramatically impacts almost every known brain system from anatomy and physiology to histology. Actually, considerable emerging evidence now documents shifts in most biological domains in the body including gut function, inflammation, pain, and immune response.

By connecting the nature of these changes, including the vast and pervasive neurological changes that occur in autism and the associated teratogens, researchers now estimate that for some cases of autism, brain changes begin by the eighth week of in utero development (Arndt, Stodgell, & Rodier, 2005). The structural brain changes relate to increases in overall brain volume and significant structural abnormalities in many brain regions, ranging from the frontal lobes to the cerebellum (Chen, Jiao, & Herskovits, 2011).

The most consistent and greatest abnormalities are found in the cerebellar vermis. Originally felt to be associated with only motor control, neuroscientists have increasingly found that the cerebellar vermis is in fact linked to a wide range of nonmotor functions. Early in my career as a medical student at the University of Arizona, I did neuroscience research as part of my interest in theories of consciousness. My final thesis in 1981 linked the cerebellum to primary cognitive control of thought based on computer modeling of brain centers. At the time it was quite speculative, but now considerable science ties the cerebellum to a central role in the processing and coordination of thought. The esteemed neuroscientist Rodolfo Llinás agrees: "Active movement is the very source and main stem of mental life. That which we call thinking is the evolutionary internalization of movement" (2001, p. 35).

I trouble you with this aside because I think that, at its heart, autism represents a breakdown in the very essence of the human mind and its primary functional core. These cerebellar abnormalities are connected not only to thinking and language but also to the range of motor abnormalities we find in autism. In fact, autistic children universally have dyspraxia (Jones & Prior, 1985), which is related to the communication in the brain between planning and executing a movement. They also usually have gait abnormalities too (Vilensky, Damasio, & Maurer, 1981). This might be why blind raters were able to distinguish autistic children from controls based only on viewing home movies before autism was suspected (Adrien et al., 1992). What all this shows is the possibility that with autism we're looking at a breakdown of the primary functional core of the mind, and indeed the brain, and that movement and thought are related more closely than we previously thought. Based on this idea, movement may offer an intriguing method to retrain the mind.

But before we go any further, let's backtrack and learn a little bit more about this perplexing disorder.

Autism spectrum disorders (ASDs) include three diagnoses: autism, Asperger's syndrome, and pervasive developmental disorder (PDD). ASDs affect boys four times as often as girls. Like many parts of autism, we don't know why. ASDs consist of three main symptomatic components: communication deficits, social impairment, and behavioral abnormalities. These are typically pervasive and ongoing. Asperger's syndrome is a milder variation in which communication and language are much less impacted. PDD describes kids who do not meet full criteria for either disorder.

The rates for autism are increasing across the board. According to a report issued by the Centers for Disease Control in March 2012, using data derived from the Autism and Developmental Disabilities Monitoring surveillance network, 1 in 88 children—1 in 54 boys and 1 in 252 girls—have an ASD diagnosis by age 8 (Baio, 2012). This represents a serious spike from the last estimate of 1 in 110. This means there's been a rise of 78% since 2002 (Baio, 2008). Wider diagnostic criteria and increased awareness have something to do with these rising numbers, but it's tough to tell how much. What we do know is that children are now also being diagnosed much earlier, sometimes by age 3, an increase from 12% for children born in 1994 to 18% for children born in 2000. Sadly, 40% of children aren't getting a diagnosis until after the age of 4. We still have a long way to go.

The prognosis, no matter the age of diagnosis, is not bright. Rates of recovery are estimated to be 3–25% in ASD. In one study of young adults with autism, only 4% were living independently (Billstedt, Gillberg, & Gillberg, 2005). For children with ASD followed into young adulthood, 17% had a good outcome and 4% a very good outcome, according to another study (Eaves & Ho, 2008). About half of children with ASD are placed on psychiatric medications for management of symptoms. There is no cure.

The cost of these disorders is extraordinary. Recent estimates put autism costs at about $60 billion per year in the United States. This amounts to a staggering $3.2 million over the course of the average life of a child with autism (Ganz, 2007). Parents face perhaps the greatest stress imaginable in caring for a child with autism. Based on a 2008 study, they also suffer a 14% loss of income simply based on the demands of incessant care and treatment (Montes & Halterman, 2008).

These parents deal with many varied issues as there's very significant comorbidity in this population. Mental retardation is found in 25–70% of children with autism. (It is often very hard to assess IQ in someone with autism, hence the huge range.) Anxiety disorders are found in 11–84%. Epilepsy occurs in about 10–30%, often appearing first in the teen years. About 30% have a problem with self-injurious behavior. Sleep issues present for two-thirds of children with ASD. As I mentioned before, motor abnormalities are so common as to be the norm. The motor issues are often related to motor planning, delayed motor milestones, toe walking, and so on. Aggression is also very often a key feature, which is usually the most difficult aspect of the disorder for many parents to manage.

One of the most interesting phenomena in all of ASD is the presence of savants. Savants are people who, like the character made famous by Dustin Hoffman in *Rain Man*, possess incredible cognitive skills in narrow areas of human functioning. For about a decade I worked as primary psychiatrist to a community agency in Greeley, Colorado, for developmental disabilities. There I encountered a number of savants, who make up about 1% of the ASD population. Two of these kids come right to mind. Rob and Tom were twin brothers who fought incessantly and had some really unique abilities. When I met Tom, he asked me my birth date. Five seconds after I told him, he said, "Saturday." Right after this exchange, his brother Rob asked what car I drove. When I told him, he recited my license plate number to me immediately. Apparently he had memorized all of the plates in the lot on his walk in.

Kim Peek, the basis for the character in *Rain Man*, died in 2009. Like Tom and Rob, he had capacities that boggle the mind. Kim permanently retained anything that he read, and he could read two books at a time, one with each eye. He knew the location for all of the zip codes in the United States and had encyclopedic knowledge on almost every topic. His brain was massively abnormal: It had neither a corpus callosum nor an anterior commissure. No one has any idea how he did what he did—and did it so effortlessly. Savants have much to teach us about the potential of the human mind.

Cause

As in many psychiatric illnesses, we know that genetics are a factor in the expression of autism. For example, siblings of an autistic child have 25 times the rate of illness as the normal population. But, as in many psychiatric illnesses, this heritable history tells us little and does nothing to impact treatment. The ever-changing landscape of the generation of genomic data coupled with the vast heterogeneity in cause and expression of ASDs (further influenced by issues of penetrance, variable expressivity, and multigenic inheritance) creates a complexity that defies simple answers. So while we might be able to predict expression based on heritability, it's neither conclusive nor informative. A. L. Beaudet puts it this way: "A substantial fraction of autism cases may be traceable to genetic causes that are heritable but not inherited. That is, a mutation that causes autism is not present in the parental genome" (2007, p. 534). Needless to say, the link is little understood. This is all complicated by the fact that we have witnessed a growing percentage of autism cases that are a regressive subtype (Stefanatos, 2008). In these cases the child looks and acts normally for a period of time, then regresses backward into full autism before the age of 30 months. The words *polygenic* and *multifactorial* feel inadequate but they may be the best summary to this section.

Given the very basic lack of understanding about autism, it should come as no surprise that a wide range of possible external triggers have been identified. They include infectious disease, heavy metals, solvents, diesel exhaust, PCBs, phthalates, phenols, pesticides, flame retardants, alcohol, smoking, illicit drugs, vaccines, and parental stress. No patently clear link has been established, however. And the issue of vaccines as a possible trigger remains controversial. The population-based studies have all but ruled it out as a consistent notable influence. In isolated cases the connection may seem more clear-cut, but thus far the hypothesis that vaccines or the mercury and thimerosal in them cause autism does not appear to hold any water (DeStefano, 2007; Schultz, 2010).

A review of the literature gives us some clue about where we need to focus our study if we're going to treat and prevent this malady. Rossignol and Frye (2012) identified four main directions in autism research related to both the physiological and metabolic abnormalities in the disorder: immune dysfunction or inflammation, oxidative stress, mitochondrial dysfunction, and environmental toxins. The research on these topics is overwhelmingly positive. The two researchers found that in each of these arenas the proportion of articles reporting positive findings ranged from 89% (170/190 positive articles on toxins) to 95% (416/437 on immune/inflammation) and 95% (145/153 on mitochondrial dysfunction) to 100% (115/115 on oxidative stress) (Rossignol & Frye, 2012). (Most—62%—of the publications are in the five years prior to 2012.) The authors then reviewed the strength of the findings. They found that 45% of all of the articles reported strong findings of an association between physiological abnormalities and autism. What this tells us is that there's a good chance that both the illness and its trigger are systemic in nature, ideas we've only recently begun to explore.

Robert Hendren, chair of child psychiatry at the University of California, San Francisco, and former director of the MIND Institute (one of the premier neurodevelopmental research settings in the U.S.) in Davis, California, invited me to join Rossignol and Frye, and 17 other researchers and clinicians in the field of autism, at a national summit in San Francisco in January 2012. The goal of this two-day meeting was to identify some possible targets for translational research into the biological foundations of autism. The first step was to identify a number of clinical or biochemical abnormalities that we treated. We then developed a list of the assessment tools we found most helpful in the care and treatment of children with autism. The interplay between researchers and clinicians was fascinating. Cutting-edge research at places like Stanford, UCSF, and the MIND Institute is merging with long-established clinical practices. This newfound unity of concern from conventional and alternative medicine over issues like immune dysfunction, micronutrient deficiency, and digestive abnormalities struck me as both ironic and inevitable.

The list of tests we agreed upon at the end of the conference is both a testament to the breadth of physiology involved in autism and a practical guide to its clinical assessment. I share this list for illustrative purposes only (this is not a recommended list):

- Basics: Metabolic panel, CBC, RBC magnesium, selenium, RBC zinc and RBC copper, vitamin D, vitamin C, fat-soluble vitamins, ferritin, TIBC, serum lead, cholesterol, RBC folate, and ceruloplasmin.
- Genetic screen: CGH array and FMR1 DNA.
- Oxidative stress: nitro tyrosine, urine porphyrins, transferrin, GSH, csyteine/cystine, and 8-OHdG.
- Mitochondrial dysfunction: lactate, pyruvate, carnitine, creatine kinase, ubiquinone, and ammonia.
- Immune function and inflammation: ANA, ESR, anticasein, antigluten, antisoy IgG, activated T cell and B cell subsets, IgM, IgA, IgE, and C-reactive protein.
- GI function: comprehensive digestive stool analysis, Bristol stool sample, GI questionnaire, and calprotectin.
- Hormones: Thyroid function—FT3, FT4, TSH, and salivary cortisol.
- Allergy: IgG and IgE food antibodies as indicated.
- Toxins: urine porphyrins.

The assessment protocol that came from this summit is complex and offers further evidence that autism represents a body-wide phenomenon. Of particular interest among these tests are those of GI function, particularly tests of gut abnormalities and digestive issues, which seem to accompany the vast majority of kids with autism. In fact, almost half of children with autism have GI complaints, typically indigestion, constipation, loose stools, or abdominal pain (Buie et al., 2010; de Magistris et al., 2010). In studies of gut function, permeability measures the difference in the absorption between lactulose and mannitol in order to ascertain if there's a leaky gut. A leaky gut is one sign of abnormal gut function and a potential cause of food allergies, as the proteins in food leak into the bloodstream and cause an adverse reaction. According to one large study, 37% of autistic children showed this abnormality versus 5% of controls (de Magistris et al., 2010). Another similar study showed that altered intestinal permeability was reported in 9 of 21 (43%) children with ASDs, and zero of 40 healthy age-matched controls (D'Eufemia et al., 1996). Beyond autism, breakdown of the tight junction in the gut lining has been implicated in other childhood illnesses such as asthma, allergies, and diabetes (Liu, Li, & Neu, 2005).

Endoscopy trials in autistic children have demonstrated a higher prevalence of nonspecific colitis, lymphoid hyperplasia, and gastritis compared with controls (Galiatsatos, Gologan, & Lamoureux, 2009). In fact, the severity of gut symptoms appears to correlate well with ASD severity, according to one study (Adams, Johansen, Powell, Quig, & Rubin, 2011). The data from this study also showed a strong positive association of autism severity with GI dysfunction. This association was evident within each subcategory of the researchers' autism assessment, including speech, social, sensory/cognitive, and physical/behavioral. Now it is unclear whether the GI symptoms are simply added pain and discomfort or if they are causative.

In related studies, researchers are now reporting microbiome abnormalities in ASD. A number of studies have documented elevations of clostridium species that are pathogenic (Parracho et al., 2005). Studies also have found abnormal gut bacteria (desulfovibrio) in children with regressive autism (Finegold, 2011). These researchers have found a pattern of abnormal phylogenetic shifts in the ASD child and some abnormality in siblings as well. A few attempts have found that treatment with the appropriate antibiotics will improve behavior in ASD for the duration of the treatment (Sandler et al., 2000). This remains speculative, but considerable interest has arisen even in the conventional GI community about the use of probiotics to address these abnormal findings (Critchfield, van Hemert, Ash, Mulder, & Ashwood, 2011).

It's likely that food allergies play an integral role in ASD. This is seen simply in the fact that a gluten-free and casein-free (GFCF) diet is perhaps the most common intervention in ASD. Even so, until recently we had very little information on the usefulness of the GFCF diet. Researchers from Penn State University published a study in March 2012 that surveyed 387 parents of autistic children on the GFCF diet. They found that strict implementation (crucial for food allergy interventions) of the GFCF diet was associated with significant improvements in ASD symptoms, social behaviors, and physiological symptoms (Pennesi & Klein,

2012). The presence of GI complaints prior to the diet also predicted response. An RCT of 55 autistic children in England followed for 24 months had similar positive findings (Whiteley et al., 2010). Isolated case reports also echo this response (Hsu, Lin, Chen, Wang, & Wong, 2009).

Another source of useful information is from the Autism Research Institute, which has been surveying parents of autistic children since 1967. Today, over 26,000 parents have responded to their surveys, which ask a simple set of questions about prior treatments: Did the child get better, worse, or no change? I frequently encourage the parents of an autistic child to look through these data and see what they think (Autism Research Institute, 2009). In the published data, each treatment is given a ratio between better/worse (a high number means most children had a good effect). Most psychiatric medications, interestingly enough, have a ratio of about 1. Notable exceptions are the antifungals, which have a ratio of about 12. No other oral prescription agent for behavior treatment, including risperidone, is above 1. Supplements like SAMe, St. John's wort, and trimethylgycine are all below one. Many of the other natural supplements, however, are between 10 and 20. Most of the specific diets score above 20, with the GFCF diet coming in around 24. Removing chocolate is 28 to 1. Removing dairy products is 32 to 1. Just talk to a parent of an autistic child—they are desperate to find what helps, and given the difficulty of introducing these diets, the advice and encouragement of thousands of other parents and their experience is worth something.

The other thing to keep in mind about food and digestion is that these kids can't tell you what they are feeling or even where it hurts. A helpful hint can be if the child rubs his belly on furniture or other household items as a sign of discomfort. If there is a change in diet, look to see if it correlates with incidents of screaming, night arousals, aggression, and so on, and adjust accordingly.

Early Identification

As you can see from the research, early identification represents our most valuable tool for managing this debilitating lifelong problem. Sadly, the average age of diagnosis for an ASD child is about 5 (Centers for

Disease Control, 2009). Yet upon closer inspection we learn that a majority of these children's office charts revealed abnormal indicators such as abnormal mood, oppositionality, delayed motor functioning, or odd responses to sensory stimuli by 36 months. The clues are there. We just need to open our eyes to them. Some indicators to pursue: no babbling, pointing, or gesturing by 12 months, no single words by 16 months, no two-word phrases (not echolalic) by 24 months, and the loss of any social or language skills at any age. The American Academy of Pediatrics recommends screens at the 9-, 18-, and 24- or 30-month visits.

Treating Autism

Conventional care focuses in on three elements: early detection, applied behavior analysis (ABA) socialization therapy, and medication management. Early intervention makes a big difference. According to the Wisconsin Early Autism Project 2006, 48% of kids identified early enter regular education by the age of 7. Using the Early Start Denver Model (which integrates ABA with developmental and relationship-based approaches), researchers have found significant social and cognitive benefits for children diagnosed under 30 months (Dawson et al., 2010). Most importantly, these kids were able to keep developmental pace with non-diagnosed controls. "Infant brains are quite malleable," says Sally Rogers, one of the study's coauthors and architects of the intervention. "With this therapy we're trying to capitalize on the potential of learning that an infant brain has in order to limit autism's deleterious effects, to help children lead better lives" (Dawson et al., 2010). This fits perfectly with a wholeness-oriented approach: It maximizes neuroplasticity and skill building by focusing on early intervention.

ABA, which seeks to modify behavior through active integration of skills and applied learning, is the most-researched psychosocial intervention in autism. This intervention appears to help in the short run, but we don't yet know if it translates into improved vocational or social functioning in adulthood (Rogers & Vismara, 2008). A review of ABA found that high-intensity work offers more benefit than low intensity work, but added, "As no definitive behavioral or developmental intervention improves all symptoms for all individuals with ASD, it is recommended that clinical management be guided by individual needs and availability of resources" (Ospina et al., 2008). The main drawbacks of ABA are the cost and its limited accessibility for many families.

Psychiatric medications are an area of expanding treatment use in ASD, despite poor evidence of efficacy and limited knowledge of their neurobiological mechanism. A review in *Pediatrics* evaluated the current use of psychiatric medications in ASD and concluded,

> Evidence supports the benefit of risperidone and aripiprazole for challenging and repetitive behaviors in children with ASDs. Evidence also supports significant adverse effects of these medications. Insufficient strength of evidence is present to evaluate the benefits or adverse effects for any other medical treatments for ASDs, including serotonin-reuptake inhibitors and stimulant medications. Although many children with ASDs are currently treated with medical interventions, strikingly little evidence exists to support benefit for most treatments. Risperidone and aripiprazole have shown benefit for challenging and repetitive behaviors, but associated adverse effects limit their use to patients with severe impairment or risk of injury. (McPheeters et al., 2011)

Not what I would call a promising endorsement.

Sir William Osler, considered the father of modern American medicine, once quipped, "When you have more than one treatment for an illness, all are inadequate." Nowhere is this more apt than in a description of autism. Survey the literature and you'll find a host of different interventions, all with about the same (poor) efficacy. Talk to doctors and you'll hear a cacophony of contentious opinions and insights. Add to this the range of possible abnormalities in ASD, and it means that it's usually left up to parents to explore and decide on treatment. Most parents end up becoming experts on autism, with expansive knowledge about the positives and potential drawbacks of all the different treatments.

Charged with the task of deciding on their child's treatment, most concerned moms and dads err on the side of safety. It should come as no surprise, then, that the vast majority of them embrace alternative approaches. One study out of Harvard found that 74% of parents with an autistic child used alternative treatments (Hanson et al., 2007). In the study, families reported alternative medicine to be either helpful or without effect, but never harmful. (The main reasons cited for choosing alternative medicine related to concerns about the safety and side effects of prescribed medications.) Another study found that 75% of parents considered alternative medicine treatments to be helpful for their child with ASD (Wong & Smith, 2006). Most parents seem to think that since all treatments are inadequate, as Osler said, then perhaps it's better just to stick to the safe ones.

But let's quickly review the evidence anyway. In 2009, a comprehensive review of the evidence for emerging and novel treatments for kids with ASD was completed (Rossignol, 2009). Each treatment was graded on a scale from A to C based on the level of evidence and the diversity of studies (A is the strongest documentation). Treatments that received an A included melatonin, acetylcholinesterase inhibitors, naltrexone, and music therapy. Grade-B treatments included carnitine, tetrahydrobiopterin, vitamin C, alpha-2 adrenergic agonists, hyperbaric oxygen treatment, immunomodulation and anti-inflammatory treatments, oxytocin, and vision therapy. The C treatments included carnosine, multivitamin/mineral complex, piracetam, polyunsaturated fatty acids, vitamin B6/magnesium, elimination diets, chelation, cyproheptadine, famotidine, glutamate antagonists, acupuncture, auditory integration training, massage, and neurofeedback.

One particularly interesting study used differences in parental treatment preference to separate a group of 88 autistic children into two arms (Mehl-Madrona, Leung, Kennedy, Paul, & Kaplan, 2010). The researcher simply asked parents whether they would like their child to be treated with psychiatric prescription medications or a vitamin-mineral supplement, EMPowerplus. The target issues were aggression, self-injurious behavior, and agitation. After the children were sorted into two arms, the researchers matched them into two equivalent groups and administered treatment for at least 3 months. Children in both groups improved on the Childhood Autism Rating Scale and the Childhood Psychiatric Rating Scale. Both groups also exhibited significant decreases in total Aberrant Behavior Checklist scores, but the micronutrient group's improvement was significantly greater ($p < 0.0001$). Self-injurious behavior was lower in the micronutrient group at the end of the study ($p = 0.005$), and improvement on the Clinical Global Impressions scale was greater for the micronutrient group ($p = 0.0029$). The micronutrient group also had lower activity levels, less social withdrawal, less anger, better spontaneity with the examiner, less irritability, lower-intensity self-injurious behavior, markedly fewer adverse events, and less weight gain. There was also the added advantage of fewer adverse side effects. Neuroleptics such as risperidone often produce significant weight gain. The authors concluded that EMPowerplus represents a reasonable and safe option for the treatment of behavioral problems in the ASD population.

Given the massive range of physiological abnormalities and the infantile nature of this field, little clear direction comes from the research alone. Also, in light of the enormous loss of human potential over a life span, various treatments should be tried, with one caveat: First, do no harm.

This principle must also be applied to how we deal with the child's parents because, as practitioners, we are also entrusted with their safety and well-being. As a parent, nothing hurts more than to see your child suffer; and the ASD child suffers greatly. But beyond the physical pain and frustration of their disorder, such children also have the added burden of never fully expressing who they are and who they can become. The pain of living that far short of human potential reverberates outward and can very well erode the spirit of those around the sufferer. Parents want their children to feel normal, to reach their potential and strive for more—they want to help.

That's why parents, particularly of ASD kids, so often become dedicated to, and even obsessed with, finding help and relief for their child. It often becomes a full-time job and a late-night fixation. They invest all of their time and energy into exploring new potential avenues for treatment; and hope is often their only guide in this landscape. As a result, they can be easily preyed upon by the unscrupulous or the misguided; they can fall into the trap of thinking that this one treatment, finally, will cure their child. Our role as practitioners, then, is to measure and temper this kind of thinking, acting as the seasoned, shrewd guide in the journey. We need to help parents make healthy long-term decisions for the suffering child, even if those decisions require a few hard doses of reality.

This is not to say that wholeness is out of reach. Little by little we are peeling back the onion that is ASD and finding new, safe avenues to promote health and wholeness. We're still in the dark, but with time and careful attention we can remove barriers and offer supports at each step along the way. These kids deserve to be happy; they deserve the ability to know and express themselves.

Treatment Plan: Step by Step

1. Comprehensive evaluation of child's six realms (see Chapter 6) and common presenting issues (see Chapter 7).
2. Identify barriers, deficiencies, strengths, and gifts.
3. Early identification and intervention are crucial. The Early Start Denver Model shows great promise. ABA or Lovaas intervention, if available and affordable, makes sense as another foundation.
4. Work with the diet. The first thing that I have parents do is move to a GFCF diet trial. If they can only do one, do one. A number of children in my care have started speaking within weeks of starting this diet. This is the single best intervention for ASD kids. Give it 4 weeks or more. Monitor symptoms and then reintroduce the offending foods. Most parents who give this trial the respect and careful attention it requires come away quite pleased. Half-hearted attempts produce minimal results. A nutritionist can be very helpful in this process. After starting the GFCF diet, explore for other food allergies, clean up the diet, and remove additives and dyes. Once gut health is improved, the typically narrow diet of the ASD kid (e.g., macaroni and cheese, ramen noodles, bread and butter) will begin to broaden naturally without effort. The selective appetite of the ASD child, in my experience, is just a symptom of dysbiosis and ill gut health. I usually refer to a naturopath for support here.
5. Examine for family conflict, depressed or overwhelmed parents, oppositional behavior, marital stress, poor communication, and sibling stress. Think about family therapy if needed. A parenting and behavior support program such as Nurtured Heart almost always makes some sense.
6. Begin biomedical assessment. This will typically mean testing urine for organic acids, a comprehensive stool analysis, and blood work. (Remember, blood work can often be extremely traumatic for these kids; so be considerate.) Good progress can usually be had with the first two, avoiding or delaying a very traumatic blood draw.
7. Start with the safest, simplest, and cheapest natural supplements to address the physiological abnormalities documented: B vitamins, magnesium, probiotics, digestive enzymes, anti-inflammatory agents (e.g., fish oil, N-acetylcysteine), and so on.

8. Explore novel modalities to engage the child: music therapy, horse therapy, time in nature, exercise, dance, and so on.

9. After trying these first steps, consider more expensive treatments, such as hyperbaric oxygen, neurofeedback, or acupuncture.

10. Continue to delve deeper into the biomedical rehabilitation with more testing and intervention.

11. For Asperger's, work aggressively with social skills and self-awareness. Many self-help programs like "How Does Your Engine Run?" (www .alertprogram.com) help to support personal growth.

12. Look for areas of talent, and think about how those abilities can be leveraged to help foster the child's engagement in the world. For example, a 15-year-old with Asperger's symptoms and an interest in electronics might become the tech coordinator for the drama department.

13. Develop a respectful, open-minded, communication-rich relationship with the parents so that they feel comfortable discussing possible treatment interventions with you. Have them keep you posted about what they are doing and the results. Monitor the child for progress. Steer the family away from the riskiest treatments, like IV chelation.

14. Save the use of antipsychotic medications as a last resort. They tend to create a new tier of physiological problems such as weight gain. Consider EMPowerplus as a stand-in for antipsychotic medications for aggressiveness or volatility.

Nathan

Nathan's pediatrician sent him to a local community mental health center for ongoing care. Although he was just 5 years old, he had already been given the following diagnosis: anxiety disorder not otherwise specified, Asperger's disorder, ADHD, mood disorder, and sensory integration disorder. This gives only a partial reflection of his early struggles. He had a normal delivery and experienced colic in his first 3 months. After that, he had completely normal development until 18 months, when he became constantly agitated and emotionally dysregulated, with constant screaming and distress. His sleep went from smooth and predictable to erratic and restless. Nathan had been starting to talk but this ground to a halt. He stopped playing and showed much less interest in cuddling his mom, Cynthia. Mom knew something was wrong and sought help.

The pediatrician shared her concerns and referred Nathan out for evaluation. They recommended formal evaluation and Head Start classes. Ear infections, which started at about 1 year of age, became chronic and necessitated almost constant antibiotics. Nathan began some hand flapping and rocking to soothe himself. He showed much less interest in the family and began to get preoccupied with his toy trains. It was all he wanted to do, and he screamed if Cynthia took them away or tried to engage him in some other activity.

By age 4, the concerns mounted. He was not yet potty trained and his language was limited, with poor speech. He underwent tonsillectomy and adenoid surgery at 27 months to address the constant infections. By the time he turned 5, he was not ready for kindergarten: He was restless and had poor focus and inconsistent effort. Mom was concerned that he had lost some academic skills learned in the previous year. He began to show excessive anxiety about separating from his mom and new places; he needed someone to lie with him at night to fall asleep; and he never seemed to be comfortable or feel safe. He was difficult to engage with other children, as he ignored them and preferred infants or young toddlers. He showed no sense of boundaries and often got into others' personal space and sometimes even licked other people or objects.

On his first visit, he walked in through the office door, stocky with a distended abdomen. His cheeks were bright red and so were his ears. His walk was somewhat stiff legged, like a little robot. His gaze was restless, and he avoided eye contact, with his glassy dark eyes. A pink ring of chapped skin surrounded his mouth. Nathan initially sat beside the couch and averted his gaze while he intently sucked his thumb. He would not respond to any questions, and seemed to be off—elsewhere. Cynthia brought in a sample of his work at school, which caused grave concern among his teachers. His writing was scrambled and geometric, without any sign of coherent lettering. "He's not ready for school, they tell me," she said.

As we shared Nathan's case at our weekly team meeting, Dr. Mullin, the boy's psychiatrist and a member of my team at the Wholeness Center, showed us the writing sample and said,

I felt that there was an underlying biomedical irritant that was exacerbating his symptoms; we had to get his gut straightened out before we could really do anything for him. The first thing I did was to order digestive enzymes and probiotics to target encopresis; I also ordered metabolic testing. At his second visit 2 weeks later, mother indicated that the encopresis and bloating had significantly improved. His testing work-up indicated a yeast dysbiosis and we commenced treatment with fluconazole (an antifungal). Within 10 days, a writing sample showed well-formed letters [see Figures 15.1 and 15.2]. He was making great eye contact, sat calmly next to his mother, and was responding normally to questions.

As of his last visit, 1 year after start of treatment, Nathan's eyes had cleared, revealing warm brown eyes. His cheeks and ears had returned to a normal skin tone, and his abdomen had flattened to reveal a ticklish soft belly. Cynthia was very pleased at his progress over that year. Whereas he was initially in danger of repeating kindergarten, he was now happily preparing to enter second grade. He was not on any psychi-

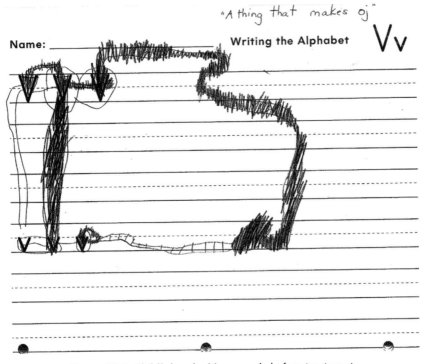

Figure 15.1. Child's handwriting sample before treatment.

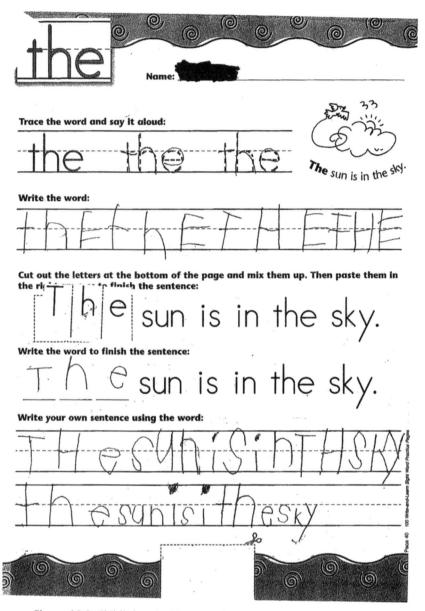

Figure 15.2. Child's handwriting sample after a few weeks of treatment.

atric medications and was much more engaged with his age group peers. Nathan still has struggles. He remains reactive at times and needs additional help to master social-emotional skills, but he is certainly better able to learn and grow.

I shared Nathan's story in particular for a few reasons. First, the writing samples vividly convey the dramatic and significant quality of his transformation. Second, he had significant conventional care that treated nothing in his diet or gut. Third, his care occurred in a community mental health care center—just imagine how much money this simple, cheap intervention saved in terms of chronic care and medications over years or decades of symptomatic management. Of course, this type of improvement is not always found in treating autism. I have been surprised both by the amount of positive change that I have seen in this type of care and the grave difficulties that often remain.

CHAPTER SIXTEEN

Trauma and PTSD

From 50% to 90% of us will experience some highly traumatic event in our lifetimes. According to federal statistics, over 6 million reports of child abuse occur each year, but only 1 million are documented. Most victims never surface and most abusers are never identified. As best we can tell, one in four girls and one in six boys are sexually abused before the age of 18. Nearly 70% of all reported sexual assaults (including those on adults) happen to children under 18 (Snyder, 2000). What's more, if we include physical and emotional abuse, the numbers skyrocket.

The sad truth is this: Traumatic events sufficient to cause PTSD may occur in upwards of 25–35% of children and, devastatingly, most of these cases go unidentified and as a result untreated.

PTSD, at least in its current diagnostic form, has existed since about 1983. The current diagnostic specifics may, and probably will, change somewhat over the next few years as we learn more about its neurobiology. The basic essence of PTSD is an event that spawns the continual reexperiencing of the threat of death or injury. The symptoms of PTSD fall into three main categories: the continual reenactment of the traumatic event; avoidance of the event or general withdrawal; and physiological hyperreactivity. PTSD keeps the brain in a state of hyperarousal, fear, and avoidance, meaning that the memory of the event cannot be properly processed by the psyche.

Interestingly, there are no specific criteria for children. The *DSM-IV* even acknowledges that the pattern in children may be quite different from that of adults. But it offers no further elucidation on what these differences might be, or what they could mean for treatment.

Each child has a variable risk of PTSD. The risk factors are hard to quantify, but there are a few prevalent patterns. Girls, for example, are more at risk than boys. Preexisting sexual abuse, as you might guess, predisposes a kid to a much higher risk. A child or teen who has experienced anxiety or depression previously has an elevated risk. Drug and alcohol abusers also carry more risk. A child that had early separation from a parent is more vulnerable, as are children from a dysfunctional marriage.

The take-away for the clinician, then, is that this illness is difficult to predict and hard to prevent, and you have to probe into children's lives to find out how they process traumatic events and if any continue to plague them. Unfortunately, there's no rubric or clinical guide here: A large group of children may be exposed to the exact same stressor—say, a car accident—but each of them will experience and process the trauma of the crash in a different way. With trauma, there is a spectrum of possible responses based on individual vulnerabilities; and, unfortunately, it's probably as wide as the spectrum of possible traumatic events.

Perhaps more than any other childhood affliction, trauma is mercurial and individualized, manifesting itself in a vast array of physical, mental, and emotional symptoms. But anxiety is the form it most often assumes. That's why I find it clinically helpful to think about trauma—and its diagnostic analogue PTSD—as a subtype of anxiety, or at least as triggers of common anxiety symptomatology. (For the sake of brevity, the terms trauma and PTSD are used interchangeably to describe the clinical presentation of stressful events.) Thus, when you see a kid with high levels of anxiety, keep in mind that there might really be some traumatic history at play. This doesn't necessarily mean there's been a history of abuse or neglect, though. Trauma, and the resulting anxiety, can come from the evening news or violent video games, car accidents or R-rated movies, or physical or sexual abuse. Many modern homes are traumatic simply as the result of the kind of chaos and aggression that they contain, even if the child is not directly abused. Any child with anxiety, depression, or hallucinations should be screened carefully for trauma in a private session. This may take time to assess and parse out.

This is made more difficult by virtue of the fact that kids are often hesitant to talk about trauma, which means it can remain hidden for years. Not only that, but researchers have long documented that children exposed to a history of trauma present not only with symptoms of PTSD and anxiety but also with a mix of behavioral disorders, phobias, depressive disorders, and even attentional issues (Famularo, Kinscherff, & Fenton, 1991; Teicher, Glod, Surrey, & Swett, 1993; Ogata, et al., 1990).

This is why it is so important to thoroughly assess for trauma, asking numerous, probing questions about the child's experience of any potentially traumatic events (e.g., abuse, violence, car accidents). One researcher found that just as many kids experience subthreshold PTSD as full PTSD, lending support to the idea that the spectrum of response is as diverse and wide as the range of possible traumatic events (Marshall et al., 2001).

In fact, researchers are now finding that children can experience PTSD merely from living in a violent, chaotic neighborhood or home. Even more interesting, one study in the Oklahoma City area on the effects of the 1995 federal building bombing found that 20% of sixth graders evaluated met criteria for PTSD up to 2 years after the bombing, despite living over 100 miles away and not knowing anyone harmed in the atrocities (Pfefferbaum et al., 2000). Based on current criteria these kids would not meet the diagnosis, as their lives were not at risk or threatened. But let us say without a doubt that their feelings were real: They were traumatized by the media exposure of the event. Not surprisingly, the authors noted that amount and duration of media exposure became a significant predictor of symptomatology. After 9/11, it has become much more clear that the nature of graphic media exposure, time spent viewing, personal connections to the trauma, and parental responses are significant factors in whether children become symptomatic or not. It's up to us to identify it.

Trauma, Media Exposure, and . . . ADHD

If we step back and really examine the signs and symptoms of trauma and PTSD—disorganization, difficulty concentrating, hypervigilance, impairment in school, and hyperarousal—it begins to look like another common ailment in our kids: ADHD. And if trauma can come from anywhere, but most predominantly from watching violent events, as we've learned from the post-9/11 studies and school-based research, it begs several questions: Are all of these things connected somehow? Is exposure to violence traumatizing our kids, giving them PTSD and manifesting itself as ADHD? Has the allostatic load (the cumulative effect of ongoing stressors on the homeostatic response) of media—TV news, violent video games, graphic movies—created some facet of our ADHD epidemic? Is ADHD just one of the many masks of trauma? Is ADHD just a form of PTSD?

Perhaps—PTSD can often present with all of the core features of ADHD. So how do you tell them apart? Often you can't—which backs up the idea that they may be connected, but doesn't really help us solve either clinically. In general, I look for significant sleep disturbance, apprehensiveness, a tendency to worry, family history of anxiety, history of traumatic events, flashbacks, signs of autonomic arousal, and specific fears. The more of these present, the more I consider PTSD the culprit. If there is some ambiguity between the two, treat the trauma and anxiety.

The scientific data, for one thing, certainly support a connection between ADHD-like altered brain functioning (disorganization, attentional problems, hyperarousal) and media exposure, particularly violent video games. Childhood exposure to violent video games, in fact, has been the subject of a heated political controversy in recent years, including a flawed Supreme Court ruling striking down a California ban on a child's ability to buy violent video games.

Politics aside, scientists know that violent video games alter brain function, and not for the good. According to Craig Anderson of Iowa State University and his counterparts in Japan, the level of violence in a game in fact predicts the level of increased aggression down the road for kids, after accounting for baseline differences in aggression (Anderson et al., 2008). One study found that playing video games for 1 week changed brain function in the dorsolateral prefrontal cortex (the center for involuntary inhibition and executive functioning) and the anterior cingulate gyrus (involved in attention) of teens and young men. This change was significant from baseline in those unexposed to violence and, more importantly, it endured for the 1-week washout period after all exposure ended (Birk, 2012). Violent video games have also been shown to desensitize the physiological response to violence (Carnagey, Anderson, & Bushman, 2007). Studies have also found alternations in cortisol and norepinephrine in response to video game exposure.

One experimenter gave subjects a math test and then had them watch either *Shrek* or the first 20 minutes of *Saving Private Ryan* and its horrifically graphic depiction of the D-Day landing. The *Saving Private Ryan* group demonstrated a significant deterioration in their performance after retesting (Beversdorf, 2005). Interestingly, this decay in performance was blocked by propranolol (a beta-blocker that inhibits the impact of epinephrine or adrenaline). The cartoon watchers, on the other hand, scored 39% higher on the retest.

The science is clear: Violent media exposure, particularly video games, alters brain function and chemistry—for the worse—in little kids.

Could the increased exposure to graphic violence, in general, over the last 30 years be a factor in the explosion of ADHD in kids? We can't answer that question definitively, but it makes enough sense, given the neurobiology of exposure to violence, to keep asking questions about it, and perhaps give a commonsense response. It makes more sense to limit kids' exposure to stressors like violent media than it does to stand by and continue to treat an ever-increasing population of highly symptomatic kids.

Adverse Childhood Experiences

The literature on adverse childhood experiences (ACE) provides clear and sobering evidence for the power of early events—no matter how seemingly small or limited—to alter life course. Vince Felitti, a Kaiser physician from San Diego, published the first ACE study in 1998; it measured ACE in seven different categories and explored the health outcomes of over 17,000 people in adulthood (Felitti et al., 1998). The seven categories included psychological abuse, physical abuse, domestic violence, living with a substance abuser, living with mental illness, and living with a felon. Felitti found that children who experienced four or more categories of ACE were four to 12 times more likely to display alcoholism, drug abuse, or suicide attempts as adults. And they were two to four times more likely to smoke, have poor health, or develop sexually transmitted diseases. In the end, the researchers documented a strong relationship between all ACE categories and multiple leading causes of death.

In later research, Felitti found a graded link between the number of ACE categories and the development of heart disease, cancer, lung disease, fractures, and liver disease as an adult (Weber & Baumann, 1988). In one ACE study, researchers explored the relationship of ACE categories to later psychiatric outcomes. They found that the risk of every one of the 18 psychiatric outcomes they selected was directly related to the number of ACE categories the child had experienced. Furthermore, the risk of affective, somatic, substance abuse, memory, sexual, and aggressive disorders increased in graded fashion with the ACE score ($p <$

0.001) (Anda et al., 2006). Other more recent research has established a link between ACE and adolescent or preteen inflammation, which is directly associated with a number of psychiatric ills including depression, as well as the presence of adult sleep disorders (Slopen, Kubzansky, McLaughlin, & Koenen, 2012; Chapman et al., 2011). ACE research is still evolving, but it seems that everywhere you look, researchers are connecting early childhood trauma to negative adult outcome.

More specifically, growing evidence ties early maltreatment to a range of neurological and genetic sequelae that deteriorate the central nervous system, which in turn can disrupt self-regulation and the nervous system's response to adverse events (McCrory et al., 2011). Given the predictable set of risks, it may make sense to screen your little patients sooner rather than later. The ACE survey is quick and easy to use with your own clients (Figure 16.1).

The Pathology of Stress and Trauma

Needless to say, the effects of ACE and PTSD, as well as extreme stress and trauma, reverberate throughout the entire body of the child. As the famous endocrinologist Hans Selye (1956) so elegantly demonstrated, stressful events create significant effects in the hypothalamic-pituitary-adrenal (HPA) axis, with the release of cortisol and epinephrine (adrenaline), which often compounds the trauma, creating a new maladaptive structure of stress response in the body. This also causes, in turn, an imbalance of sympathetic versus parasympathetic response in the autonomic nervous system.

Perhaps the most devastating facet of traumatic events is the potential duration of suffering—the reexperience of trauma can often last the rest of a victim's life. Epigenetic changes in the HPA axis may be to blame. A Canadian researcher, Patrick McGowan, examined suicide victims' brains looking for receptor changes related to the HPA axis. He divided this group into those who had experienced abuse of some kind versus controls with no abuse history. The results found that the abuse group had structural changes in the NR 3CI receptor (McGowan et al., 2009). It appears, the researchers concluded, that abuse creates lifelong epigenetic changes to the receptor deactivating the HPA axis, crucial to neuroendocrine health.

Finding Your ACE Score

While you were growing up, during your first 18 years of life:

1. Did a parent or other adult in the household **often** ...
   Swear at you, insult you, put you down, or humiliate you?
   or
   Act in a way that made you afraid that you might be physically hurt?
   Yes No   If yes enter 1 _____

2. Did a parent or other adult in the household **often** ...
   Push, grab, slap, or throw something at you?
   or
   Ever hit you so hard that you had marks or were injured?
   Yes No   If yes enter 1 _____

3. Did an adult or person at least 5 years older than you **ever** ...
   Touch or fondle you or have you touch their body in a sexual way?
   or
   Try to or actually have oral, anal, or vaginal sex with you?
   Yes No   If yes enter 1 _____

4. Did you **often** feel that ...
   No one in your family loved you or thought you were important or special?
   or
   Your family didn't look out for each other, feel close to each other, or support each other?
   Yes No   If yes enter 1 _____

5. Did you **often** feel that ...
   You didn't have enough to eat, had to wear dirty clothes, and had no one to protect you?
   or
   Your parents were too drunk or high to take care of you or take you to the doctor if you needed it?
   Yes No   If yes enter 1 _____

6. Were your parents **ever** separated or divorced?
   Yes No   If yes enter 1 _____

7. Was your mother or stepmother:
   Often pushed, grabbed, slapped, or had something thrown at her?
   or
   Sometimes or often kicked, bitten, hit with a fist, or hit with something hard?
   or
   Ever repeatedly hit over at least a few minutes or threatened with a gun or knife?
   Yes No   If yes enter 1 _____

8. Did you live with anyone who was a problem drinker or alcoholic or who used street drugs?
   Yes No   If yes enter 1 _____

9. Was a household member depressed or mentally ill or did a household member attempt suicide?
   Yes No   If yes enter 1 _____

10. Did a household member go to prison?
    Yes No   If yes enter 1 _____

Now add up your "Yes" answers: _____ This is your ACE Score.

Figure 16.1. Adverse Childhood Experience Questionnaire.

(Courtesy of Kaiser Permanente and the Centers for Disease Control and Prevention)

Research like this demonstrates the way in which childhood abuse can trigger enduring dysregulation of the stress hormone response system. Moreover, perturbations of this system are one of the most common neurobiological abnormalities found in PTSD sufferers, and the research offers insight into why the effects often last for decades. Early life stress in childhood has also been linked to increased risk of PTSD. Epigenetic changes making the child more susceptible to a poor stress response may be responsible.

Trauma in utero may also create lasting change via epigenetics. In 1998, Quebec endured a heinous ice storm, leaving the region under an impassable sheet of ice two and a half inches thick in some places. The area was crippled for weeks and many suffered injury and death. Researchers isolated and studied a group of pregnant women who endured the storm (Laplante et al., 2004). After they gave birth, the researchers identified a 10-point loss in IQ in the group's children at the age of 5. Those mothers who experienced the ice storm during the first half of their pregnancy had children with higher anxiety, depression, and aggression.

Bruce Perry has documented the devastating effects of severe childhood trauma and abuse on children's brains. His work details the neuroanatomical effects of trauma and abuse. According to Perry, it distorts and inhibits the development of the amygdala (modulation of emotional tone), the corpus callosum (communication between the right and left hemispheres), and the neocortex (abstract thinking) (Perry & Pollard, 1998; Perry, 2006). Perhaps the most profound damage occurs in the hippocampus, crucial for new memory formation. Much of the damage comes from chronically elevated levels of cortisol, which acts as a neurotoxin in the developing brain.

These structural changes alter the learning, experience, and attachment of the affected child. All in all, the crucial take-away is that while trauma and abuse in an adult may alter the developed brain in significant and damaging ways, those experiences in a child alter the more plastic, receptive developing brain. This sad truth must be appreciated if we are to help affected kids.

Trauma damages all developmental tracts: speech, motor, social, emotional, and behavioral. Each brain region, of course, has its own separate timeline of development, and, because synaptogenesis and other microdevelopmental processes are most active in different brain regions at different times, the disruptive effects of trauma can occur during sensitive developmental periods. In this way, for the young child, the timing of stress and trauma are very important. If a traumatic event occurs during a time of critical motor and speech development, for instance, those areas will be most affected.

The brain largely develops in four anatomical regions: from the bottom (brain stem) to the top (cortex), and from the inside (midbrain) out (limbic system). It is 80% organized by the age of 3.

Bruce Perry has created a brain map that outlines the damage and consequent impact of trauma on the growing child. He calls this the neurosequential model (Perry, 2006). In this model, Perry lays out a four-step process for normal brain development for the first decade of life, each step building on the previous one:

1. Brain stem: Establish physiological regulation.
2. Midbrain: Establish somatosensory integration.
3. Limbic system: Establish emotional regulation.
4. Neocortex: Encourage problem solving and abstract thinking.

Trauma or extreme stress can derail any of these steps and leave the child's brain damaged. These events can be a specific episode of trauma or a series of events. Family conflict, for instance, whether episodic or consistent, can qualify. Surprisingly unpredictable events may predispose the child even more to a traumatic reaction. Luckily, there is hope.

Treating Trauma

In my career, I have spent about 20 years working as medical director and child psychiatrist for various residential treatment centers (RTCs) for children, teens, and young adults. About 15 years of that time was spent in RCTs for severely abused young children aged 3 to 12. Most of these children had severe PTSD, often from experiences at the hands of their drug-addicted, criminal parents.

The children typically arrived from a hospital where they had been admitted for severe aggression or out-of-control behavior. Each child carried a long list of diagnostic labels: bipolar, depression, ADHD, reactive attachment disorder, intermittent explosive disorder, anxiety, disruptive disorder, and so on. The average child arrived with four or five labels, but some had as many as 12 or 15. These kids were typically on neuroleptics to control aggression and violence, but many were also on mood stabilizers and stimulants. It was rare that any child arrived without a long list of medication trials and current medications.

Most often, on arrival from the hospital the child would be heavily sedated on antipsychotics, even though there were no psychotic symptoms or diagnosis. As numerous studies have demonstrated, the vast majority of neuroleptic use in children is for nonpsychotic presentations. Why? The short answer is that these medications are sedative; they make these tough kids easier to manage.

The medications were only really effective in sedating the kids, which simply buried their trauma. They slept and ate excessively, yet failed to learn, develop, or communicate—in short, heal—in any substantive way. After a period of time, the medications would wear off and the target problems—aggression, rage, irritability, mood swings, overarousal—would inevitably return.

As the research demonstrates, we have no effective psychopharmacological intervention for kids suffering from trauma. It is not a simple neurochemical problem; it is a complex, relational, personal, whole-body problem. In fact, there is a relatively small reservoir of research on the topic of childhood PTSD, and there seem to be few interventions that actually work.

One day, the director of Child and Family Services at North Range Behavioral Health (the community mental health center for Weld County, Colorado), Dave Rastatter, asked me to take over as medical director for a residential treatment center that was at risk of losing its funding over complaints of excessive restraint use, seclusion practices, and overuse of medications. I agreed, but with one caveat. I had to have free rein to design a new treatment model for the traumatized kids.

At this RTC (and another in Larimer County), I worked with an enlightened group of women, Joanna Martinson, Cyndi Dodds, and Sheryl Zeigler, among others, to dramatically shift our approach to traumatized kids. In a challenging transition, we converted the program from an old-school power and control model in which transgressions were punished with seclusion, restraint, and medication to an approach built on Bruce Perry's neuroanatomical work. Its basis was secure, warm relationships with staff and the promotion of self-regulation. We quickly put in place a four-tiered program based on developmental stages:

1. Establish physiological regulation (brain stem): In this step, we focus on calming human touch, breath work, calming music, relaxation exercises, and other soothing techniques.
2. Establish somatosensory integration (midbrain): We work with movement therapy, Brain Gym, drumming, yoga, acupuncture, and EMDR.
3. Facilitate emotional regulation (limbic system): We employ art therapy, playtime, nature walks, and a practice we called "time-in," where each kid gets one-on-one time with an adult.
4. Encourage abstract thought (neocortex): Here, we utilize things like storytelling, role modeling, and problem solving.

We adapted this model to the needs of each kid. The biggest challenge was shifting away from a model of punishment. "You mean we can't hold them responsible for their actions?" was a common response from the staff during the implementation of my program. It wasn't that we were no longer holding children responsible for their behavior—we were, in some sense—but it was more important to discontinue punishing action.

Typically, punishment for these kids just perpetuates their cycle of trauma, dysregulation, and suffering. Traumatized kids can barely self-regulate, in any sense of the word, let alone internalize and process punishment as a lesson. So the first step had to be geared toward self-regulation, and that meant spending many hours in intimate contact with them, calming them down and helping them slowly process their aggressions or outbursts, instead of just isolating and punishing them. We learned that when these kids were agitated they could not process any information or learn. So we waited and calmed them down.

Another important step was changing nutrition. All of the kids subsisted on junk food, candy, and processed meals. So I implemented a nutritional plan based on a whole foods and high-protein intake shown to improve school performance.

Finally, we de-emphasized medications progressively, slowly reducing all the kids' intake. Over time, we were able to achieve incredible results. Our seclusion and restraint numbers fell from around 90 a month in our 24-bed facility to between five and eight. Our use of medications fell to around 30% of prior numbers. In the new program, kids were finally learning; they were developing and growing like they should. Ultimately, the new program was much more satisfying for our staff, but it was not without its many challenges. In this model, you do have less control; at times you have to tolerate a lot of chaos.

The RTC, in a relatively short window of time, went from nearly shutting down to being recognized by the state of Colorado for our therapeutic achievements. The program worked; kids got better; they were healing from their trauma. We had shorter and shorter durations of stay as we fine-tuned and streamlined the program. It was a success in every sense of the word.

Except for one.

In a sad twist of irony, since kids were getting healthier quicker, and keeping our beds in rotation, our per diem payments from the state dwindled. On top of that, decreases in Medicaid reimbursement and state budget cuts put pressure on mental health centers all around the state. And with that, the vast majority of children's RTCs in Colorado, including ours, closed.

Nevertheless, we had found a program that worked: We recognized the barriers presented by stress and trauma and supported kids' development, and so got them better. We helped them move through their trauma, and most of them went on to live happy and healthy lives.

As our work demonstrates, trauma creates a body-wide problem that cannot be solved by a solitary mental (talk therapy) or neuronal (medication) approach. Consistent with PTSD, the approach needs to honor wholeness and treat the sufferer's body, mind, and soul with an integrative approach.

First, work to reduce anxiety and manage stress in the home. Does it make sense to treat the child with inositol if the home is a chaotic mess of turmoil and conflict? Not really. The treatment will be fighting an uphill battle. Start with family dynamics and move out to each individual relationship from there. Address the mental health of the parents and help them to reduce stress: A child's ability to manage a traumatic event is directly related to how well the parents manage traumatic events. In fact, a parent's mental health and coping responses are directly tied to the response of children and the development of posttraumatic symptoms (Wilson, Lengua, Meltzoff, & Smith, 2010). This is either very good news or very bad news, depending on the family. Whatever is the case, if trauma is found in the child's history, family-wide support needs to be buttressed.

Teach the child. Children with PTSD need to be in a counseling environment. This should be evocative and psychoeducational. The child needs to learn about stress and needs to learn how to handle conflict. Trauma-based CBT is a great cognitive tool to manage the effects of trauma.

Treat the HPA axis. Yoga, biofeedback, meditation, and guided imagery are all excellent tools to reset the child's strained HPA axis. Acupuncture is proven to address the physiological disruptions of PTSD, but should really be used only on older kids (12 and up), if the child is inclined.

Consider EMDR to help process the stressful event. It's a well-proven tool that helps children digest their trauma and stop reexperiencing the event in a loop of nightmares, fear, and paranoia. Also consider a somatic-oriented therapy that bridges body and mind and helps soothe the soul. Somatic Experiencing or Hakomi are two emerging psychotherapies that I have found very helpful. Monitor and remove media violence from the child's daily experience, as it will help to clear the child's mind of traumatic imagery. For those moving into the teen years, a thoughtful discussion about violence and regular exposure is an important detail.

Clean up the diet with whole foods; eliminate caffeine; reduce sugar and glycemic load. Explore for food allergies that may magnify symptoms. For additional dietary support, supplement with inositol (3–6 g daily) and L-theanine (200–400 mg three times daily). Lemon balm, valerian, or California poppy are three herbals that may help this process as well. If sleep is a problem, consider melatonin (0.5–1 mg at night) or magnesium (100–300 mg twice daily), which can help agitation and sleep.

In war-torn Kosovo, Jim Gordon developed a clinically useful program for teens with PTSD. He studied the value of a 12-session group protocol that employed training in meditation, guided imagery, breath work, and self-expression through words, drawing, music, or movement as well as biofeedback and genograms. Trained high school teachers taught the program to the teens. The effect on PTSD symptom scores was significant compared to controls and was maintained at 3 months postintervention (Gordon, Staples, Blyta, Bytyqi, & Wilson, 2008). This is but one example of what can be done to help the most severe cases of pediatric PTSD. It's a program that builds on education and skills. And it's teachable. Our kids can get over PTSD, but only if we provide the skills. Wholeness will take it from there.

Treatment Plan: Step by Step

1. Comprehensive evaluation of child's six realms (see Chapter 6) and common presenting issues (see Chapter 7).
2. Identify barriers, deficiencies, strengths, and gifts. Consider ACE Screen (see Figure 16.1) if suspicious of traumatic events.
3. Examine the child for diet issues, food quality, food allergies, or gut issues. Consider a gluten-free trial. Remove all caffeine. Refer to a nutritionist or naturopath as needed.
4. Examine for family conflict, depressed or overwhelmed parents, oppositional behavior, marital stress, or poor communication. Consider family therapy or a Nurtured Heart–type program.
5. If the child is depressed, anxious, or traumatized refer for individual therapy. If already in therapy, contact prior or current therapist for background and collaboration.
6. Lab testing: Check TSH, vitamin D (25 OH), ferritin, lipid profile (low cholesterol), and HS CRP. Treat abnormalities as they appear. Consider DHEA-sulfate and salivary cortisols for adrenal assessment.
7. Explore sleep issues. Most traumatized children sleep poorly and may need help from melatonin and/or other agents. Rule out sleep apnea.
8. Consider EMDR and/or trauma-based CBT.
9. Add supplements to reduce ambient anxiety such as inositol and L-theanine and/or herbals.
10. Consider adding biofeedback using heart rate variability to calm.
11. Add mind-body skills such as meditation or yoga for lifelong stress reduction and autonomic balance.
12. If older, consider acupuncture.

Daniel

Daniel came to my office over 20 years ago when I was fresh out of my child psychiatry fellowship and he was 10. He had all the hallmarks of pediatric bipolar disorder: episodes of rage, sleep dysregulation, high energy, irritability, labile mood, extreme aggression, and hypersexuality. His behavior drove his single mom, Pam, to my office after he chased her through the house with a kitchen knife. At wits' end, his school also pleaded with me to do something to stop him from throwing chairs. Pam appeared exhausted from the strain of protecting her 7-year-old daughter, Chloe, from Daniel's wild aggression and unpredictability.

In my interview with Daniel, he radiated excitement as he explored my office, leaving a wake of clutter and disarray behind him. The dark-haired boy was so distracted that it was difficult to engage him in any way. Daniel seemed to be two steps ahead of whatever we did or discussed. His mood, at that time, was almost euphoric. There was no evidence of sadness, trauma, bullying, or abuse. The family history was positive for mood disorders in two close relatives; his father had a history of mood swings but had been out of the picture for many years. At the end of our time together, I was exhausted and immediately empathized with his mother and her Sisyphean task of managing this young, wild boy.

At that time in my career, I felt comfortable with the diagnosis of pediatric bipolar disorder. (I have since grown much more cautious.) Daniel responded well to Depakote and Mellaril. His behavior improved dramatically: He began to sleep well, lost his aggression, and turned his school performance around. After 3 months, I felt satisfied that Daniel was on the road to recovery.

One morning a month or two later, however, I got a disturbing phone call from Daniel's mom. "Daniel was sexually abused by a neighbor kid who is 8 years older," she told me. "A few days ago, the kid was caught abusing another boy in the neighborhood and was arrested. When I heard about this I remembered that some time back the same kid had taken an interest in Daniel and spent some time with him. So I asked Daniel about the kid. Daniel started crying when I mentioned his name and told me that the kid sexually abused and threatened him. I don't know what to do—I'm devastated, Dr. Shannon."

Over the next 5 months, the entire story came out in the open bit by bit. It became clear to me through the details of Daniel's story that many, or perhaps all, of his symptoms were related to the horrific series of events that had befallen him. He was a wounded little boy. So I weaned Daniel off his medications over the next 9 months while he went into trauma-focused care.

Daniel was pivotal. He shifted my awareness. Daniel was not bipolar; he was traumatized. Trauma can and does manifest as any psychiatric illness. Because of this, I call it the great masquerader. I shudder to think how Daniel's case would have turned out had his abuser not been identified.

EPILOGUE

The complexity of the human brain creates an awareness, behavior, and psychology that vary enormously from person to person. Our nutrition, neuroplasticity, and epigenetic machinery create an individual biochemistry that becomes more unique as we age. In some ways it would seem that the depth of knowledge required to address mental illness would be prohibitively expansive. However, thanks to the innate wisdom found in the idea of "wholeness," a different path is available to all of us.

As this book has shown, the paradigm of wholeness carries with it a few valuable lessons that serve our children well.

First, this perspective empowers parents and families. Contrary to the notion that the most valuable tools of mental health are secrets of technology, medicine, or arcane psychology or psychiatric teachings, we can view mental wellness as being grounded in the commonsense wisdom that most of our grandmothers possessed: good food, sleep, exercise, loving relationships, and balance in all things. This is not to say that wholeness implies a Luddite-like avoidance of technology or a nihilistic attitude toward invasive treatment; it merely tempers the enthusiasm of psychopharmacology with some perspective and embraces the benefits of alternative approaches, like neurofeedback, that enhance the growth of a "plastic" brain. Showing children and their families a range of ways to embrace well-being is the ultimate goal. Once we begin to share this approach more widely, parents will have a better sense of the lifestyle choices that will best launch their young ones.

A second beneficial consequence of the wholeness approach is its overarching emphasis on inclusion and integration. Wholeness makes room for all of the existing knowledge and data that we have accumulated on psychodynamics, psychopharmacology, development, and neurobiology. It merely offers context and perspective to guide clinical assessment and decision making. In some ways, wholeness provides an attitude and philosophy from which to filter all of the science and research every time we evaluate a young person sitting in front of us. It is clearly not a cure-all but rather a guidance system to operate from. It helps us better organize and apply the information that we already possess.

Last, a perspective of wholeness allows us to more easily identify the triggers at the root of many mental illnesses: adverse childhood experiences, stress, poor nutrition, and so on. Understanding an individual's triggers and barriers to mental wellness is invaluable, as is the need to address them preventatively so we don't end up offering treatments purely as damage control.

We face a new reality: The complexity of our biological intelligence far outstrips our feeble attempts to understand, much less master it. If we take a step back, we can see the "ecological" web—the myriad factors that influence and form who we are and how we behave. In our quest to treat and heal our patients as best we can, this is a step toward humility, but also optimism. The truth is, as mental heath practitioners, our job is not to cure the disordered complexities of the brain or to know better than biology but to remove barriers to health, add support, and foster the biological intelligence found in each and every child.

Love is what brought us to this work. We remain enamored of the beauty, purity, and potential found in each and every young person we encounter. However, love alone is not sufficient for the challenges of mental health. Unconditional love may be the most powerful healing force on earth, but many things can undermine its power and potential. Otherwise, grandparents might put us out of work. We may love the child in front of us, but we must also learn to appreciate the nature of wholeness, for that allows us to be of greatest service to each child, to each person that we encounter.

On one level this book is about children and mental health, on another it is about wholeness—the intelligence of nature. We must leverage our love with the insights of wholeness. Only that can heal our children. Just as consciousness springs forth as a natural extension of the life force, so too does unconditional love manifest all that we are and the nature of our universe. Our deepest challenge is to appreciate that complexity, embrace our nature, and love it most fully. We all walk together on this journey.

Sample Intake and Assessment Form

Tell Me About Your Child

Please list your child's strengths: _____
_____
_____

Diagnoses or explanations given to you about your child: _____
_____
_____

Being as descriptive as possible, please describe your child to me (attach a sheet if necessary): _____
_____
_____

When did you first notice your child's problems: _____
_____

What things did you first notice: _____
_____
_____

Was the onset of your child's problem sudden or gradual: _____
Was there any event or action that you or others think might have contributed to your child's symptoms (be as detailed as possible): _____
_____
_____
_____
_____

Current Living Situation

Who is the child presently living with (e.g., biological mother, stepfather): _____
_____

How many people currently live in the household? _____
Are there currently any significant marital stressors? Yes / No *If so, please briefly explain:*

_____
_____

Is this child adopted? Yes / No *If so, please briefly describe the age of the child when adopted and the circumstances of the adoption:* _____

_____

Parents

How long have the child's parents been: Married:_____ Separated: _____
Divorced: _____ Living together: _____
If the parents are separated or divorced, please describe custody (physical and legal) and visitation rights: _____

_____

If married, describe current relationship (e.g., supportive, conflictual): _____

_____

Please list any previous marriages: _____

_____

Biological Mother

Name: _____ Age: _____
Highest grade completed: _____ Occupation: _____
Do any medical illnesses run in the biological mother's family (e.g., thyroid, diabetes, seizures, movement problems such as tics or other neurological problems, allergies)?_____

_____

_____

Has the biological mother or any of her relatives experienced any of the following psychological or emotional difficulties? *Please circle the difficulty and then list the person who has or had the problem.*

Depression _____ Autism_____
Suicide or attempt(s) _____ Mental retardation_____
Anxiety disorders _____ Attention difficulties_____
Psychosis or thought problems _____ Learning disabilities_____
Aggressive or violent behaviors _____ Physical or sexual abuse_____
Alcohol abuse _____ Other substance abuse_____
Social difficulties _____ Legal trouble_____
Other _____

Biological Father

Name: _____ Age: _____
Highest grade completed: _____ Occupation: _____
Has the biological father or any of his relatives experienced any of the following psychological or emotional difficulties? *Please circle the difficulty and then list the person who has or had the problem.*

Depression _____ Autism_____
Suicide or attempt(s) _____ Mental retardation_____
Anxiety disorders_____Attention difficulties_____
Psychosis or thought problems _____ Learning disabilities_____
Aggressive or violent behaviors _____ Physical or sexual abbuse_____
Alcohol abuse _____ Other substance abuse_____
Social difficulties _____ Legal trouble_____
Other _____

Siblings

Name	Age	Blood or Step Sibling	In Home?
_____	____	_____	Yes / No
_____	____	_____	Yes / No
_____	____	_____	Yes / No
_____	____	_____	Yes / No
_____	____	_____	Yes / No

Have any of the siblings experienced psychological or emotional problems (suicide or suicide attempts, attention or learning difficulties, legal problems, alcohol or substance abuse, social difficulties, or medical problems)? If so, please state who and the nature of the problem. _____
_____

Please list (current or past) significant areas of conflict in the home between this child and others. _____
_____
_____

Birth History

Mother's age at time of birth: ___ Years   Father's age at time of birth: ___ Years

Did the mother smoke during the pregnancy? Yes / No *If so, how many cigarettes per day?*_____

Was alcohol consumed during pregnancy? Yes / No *If so, what was the amount per day?*_____

Were any drugs used during the pregnancy? Yes / No *If so, list the name of the drug and amount:*_____

How many ultrasounds during pregnancy: _____

Was the child premature? Yes / No   Number of weeks late:_____ Number of weeks early:_____

Was the biological mother under anesthesia during childbirth? Yes / No

If yes, local, spinal, or general: _____

Was the delivery unusual in any way? Yes / No *If yes, please explain:* _____

_____

_____

Did the biological mother have a cesarean? Yes / No *If yes, please describe complications:* _____

_____

Was this baby normally active? Yes / No   Baby's birth weight: _____

Apgar scores_____

Were any birth defects evident? Yes / No *If yes, please describe:* _____

_____

How many days was the infant in the hospital after delivery? _____

Any dietary restrictions during pregnancy: Yes / No *If yes, please explain:* _____

_____

Please add any comments regarding your pregnancy or delivery: _____

_____

Infancy Period

Child Breast-fed: Yes / No For how long: _____ When put on formula: _____

Did the mother have problems with depression after birth? Yes / No *If yes, please briefly describe:* _____

_____

_____

Did either parent have significant problems adjusting after the birth? Yes / No

If yes, please briefly describe: _____

_____

Describe any physical or emotional separations from the caregivers in the first few years of life:

_____

_____

Circle all that apply:

Jaundice as a baby	Y / N	Colic	Y / N
Cradle cap	Y / N	Anemia	Y / N
Eczema or psoriasis	Y / N	Stomachaches	Y / N
Diarrhea	Y / N	Asthma	Y / N
Constipation	Y / N	Warts	Y / N
Finicky eating	Y / N	Nightmares	Y / N
Poor teeth	Y / N	Bed-wetting	Y / N
Chronic sniffles	Y / N	Excessive tantrums	Y / N
Bad foot odor	Y / N	Defiant	Y / N
Very sweaty	Y / N	Fears/phobias	Y / N
Hyperactivity	Y / N	Diaper rash	Y / N
Growing pains	Y / N	Early puberty	Y / N

Developmental History

Motor development (sitting, crawling, walking)	Average	Early	Late
Speech and language	Average	Early	Late
Self-help skills (dressing, brushing, hygiene, etc.)	Average	Early	Late
Bowel trained	Average	Early	Late
Bladder trained	Average	Early	Late
Started to read	Average	Early	Late

First words: _____

First phrases or sentences, give age as well: _____

Coordination

Handedness: Left / Right / Both

Rate this child on the following skills: Good / Average / Poor

Writing: _____ _____ _____

Athletic abilities: _____ _____ _____

Does this child have an excessive number of accidents compared to other children? Yes / No *If yes, please describe:*

_____

_____

_____

Environmental Exposures

Has the child ever lived near a refinery, polluted area, or in a home with lead paint? If so, what sort of pollution was the child exposed to: _____

_____

_____

Has the child ever lived in a house that had new carpeting, paint, cabinets, or any other refurbishing that seemed to affect the child's health? _____

_____

Does the child seem particularly sensitive to perfumes, gasoline, or other vapors?

_____

Do you spray pesticides, herbicides, or other chemicals around your home? ____

_____

What year was your home/apartment built? _____

Do you have vinyl blinds, and what year were they put in? _____

Water: City / Well   H2O Purification System: Yes / No   Air Purifiers: Yes / No

Type of heat: Gas / Electric If other please describe: _____

If you live near water list type: Swamp / River / Ocean If other please describe:

_____

Do you live near: High Voltage Power Lines / Refinery / Woods / Industrial Area:

_____

Describe child's bedroom (curtains, blinds, carpet, feather pillows, etc.): _____

_____

_____

Flooring in other rooms your child spends time in: _____

_____

_____

Behaviors, Moods, and Attitudes
(Infancy, Toddler, Preschool)

Circle all that apply:

Adaptable	Sleeping difficulties	Curious
Rocking	Responds well to challenges	Temper outbursts
Able to play alone	Moody	Overactive/into everything
Difficulty with attention	Easily frustrated	Angry
Impulsive	Aggressive/violent	Staring spells
Easy to manage	Obsessive or compulsive	Breath-holding spells
Underactive/passive	Sensitive or empathic	Difficulties in interactions with others

Deals well with frustration	Wants to be left alone	Happy
Stubborn	More interested in things than people	Affectionate
Daredevil	Playful	Head banging
Eating difficulties	Severe tantrums	Stuttering/speech problems
Difficulty with changes	Slow to warm up	Sad
Cautious	Overwhelmed by challenges	Irritable
Shy or timid	Fearful	

Were any of the following present, to a significant degree, during the first year of life? *If so, please describe:*

Did not enjoy cuddling: _____

Was not calmed by being held: _____

Was difficult to comfort: _____

Was colicky: _____

Was excessively restless: _____

Was excessively irritable: _____

Experienced sleep difficulties: _____

Experienced difficulty with nursing or food: _____

Current Behaviors, Moods, Attitudes

How would you describe this child's conscience? Normal / Lax / Harsh / Preoccupied with issues

Do you have any concerns about this child's: (*If yes, please describe*)

Self-esteem? Yes / No _____

Sexual knowledge or awareness? Yes / No _____

Gender identity? Yes / No _____

Sexual orientation? Yes / No _____

Please circle any of the following that this child has problems with (currently or in the past):

Bed-wetting	Immaturity	Hallucinations
Involuntary vocalizations	Secretive	Alcohol abuse
Obsessive-compulsive behaviors	Crying episodes	Other substance abuse
Depression	Sexual problems	Strange ideas or behaviors
Soiling	Anxiety	Impulsiveness
Significant weight change	Panic	Explosive episodes
Self-conscious	Extreme moodiness	Property destruction

Embarrassed	Irritability	Self-destructive behaviors
Shy	Anger	Running away
Withdrawn	Lying	Aggression
Sleep problems	Stealing	Violence
Oppositional defiant	Cruelty to animals	Frequent accidents
Frequent arguing	Setting fires	Suicidal talk or behaviors
Fearful	Poor motivation	Guilt
Eating problems	Change in personality	Hopelessness
Suspicious	Distrustful	Other:_____

Please list the types of discipline you have tried with this child and their effectiveness: _____

_____

_____

_____

Please note any of the following significant events that have occurred within your family and briefly describe:

Death of a family member or significant person: _____

_____

Significant move: _____

_____

Comprehension and Understanding

Do you consider this child to understand directions and situations as well as other children his/her age? Yes / No *If not, please explain:* _____

_____

If this child tells a story about a show, event, etc., do you or others have difficulty understanding him/her? Yes / No *If yes, is it because he/she (circle all that apply):*

Appears confused   Leaves out important information   Has trouble finding the right
Is disorganized   Loses train of thought   words

Does this child have trouble remembering things that he/she really cares about? Yes / No

Please describe: _____

_____

_____

Does this child have difficulty following routines (bedtime, dressing, etc.)?
Yes / No
Please describe: _____

_____

_____

Does this child frequently lose things or have trouble being organized?
Yes / No
Please describe: _____

_____

_____

How would you rate this child's overall level of intelligence compared to other children?   Above average / Average / Below average

Free Time

Please describe how this child generally spends her/his free time (e.g., plays alone, plays with friends, plays sports, watches TV, plays video games): _____

_____

Please list the approximate number of hours per day that this child watches TV and list the type(s) of shows watched: _____

_____

Please list the approximate number of hours per day that this child plays video games and list the type(s) of games played: _____

_____

Independent Activities

Please describe this child's ability to function in an independent manner:

_____

_____

School History

Did this child attend day care or preschool? Yes / No *If yes, please estimate approximately how many hours per week:* _____
What are your current care arrangements for this child before and after school?

_____

_____

Beginning with kindergarten, list school and indicate performance:

		Academic Performance			Behavioral Performance		
Grade	School	Good	Fair	Poor	Good	Fair	Poor
KG	_____						
1st	_____						
2nd	_____						
3rd	_____						
4th	_____						
5th	_____						
6th	_____						
7th	_____						
8th	_____						
9th	_____						
10th	_____						
11th	_____						
12th	_____						

Are there any known learning disabilities?   Yes / No *If yes, please list:*_____

_____

_____

Has this child been in any special programs (speech, reading, occupational therapy, etc.)? Yes / No *If yes, please explain and list grades:* _____

_____

_____

Has this child ever had to repeat a grade? Yes / No *If yes, please explain:* _____

_____

_____

Current Academic Performance

Excellent   Good   Satisfactory   Unsatisfactory   Failing

Does this child enjoy school?   Yes / No

School subject strengths: _____

_____

School subject weaknesses: _____

_____

Circle any of the following problems this child has with school:

Problems with written language	Difficulty being quiet	Does not complete classroom work
Poor handwriting	Interferes with others' tasks	Fails to check homework

Poor at spelling	Poor at math	Difficulties in groups
Poor reader	Requires additional supervision	Test anxiety
Does not remain seated	Talks inappropriately	Does not do homework
Frequently sent out of class	Makes careless mistakes	Difficulties with peers
Too withdrawn or passive	Daydreams	Poor attention
Impulsive	Messy and disorganized	Excessive time to complete assignments
Forgets instructions	Noncompliant in class	Oppositional with teachers
Skips school		

Is this child involved in extracurricular activities? Yes / No *If yes, please describe:* ___

_____

_____

Any additional comments regarding school functions? _____

_____

_____

_____

_____

_____

Peer Relationships

Does this child seek friendships with peers?   Yes / No

Is this child sought by peers for friendship?   Yes / No

Circle any of the following which describes this child's interactions with peers:

Plays well in groups	Trouble making friends	Bossy and controlling, teasing
Teased by other kids	Loses friends	Jealous
No problems	No friends	Bragging/boastful
Cooperative	Few friends	Uncooperative
Supportive	Rejected by other kids	Feelings get hurt easily
Shares well	Easily led by others	Involved in risky or dangerous behavior
Plays primarily with younger	Aggressive or mean	Involved in alcohol or substance abuse
Plays primarily with older	Frequent arguments	Involved in delinquent behavior
	Frequent fights	

Child's Medical History

If this child's medical history includes any of the following, please note the age when the incident or illness occurred and any other pertinent information.

Hospitalizations: _____   Encephalitis: _____
Operations: _____   Eye problems: _____
Handicaps or deformities: _____   Hearing problems: _____
Failure to grow: _____   Anemia: _____
Pneumonia: _____   Stomach problems: _____
Asthma: _____   Constipation: _____
Allergies: _____   Poisoning: _____
Diabetes: _____   Whooping cough: _____
Skin problems: _____   Rubeola: _____
Multiple ear infections: _____   Bronchitis:_____
Tubes placed: _____   Rubella: _____
Seizures: _____   Chicken pox: _____
Persistent high fevers: _____   Mumps:_____
Obesity: _____   Mono: _____
Movement problems (tics, repetitive   Thrush: _____
movements, etc.): _____   Sinus infection: _____
Head injury: _____   Frequent colds: _____
Other physical trauma: _____   Strep throat: _____
Coma: _____   Other: _____

Has this child ever had a neurological evaluation (exam, MRI, CAT scan, EEG, etc.)? Yes / No *If so, please describe:*_____

_____

Has this child's vision been tested?   Normal Date: _____
Has this child's hearing been tested?   Normal Date: _____

Vaccination History

Yes, has had; No, has not; Some, did not finish all shots
If possible please include a copy of your child's vaccination papers
MMR: Yes No Some   DPT: Yes No Some   Hep B: Yes No Some
Hib: Yes No Some   Chicken Pox: Yes No Some   Polio: Yes No Some

Child's Present Nutrition Status

Height: _____ Weight: _____
Describe this child's appetite and diet: _____

_____

_____

_____

Check the most appropriate description below of your child's diet:

____ Mostly baby foods   ____ Mostly meat

____ Mostly carbohydrates (bread, pasta, etc.)   ____ Mostly vegetarian

____ Mostly dairy (cheese, milk, yogurt)   ____ Other: _____

Have you tried any dietary modifications with your child, and what were the results?_____

_____

_____

Any known allergies to food: Y / N *If yes, what foods and when were they tested?*_____

_____

Please describe your child's stool pattern, frequency, and consistency (e.g., daily, foul, large, mushy, brown): _____

_____

Child's Present Medical Status

Present care doctor: _____

May we contact him/her if needed?   Yes / No

List any present illness(es) for which this child is being treated:_____

_____

_____

What was the date of this child's last physical exam? _____

Was blood work done?   Y / N _____

List all medications (from drugstore or prescription) child is on now and dosages if known:

1) _____   4) _____

2) _____   5) _____

3) _____   6) _____

List all supplements child is now taking, and dosages if known:

1) _____   4) _____

2) _____   5) _____

3) _____   6) _____

Any known allergies to drugs, environment, animals: _____

_____

Does this child frequently complain of: (*Please check all that apply.*)

Headaches	Tiredness	Trouble with vision
Dizziness	Difficulty breathing	Trouble hearing
Sleep problems	Painful urination	Menstrual problems
Nightmares	Chest pain	Skin problems
Stomachaches	Palpitations	

How does this child sleep at night? _____

_____

_____

Previous Treatments

Has this child ever received any type of psychiatric, psychological, or academic evaluation or treatment?   Yes / No *If so, please fill in the following:*

Person or Institution   Dates   Address   Telephone

_____   _____   _____   _____

_____   _____   _____   _____

_____   _____   _____   _____

Signs and Symptoms of Your Child

Please check the box that applies

Description	Mild	Moderate	Severe	Duration	Details
Repetitive movements					
Rocking					
Head banging					
Self-mutilation					
Nail biting					
Skin picking					
Aggressiveness					
Mood swings					
Tantrums					
Fears/anxieties					
Hyperactivity					
Lack of concen-tration					
Fidgety in seat					
Impulsive					

Breath holding					
Dizziness					
Seizures					
Poor coordination					
Social problems					
Sensitive to crowds					
Weak memory					
Low self-esteem					
Fatigue					
Cold hands/feet					
Cold intolerant					
Heat intolerant					
Frequent fever					
Flushing					
Insomnia					
Nightmares					
Difficulty waking					
Bed-wetting					
Daytime wetting/soiling					
Numbness in extremities					
Headache					
Blinking					
Tics					
Eye discharge					
Dark circles around eyes					
Congestion					
Dripping nose					
Sensitive to light					

Difficult eating					
Food cravings					
Grinding teeth					
Mucus in stools					
Blood in stools					
Anal itching					
Tremors					
Calf cramps					
Stiffness					
Eczema					
Hives					
Acne					
Rashes					
Easy bruising					
Itchy scalp					
Dry skin					
Oily skin					
Strong body odor					
Soft nails					
White spots on nails					
OCD					
Reflux					
Persistent colic					
Toe walking					
Nosebleeds					
Bad breath					
Sore throats					
Hoarseness					
Cough					
Wheezing					
Geographic tongue					

Psoriasis					
Rough skin					

Spiritual Orientation

Please list your family's spiritual orientation or religion: _____

_____

How active are these beliefs in your life? Very active / Somewhat active / Not very active

If you like, share some of your thoughts on your spiritual practice/religion: _____

_____
_____
_____
_____
_____
_____

Other Questions

Please list any questions you would like the physician to address during this appointment:

_____
_____
_____
_____
_____
_____

Assessment Sheet:
Collaborative Treatment

Date:_____

Patient:_____ Age_____

Chief complaint:_____

Potential tools_____

Current barriers_____

Severity (rate 1 to 4)_____

Safety issues (rate 1 to 4)_____

Engagement (rate 1 to 4)_____

Resources (rate 1 to 4)_____

Treatment foci (circle all relevant)

     1. Family harmony

     2. Relationships and social skills

     3. Stress management

     4. Healthy diet

     5. Active lifestyle

     6. Sound sleep

     7. Peace and serenity

     8. Joy and satisfaction

     9. Ease of learning

    10. Ideal weight

    11. Spirituality

    12. Gut health

    13. Focus and concentration

    14. Trauma recovery

    15. Thought clarity

    16. Nonaddictive lifestyle

    17. Pain-free living

    18. Inflammation and toxic overload

    19. Obsession and compulsion free

    20. Metabolic concerns

    21. Mood regulation

    22. Behavioral cooperation

    23. Other health concerns

Primary Focus: mental health_____Primary Focus: medical_____

Primary diagnosis code for chart:_____

Follow-up (circle best fit): 1. Psychiatrist 2. Naturopath 3. Both 4. Physician
                                                                        Assistant

Follow-up visit: _____ weeks

Other referrals:_____

GLOSSARY

5-HTP (5-hydroxytryptophan): The metabolite of L-tryptophan and the precursor of serotonin in the central nervous system. A natural supplement used for anxiety and depression.

504 Plan: A plan developed to ensure that a child who has a disability receives accommodations in school. Less formal than an IEP for children who do not require specialized instruction.

ACE: adverse childhood experiences. A list of nine potential traumas or stressors experienced by children that alter the risk for long-term mental and physical health.

ADHD: attention-deficit/hyperactivity disorder. A final common pathway of symptoms frequently observed in children that consists of hyperactivity, impulsivity, and inattention. This syndrome can be caused by many different triggers. The current conventional treatment is primarily stimulant medication, as it effectively reduces the behavioral elements of this problem, especially in the classroom. Long-term evidence of academic benefits for stimulant medication is lacking. This syndrome leads to an elevated risk of a variety of problems emerging in later life.

allostatic load: A term coined in 1993 by McEwen and Stellar that describes the physiological consequences of long-term exposure to stress. The response of the human body to long-term stress is calculated to maintain a state of balance or homeostasis, in a process of adaptation called "allostasis." Cortisol and epinephrine (adrenaline), the two main hormones released in response to stress, are essential in the short term but have negative physiological effects when the stress becomes chronic, resulting in an "allostatic load" that begins to break down the body. This biological burden exacts a cost on system and speeds up the aging process.

antidepressant medication: A type of medication used in psychiatry with a particularly strong enhancement of the placebo effect.

ASD: autism spectrum disorder. This term refers to the range of learning, behavior, social, and language problems that afflict those diagnosed with some elements of autism from the most severe to the more restricted limitations found in Aspergers.

BDNF: brain-derived neurotrophic factor. A growth-inducing protein found in the central nervous system that enhances neuronal growth and survival crucial to learning, memory, and brain health.

BMPT: behavioral management and parenting training. A type of psychoeducational program that trains parents in behavior management and parenting skills to help children with externalizing disorders.

CAM: complementary and alternative medicine. At one time this definition referred to the forms of health care that were not taught in medical school. The term "complementary" denotes health-care treatments that accompany conventional care, while alternative medicine is less likely to be used in conjunction with conventional care. Integrative medicine is a new specialty within conventional medicine that seeks to provide the best of CAM and conventional medicine.

CBT: cognitive behavioral therapy. This is a type of psychotherapy that helps individuals understand the link between their thoughts, feeling, and behaviors. Current research documents that CBT is effective in addressing a wide range of disorders, including phobias, addictions, depression, and anxiety. The treatment uses a psycho-educational approach to teach patients techniques for recognizing negative thought patterns and understanding how to interrupt them. This is the most researched and proven form of psychotherapy.

comorbidity: The occurrence of more than one illness at a time.

DBT: dialectical behavior therapy. This type of psychotherapy combines techniques from CBT that enhance emotion regulation with skills drawn from meditative practice, such as distress tolerance, acceptance, and mindful awareness.

DHA: docosahexaenoic acid. An omega-3 metabolite crucial for brain development.

DHEA: dehydroepiandrosterone. This steroid hormone is produced mainly by the adrenal gland and to a lesser degree by the brain and gonads, with the highest rate of circulation of any steroid in the human body. It functions as a metabolic intermediate in the production of male and female sex hormones. DHEA levels reflect the health of the adrenal gland and fall with chronic stress. It is one of the best biological indicators of the aging process.

DMAE: dimethylaminoethanol. This compound is the precursor of neurotransmitter acetylcholine and appears to enhance alertness, mood, and vigilance. Previously a prescription medication, it is now available over the counter.

dysbiosis: A stable but unhealthy mix of various bacterial strains and/or yeast, in the gut, resulting in ill health.

EFA: essential fatty acid. Fatty acids are lipids essential to the structure and function of cells which are not created by the body and therefore must be ingested. EFAs are particularly important for children—they aid in brain development, and omega-3 (anti-inflammatory) and omega-6 (pro-inflammatory) EFAs in particular are necessary for normal growth and development.

EMDR: eye movement desensitization and reprocessing. A technique utilizing eye movements or bilateral motor activity that has been shown to be useful in trauma and PTSD.

EMPowerplus: A proprietary multivitamin, multimineral supplement originally designed to treat bipolar disorder that has been the subject of 20 peer-reviewed articles in the psychiatric literature.

EPA: eicosapentaenoic acid. An omega-3 metabolite crucial for brain development.

epigenetics: The study of heritable changes in gene expression by means other than changes in DNA structure. Increasingly, this describes the power of environmental and external influences such as diet to alter human biology in a manner that persists and can be passed to offspring.

ERP: exposure response prevention. An evidence-based form of cognitive-behavior therapy used to treat obsessive-compulsive disorder.

GFCF: gluten-free and casein-free. A commonly used dietary modification that removes all dairy and wheat products from the diet.

gluten: A protein composite found in some grains (wheat, rye, barley, and others) that can cause immune or allergic reactivity. The protein is also the trigger for celiac disorder.

HPA axis: hypothalamic-pituitary-adrenal axis. This is one central component of the crucial neuroendocrine web that manages stress and many of the body's other functions.

IEP: Individualized Education Plan. A program mandated by the Individuals With Disabilities Education Act (IDEA) that attempts to meet the special education needs of a special child.

MDD: major depressive disorder. This is a severe mood disorder characterized by depressed mood and disturbances in sleep, appetite, and energy. Previously thought to be rare in children, the disorder is becoming increasingly common in younger and younger patients, though the reasons for this change are still unknown.

microbiome: An inclusive term for all of the bacteria that populate the human gut, providing essential contributions to digestion and health.

MTHFR: methylenetetrahydrofolate reductase. An enzyme in humans encoded by the MTHFR gene that plays a key role in folate metabolism. Alterations in this gene have been connected with a wide range of medical and psychiatric problems.

neurofeedback: A type of biofeedback that allows the participant to learn to control his or her own brain waves by using real-time EEG feedback via operant conditioning.

neuroplasticity: The responsiveness of the central nervous system on all levels to external influences that create changes in the neural pathways or synapses that drive learning, memory, and adaptation.

NMUPD: The nonmedical use of prescription drugs; a growing form of substance abuse.

Nurtured Heart Approach: A behavioral management and parenting training program that focuses on positive behavior and improved parent-child connectivity as developed by Howard Glasser for treating behavior issues in children.

OCD: obsessive-compulsive disorder. An anxiety disorder causing the individual to experience fear and apprehension, giving rise to repetitive thoughts (obsessions) or behaviors (compulsions) designed to reduce that fear. The disorder may take many different forms, such as violent or sexual fantasies, cleaning, hoarding, hand washing, and other rituals. In severe forms of the disorder the person becomes severely impaired by the repetitive process to the point of paralysis. While the thoughts and acts often appear to verge on psychotic, the suffering individual typically recognizes the absurdity of his or her behavior.

ODD: oppositional defiant disorder. A psychiatric disorder characterized by an ongoing pattern of disobedience, resistance, and animosity toward authority figures. Children with this disorder may appear extremely angry and experience explosive rages.

PANDAS: pediatric autoimmune neuropsychiatric disorders, arising as a result of streptococcal infections.The immunological result of this bacterial infection may drive a broad range of of neurological and psychiatric consequences.

PCP: primary care physician. A physician who provides basic health care for all aspects of an individual's medical needs.

PBD: pediatric bipolar disorder. A severe mental illness characterized by labile mood, irritability, rage, sleep disturbance, and agitation. This disorder manifests very differently in children than in adults: Most children seem to experience chronic rapid mood instability, rather than clear alteration of moods. The illness generates a great deal of controversy, as the frequency of diagnosis in the U.S. has exploded over the last two decades, while remaining low outside of North America.

PET: positron-emission tomography. A nuclear medical imaging process that creates an image or picture of metabolic processes in the body. The child ingests a radioactive nucleotide, which then emits gamma rays measured by the PET.

SAMe: S-adenosylmethionine. A naturally occurring component of the methylation process in each cell. A proven antidepressant.

SNP: single-nucleotide polymorphism. An inherited genetic abnormality that can reduce the effectiveness of an enzyme and create metabolic inefficiencies requiring nutrient support.

social-emotional education: A growing movement that supports the incorporation of nonacademic skills development into school curriculums.

SSRI: selective serotonin reuptake inhibitor. These are medications that increase the level of serotonin in the synaptic cleft. Used to treat depression, anxiety and OCD.

TSH: thyroid-stimulating hormone. An endocrine hormone secreted by the pituitary gland that induces the thyroid gland to produce thyroxine (T_4) and triiodothyronine (T_3), which then increase the body's metabolism.

REFERENCES

Abenavoli, L. (2010). Brain hypoperfusion and neurological symptoms in celiac disease. *Movement Disorders, 25*(6), 792–93.

Achenbach, T. M. (1978). The child behavior profile: I. boys aged 6–11. *Journal of Consulting and Clinical Psychology, 46*(3), 478–88.

Adams, J. B., Johansen, L. J., Powell, L. D., Quig, D., & Rubin, R. A. (2011). Gastrointestinal flora and gastrointestinal status in children with autism—comparisons to typical children and correlation with autism severity. *BMC Gastroenterology, 11*(22).

Addolorato, G., Capristo, E., Ghittoni, G., Valeri, C., Masciana, R., Ancona, C., & Gasbarrini, G. (2001). Anxiety but not depression decreases in coeliac patients after one-year gluten-free diet: A longitudinal study. *Scandinavian Journal of Gastroenterology, 36*(5), 502–6.

Addolorato, G., Leggio, L., D'Angelo, C., Mirijello, A., Ferrulli, A., Cardone, S., . . . Gasbarrini, G. (2008). Affective and psychiatric disorders in celiac disease. *Digestive Diseases, 26*(2), 140–48.

Ader, R., Felten, D., & Cohen, N. C. (2000). *Psycho-neuro-immunology* (3rd ed.). New York: Academic Press.

Adesman, A. R., Altshuler, L. A., Lipkin, P. H., & Walco, G. A. (1990). Otitis media in children with learning disabilities and in children with attention deficit disorder with hyperactivity. *Pediatrics, 85*(3, Pt. 2), 442–46.

Adrien, J. L., Perrot, A., Sauvage, D., Leddet, E., Larmande, C., Hameury, L., & Barthélémy, C. (1992). Early symptoms in autism from family home movies: Evaluation and comparison between 1st and 2nd year of life using I.B.S.E. scale. *Acta Paedopsychiatrica, 55*(2), 71–75.

Agrawal, R., & Gomez-Pinilla, F. (2012). "Metabolic syndrome" in the brain: Deficiency in omega-3 fatty acid exacerbates dysfunctions in insulin receptor signaling and cognition. *Journal of Physiology, 590*(10), 2484–99.

Akhondzadeh, S., Mohammadi, M. R., & Khademi, M. (2004). Zinc sulfate as an adjunct to methylphenidate for the treatment of attention deficit hyperactivity disorder in children: A double blind and randomized trial. *BMC Psychiatry, 4*(9).

Alfano, C. A., Ginsburg, G. S., & Kingery, J. N. (2007). Sleep-related problems among children and adolescents with anxiety disorders. *Journal of the American Academy of Child and Adolescent Psychiatry, 46*(2), 224–32.

American Psychiatric Association. (2010). DSM-5: Options being considered for ADHD. Retrieved from dsm5.org/Proposed%20Revision%20Attachments/ APA%20Options%20for%20ADHD.pdf

Ames, B. N. (2004). Supplements and tuning up metabolism. *Journal of Nutrition, 134*(11): 3164–68.

Ames, B. N. (2005). Increasing longevity by tuning up metabolism. *EMBO Reports, 6*, S20–S24.

Anda, R. F., Felitti, V. J., Bremner, J. D., Walker, J. D., Whitfield, C., Perry, B. D., . . . Giles, W. H. (2006). The enduring effects of abuse and related adverse experiences in childhood: A convergence of evidence from neurobiology and epidemiology. *European Archives of Psychiatry and Clinical Neuroscience, 256*(3), 174–86.

Anderson, A. R., & Henry, C. S. (1994). Family system characteristics and parental behaviors as predictors of adolescent substance use. *Adolescence, 29*(114), 405–20.

Anderson, C. A., Sakamoto, A., Gentile, D. A., Ihori, N., Shibuya, A., Yukawa, S., . . . Kobayashi, K. (2008). Longitudinal effects of violent video games on aggression in Japan and the United States. *Pediatrics, 122*(5), e1067–72.

Anghelescu, I. G., Kohnen, R., Szegedi, A., Klement, S., & Kieser, M. (2006). Comparison of hypericum extract WS 5570 and paroxetine in ongoing treatment after recovery from an episode of moderate to severe depression: Results from a randomized multicenter study. *Pharmacopsychiatry, 39*(6), 213–9.

Angold, A., Erkanli, A., Egger, H. L., & Costello, E. J. (2000). Stimulant treatment for children: A community perspective. *Journal of the American Academy of Child and Adolescent Psychiatry, 38*(8), 975–84.

Anthony, E. J. (1987). *The invulnerable child.* New York: Guilford.

APA Commission on Psychotherapies. (1982). Psychotherapy research: Methodological and efficacy issues. Presented in Washington, DC, by the American Psychiatric Association at the annual meeting of the American Psychiatric Association.

Armstrong, D. J., Meenagh, G. K., Bickle, I., Lee, A. S., Curran, E. S., & Finch, M. B. (2007). Vitamin D deficiency is associated with anxiety and depression in fibromyalgia. *Clinical Rheumatology, 26*(4), 551–54.

Arndt, T. L., Stodgell, C. J., & Rodier, P. M. (2005). The teratology of autism. *International Journal of Developmental Neuroscience, 23*(2–3), 189–99.

Arns, M., Drinkenburg, W., & Leon Kenemans, J. (2012). The effects of QEEG-informed neurofeedback in ADHD: An open-label pilot study. *Applied Psychophysiology and Biofeedback, 37*(3), 171–80.

Ashman, S. B., Dawson, G., & Panagiotides, H. (2008). Trajectories of maternal depression over 7 years: Relations with child psychophysiology and behavior and role of contextual risks. *Development and Psychopathology, 20*(1), 55–77.

Astin, J. A. (1998). Why patients use alternative medicine: Results of a national study. *Journal of the American Medical Association, 279*(19), 1548–53.

Autism Research Institute. (2009). Parent ratings of behavioral effects of biomedical interventions. Retrieved from autism.com/pdf/providers/ParentRatings2009.pdf

Awad, R., Levac, D., Cybulska, P., Merali, Z., Trudeau, V. L., & Arnason, J. T. (2007). Effects of traditionally used anxiolytic botanicals on enzymes of the gamma-aminobutyric acid (GABA) system. *Canadian Journal of Physiology and Pharmacology, 85*(9), 933–42.

Baio, J. (2012). Prevalence of autism spectrum disorders—autism and developmental disabilities monitoring network, 14 sites, United States. *Morbidity and Mortality Weekly Report, 61*(SS03), 1–19.

Barbaresi, W., Katusic, S., Colligan, R., Weaver, A., Pankratz, V., Mrazek, D., & Jacobsen, S. (2004). How common is attention-deficit/hyperactivity disorder? Towards resolution of the controversy: Results from a population-based study. *Acta Paediatrica, 93*(445), 55–59.

Barbaresi, W. J., Katusic, S. K., Colligan, R. C., Pankratz, V. S., Weaver, A. L., Weber, K. J., Mrazek, D. A., & Jacobsen, S. J. (2002). How common is attention-deficit/hyperactivity disorder? Incidence in a population-based birth cohort in Rochester, Minn. *Archives of Pediatrics and Adolescent Medicine, 156*(3), 217–24.

Barker, D. J. (1998). In utero programming of chronic disease. *Clinical Science, 95*(2), 115–28.

Barlow, J., & Coren, E. (2004). Parent-training programmes for improving maternal psychosocial health. *Cochrane Database of Systematic Reviews, 1*, CD002020.

Barlow, J., & Stewart-Brown, S. (2000). Behavior problems and group-based parent education programs. *Journal of Developmental and Behavioral Pediatrics, 21*(5), 356–70.

Bateman, B., Warner, J. O., Hutchinson, E., Dean, T., Rowlandson, P., Gant, C., . . . Stevenson, J. (2004). The effects of a double blind, placebo controlled, artificial food colourings and benzoate preservative challenge on hyperactivity in a general population sample of preschool children. *Archives of Disease in Childhood, 89*(6), 506–11.

Baxter, L. R., Jr., Schwartz, J. M., Bergman, K. S., Szuba, M. P., Guze, B. H., Mazziotta, J. C., Alazraki, A., . . . Munford, P. (1992). Caudate glucose metabolic rate changes with both drug and behavior therapy for obsessive-compulsive disorder. *Archives of General Psychiatry, 49*(9), 681–89.

Beaudet, A. L. (2007). Autism: Highly heritable but not inherited. *Natural Medicine, 13*(5), 534–36.

Beecher, H. K. (1955). The powerful placebo. *Journal of the American Medical Association, 159*(17), 1602–1606 .

Beider, S., Mahrer, N. E., & Gold, J. I. (2007). Pediatric massage therapy: An overview for clinicians. *Pediatric Clinics of North America, 54*(6), 1025–41; xii–xiii.

Beider, S., & Moyer, C. A. (2007). Randomized controlled trials of pediatric massage: A review. *Evidence-Based Complementary and Alternative Medicine, 4*(1), 23–34.

Bell, C. C., & McBride, D. F. (2010). Affect regulation and prevention of risky behaviors. *Journal of the American Medical Association, 304*(5), 565–66.

Bellinger, D. C. (2012). Comparing the population neurodevelopmental burdens associated with children's exposures to environmental chemicals and other risk factors. *Neurotoxicology, 33*(4), 641–43.

Belmaker, R. H., & Agam, G. (2008). Major depressive disorder. *New England Journal of Medicine, 358*(1), 55–68.

Benedetti, F., Colombo, C., Barbini, B., Campori, E., & Smeraldi, E. (2001). Morning sunlight reduces length of hospitalization in bipolar depression. *Journal of Affective Disorders, 62*(3), 221–23.

Bercik, P., Denou, E., Collins, J., Jackson, W., Lu, J., Jury, J., . . . Collins, S. M. (2011). The intestinal microbiota affect central levels of brain-derived neurotropic factor and behavior in mice. *Gastroenterology, 141*(2), 599–609.e3.

Berk, M., Copolov, D. L., Dean, O., Lu, K., Jeavons, S., Schapkaitz, I., . . . Bush, A. I. (2008). N-acetyl cysteine for depressive symptoms in bipolar disorder: A double-blind randomized placebo-controlled trial. *Biological Psychiatry, 64*(6), 468–75.

Berman, S. M., Kuczenski, R., McCracken, J. T., & London, E. D. (2009). Potential adverse effects of amphetamine treatment on brain and behavior: A review. *Molecular Psychiatry, 14*(2), 123–42.

Bernstein, G. A., Victor, A. M., Pipal, A. J., & Williams, K. A. (2010). Comparison of clinical characteristics of pediatric autoimmune neuropsychiatric disorders associated with streptococcal infections and childhood obsessive-compulsive disorder. *Journal of Child and Adolescent Psychopharmacology, 20*(4), 333–40.

Beversdorf, D. (2005, November). Stress interferes wth problem-solving; beta blockers may help. Presentation to the Society for Neuroscience, Washington, DC.

Biederman, J. (2005, October). Informal commentary at the annual meeting of American Academy of Child and Adolescent Psychiatry, San Francisco, CA.

Billstedt, E., Gillberg, I. C., & Gillberg, C. (2005). Autism after adolescence: Population-based 13- to 22-year follow-up study of 120 individuals with autism diagnosed in childhood. *Journal of Autism and Developmental Disorders, 35*(3), 351–60.

Birdee, G. S., Phillips, R. S., Davis, R. B., & Gardiner, P. (2010). Factors associated with pediatric use of complementary and alternative medicine. *Pediatrics, 125*(2), 249–56.

Birk, S. (2012, December 1). Violent video games alter brain activity. *Clinical Psychiatry News*. Retrieved from http://www.clinicalpsychiatrynews.com/news/adult-psychiatry/single-article/violent-video-games-alter-brain-activity/7529d40ba4.html

Black, M. M., Quigg, A. M., Hurley, K. M., & Pepper, M. R. (2011). Iron deficiency and iron-deficiency anemia in the first two years of life: Strategies to prevent loss of developmental potential. *Nutritional Review, 69*(Suppl 1), S64–S70.

Blader, J. C., & Carlson, G. A. (2007). Increased rates of bipolar disorder diagnoses among U.S. child, adolescent, and adult inpatients, 1996–2004. *Biological Psychiatry, 62*(2), 107–14.

Blair, S. N., Kohl, H. W., Paffenbarger, R. S., Jr., Clark, D. G., Cooper, K. H., & Gibbons, L. W. (1989). Physical fitness and all-cause mortality: A prospective study of healthy men and women. *Journal of the American Medical Association, 262*(17), 2395–401.

Bloch, M. H., & Qawasmi, A. (2011). Omega-3 fatty acid supplementation for the treatment of children with attention-deficit/hyperactivity disorder symptomatology: Systematic review and meta-analysis. *Journal of the American Academy of Child and Adolescent Psychiatry, 50*(10), 991–1000.

Bohnert, A. M., Crnic, K. A., & Lim, K. G. (2003). Emotional competence and aggressive behavior in school-age children. *Journal of Abnormal Child Psychology, 31*(1), 79–91.

Born, J., Rasch, B., & Gais, S. (2006). Sleep to Remember. *Neuroscientist, 12*(5), 410–24.

Bosquet Enlow, M., Kitts, R. L., Blood, E., Bizarro, A., Hofmeister, M., & Wright, R. J. (2011). Maternal posttraumatic stress symptoms and infant emotional reactivity and emotion regulation. *Infant Behavior and Development, 34*(4), 487–503.

Bottaro, G., Cataldo, F., Rotolo, N., Spina, M., & Corazza, G. R. (1999). The clinical pattern of subclinical/silent celiac disease: An analysis on 1026 consecutive cases. *American Journal of Gastroenterology, 94*(3), 691–96.

Bouchard, M. F., Bellinger, D. C., Wright, R. O., & Weisskopf, M. G. (2010). Attention-deficit/hyperactivity disorder and urinary metabolites of organophosphate pesticides. *Pediatrics, 125*(6), e1270–77.

Bowen, S., Witkiewitz, K., & Dillworth, T. M. (2006). Mindfulness meditation and substance use in an incarcerated population. *Psychology of Addictive Behaviors, 20*(3), 343–47.

Bowlby, J. (1988). *A secure base: Parent-child attachment and healthy human development.* New York: Basic Books.

Brattstrom, A. (2009). Long-term effects of St. John's wort (hypericum perforatum) treatment: A 1-year safety study in mild to moderate depression. *Phytomedicine, 16*(4), 277–83.

Bridge, J. A., Iyengar, S., Salary, C. B., Barbe, R. P., Birmaher, B., Pincus, H. A., . . . Brent, D. A. (2007). Clinical response and risk for reported suicidal ideation and suicide attempts in pediatric antidepressant treatment: A meta-analysis of randomized controlled trials. *Journal of the American Medical Association, 297*(15), 1683–96.

Briggs Myers, I. (1990). *Gifts differing: Understanding personality type.* Palo Alto, CA: Consulting Psychologists Press.

Bronfenbrenner, U. (1977). Doing your own thing—our undoing. *Child Psychiatry and Human Development, 8*(1), 3–10.

Bronfenbrenner, U. (1979). *Ecology of human development.* Cambridge, MA: Harvard University Press.

Brook, J. S., Zhang, C., Balka, E. B., & Brook, D. W. (2012). Pathways to children's externalizing behavior: A three-generation study. *Journal of Genetic Psychology, 173*(2), 175–97.

Brooks, M. (2012, February 12). Death, cancer increased with hypnotics. *Medscape Medical News.* Retrieved from http://www.medscape.com/viewarticle/759336?src

Brotman, M. A., Kassem, L., Reising, M. M., Guyer, A. E., Dickstein, D. P., Rich, B. A., . . . Leibenluft, E. (2007). Parental diagnoses in youth with narrow phenotype bipolar disorder or severe mood dysregulation. *American Journal of Psychiatry, 164*(8), 1238–41.

Brown, R. P., & Gerbarg, P. L. (2001). Herbs and nutrients in the treatment of depression, anxiety, insomnia, migraine, and obesity. *Journal of Psychiatric Practice, 7*(2), 75–91.

Brown, R. T., Slimmer, L. W., & Wynne, M. E. (1984). How much stimulant medication is appropriate for hyperactive school children? *Journal of School Health, 54*(3), 128–30.

Buie, T., Campbell, D. B., Fuchs, G. J., 3rd, Furuta, G. T., Levy, J., Vandewater, J., . . . Winter, H. (2010). Evaluation, diagnosis, and treatment of gastrointestinal disorders in individuals with ASDs: A consensus report. *Pediatrics, 125*(Suppl.1), s1–s18.

Bullock, M. L., Culliton, P. D., & Olander, R. T. (1989). Controlled trial of acupuncture for severe recidivist alcoholism. *Lancet, 1*(8652), 1435–9.

Burcusa, S. L., Iacono, W. G., & McGue, M. (2003). Adolescent twins discordant for major depressive disorder: Shared familial liability to externalizing and other internalizing disorders. *Journal of Child Psychology and Psychiatry, and Allied Disciplines, 44*(7), 997–1005.

Burstein, M., Ameli-Grillon, L., & Merikangas, K. R. (2011). Shyness versus social phobia in US youth. *Pediatrics, 128*(5), 917–25.

Burt, S. A., Krueger, R. F., McGue, M., & Iacono, W. (2003). Parent-child conflict and the comorbidity among childhood externalizing disorders. *Archive of General Psychiatry, 60*(5), 505–13.

Bushara, K. O. (2005). Neurologic presentation of celiac disease. *Gastroenterology, 128*(4, suppl. 1), s92–s97.

Calestro, K. (1972). Psychotherapy, faith healing and suggestion. *International Journal of Psychiatry, 10*(2), 83–128.

Camfield, D. A., Sarris, J., & Berk, M. (2011). Nutraceuticals in the treatment of obsessive compulsive disorder (OCD): A review of mechanistic and clinical evidence. *Progress in Neuro-Psychopharmacology and Biological Psychiatry, 35*(4), 887–95.

Campbell, S. B., Shaw, D. S., & Gilliom, M. (2000). Early externalizing behavior problems: Toddlers and preschoolers at risk for later maladjustment. *Development and Psychopathology, 12*(3), 467–88.

Campo, J. V., Bridge, J., Ehmann, M., Altman, S., Lucas, A., Birmaher, B., . . . Brent,

D. A. (2004). Recurrent abdominal pain, anxiety, and depression in primary care. *Pediatrics, 113*(4), 817–24.

Canavera, K. E., Wilkins, K. C., Pincus, D. B., & Ehrenreich-May, J. T. (2009). Parent-child agreement in the assessment of obsessive-compulsive disorder. *Journal of Clinical Child and Adolescent Psychology, 28*(6), 909–15.

Cannon, W. (1963). *The wisdom of the body*. New York: Norton. (Original work published 1932)

Capra, F. (1996). *The web of life: A new scientific understanding of living systems*. New York: Anchor.

Carlson, G. A. (1999). Juvenile mania versus ADHD. *Journal of the American Academy of Child and Adolescent Psychiatry, 38*(4), 353–54.

Carlson, G. A., Potegal, M., Margulies, D., Gutkovich, Z., & Basile, J. (2009). Rages—what are they and who has them? *Journal of Child and Adolescent Psychopharmacology, 19*(3), 281–88.

Carnagey, N. L., Anderson, C. A., & Bushman, B. J. (2007). The effect of video game violence on physiological desensitization to real-life violence. *Journal of Experimental Social Psychology, 43*(3), 489–496

Carr, A. (2009). The effectiveness of family therapy and systemic interventions for child-focused problems. *Journal of Family Therapy, 31*(1), 3–45.

Carter, A. S., Wagmiller, R. J., Gray, S. A., McCarthy, K. J., Horwitz, S. M., & Briggs-Gowan, M. J. (2010). Prevalence of DSM-IV disorder in a representative, healthy birth cohort at school entry: Sociodemographic risks and social adaptation. *Journal of the American Academy of Child and Adolescent Psychiatry, 49*(7), 686–98.

"The case against antidepressants: A growing chorus of critics is challenging the widespread use of antidepressants. Why?" (2011, July 22). *The Week*. Retrieved from http://theweek.com/article/index/217444/the-case-against-antidepressants

Castelli, D. M., Hillman, C. H., Buck, S. M., & Erwin, H. E. (2007). Physical fitness and academic achievement in third- and fifth-grade students. *Journal of Sport and Exercise Psychology, 29*(2), 239–52.

Centers for Disease Control. (2009). Prevalence of autism spectrum disorders—autism and developmental disabilities monitoring network, United States, 2006. *Morbidity and Mortality Weekly Report, Surveillance Summaries, 58*(100), 1–20.

Centers for Disease Control. (2011). *Morbidity and Mortality Weekly Report, 60*(43), 1477–1512.

Chai, G., Governale, L., McMahon, A. W., Trinidad, J. P., Staffa, J., & Murphy, D. (2012). Trends of outpatient prescription drug utilization in US children, 2002–2010. *Pediatrics, 130*(1), 23–31.

Chalon, S., Vancassel, S., Zimmer, L., Guilloteau, D., & Durand, G. (2001). Polyunsaturated fatty acids and cerebral function: Focus on monoaminergic neurotransmission. *Lipids, 36*(9), 937–44.

Chapman, D. P., Wheaton, A. G., Anda, R. F., Croft, J. B., Edwards, V. J., Liu, Y., . . .

Perry, G. S. (2011). Adverse childhood experiences and sleep disturbances in adults. *Sleep Medicine, 12*(8), 773–79.

Chavira, D. A., Garland, A. F., Daley, S., & Hough, R. (2008). The impact of medical comorbidity on mental health and functional health outcomes among children with anxiety disorders. *Journal of Developmental and Behavioral Pediatrics, 29*(5), 394–202.

Chavira, D. A., Stein, M. B., Bailey, K., & Stein, M. T. (2004). Child anxiety in primary care: Prevalent but untreated. *Depression and Anxiety, 20*(4), 155–64.

Chen, R., Jiao, Y., & Herskovits, E. H. (2011). Structural MRI in autism spectrum disorder. *Pediatric Research, 69*(5.2), 63R–8R.

Cherland, E., & Fitzpatrick, R. (1999). Psychotic side effects of psychostimulants: A 5-year review. *Canadian Journal of Psychiatry, 44*(8), 811–13.

Chess, S., & Thomas, A. (1977). Temperament and the parent-child interaction. *Pediatric Annals, 6*(9), 574–82.

Chiesa, A., & Serretti, A. (2011). Mindfulness based cognitive therapy for psychiatric disorders: A systematic review and meta-analysis. *Psychiatry Research, 187*(3), 441–53.

Chronis-Tuscano, A., O'Brien, K. A., Johnston, C., Jones, H. A., Clarke, T. L., Raggi, V. L., . . . Seymour, K. E. (2011). The relation between maternal ADHD symptoms and improvement in child behavior following brief behavioral parent training is mediated by change in negative parenting. *Journal of Abnormal Child Psychology, 39*(7), 1047–57.

Cilleruelo Pascual, M. L., Roman Riechmann, E., Jimenez Jimenez, J., Rivero Martin, M. J., Barrio Torres, J., Castano Pascual, A., . . . Fernandez Rincon, A. (2002). Silent celiac disease: Exploring the iceberg in the school-aged population. *Anales Espanoles de Pediatria, 57*(4), 321–26.

Cohen, S., Doyle, W. J., Skoner, D. P., Rabin, B. S., & Gwaltney, J. M., Jr. (1997). Social ties and susceptibility to the common cold. *Journal of the American Medical Association, 277*(24), 1940–44.

Coles, R. (1990). *The spiritual life of children.* New York: Houghton Mifflin.

Compton, S. N., Walkup, J. T., Albano, A. M., Piacentini, J. C., Birmaher, B., Sherrill, J. T., . . . March, J. S. (2010). Child/adolescent anxiety multimodal study (CAMS): Rationale, design, and methods. *Child and Adolescent Psychiatry and Mental Health, 1*, 1.

Corsetti, G., Stacchiotti, A., Tedesco, L., D'Antona, G., Pasini, E., Dioguardi, F. S., . . . Rezzani, R. (2011). Essential amino acid supplementation decreases liver damage induced by chronic ethanol consumption in rats. *International Journal of Immunopathology and Pharmacology, 24*(3), 611–19.

Cosgrove, L., & Bursztajn, H. J. (2010, March 6). Pharmaceutical philanthropic shell games: Has industry removed the transparent and replaced it with the opaque? *Psychiatric Times, 27*(3).

Costello, E. J., Erkanli, A., & Angold, A. (2006). Is there an epidemic of child or adolescent depression? *Journal of Child Psychology and Psychiatry, 47*(12), 1263–71.

Courbasson, C. M., de Sorkin, A. A., Dullerud, B., & Van Wyk, L. (2007). Acupuncture treatment for women with concurrent substance use and anxiety/depression: An effective alternative therapy? *Family and Community Health, 30*(2), 112–20.

Craft, L. L., & Perna, F. M. (2004). The benefits of exercise for the clinically depressed. *Primary Care Companion to the Journal of Clinical Psychiatry, 6*(3), 104–11.

Critchfield, J. W., van Hemert, S., Ash, M., Mulder, L., & Ashwood, P. (2011). The potential role of probiotics in the management of childhood autism spectrum disorder. *Gastroenterology Research and Practice*, 161358. doi:10.1155/2011/161358. [Epub ahead of print.]

Croen, L. A., Grether, J. K., Yoshida, C. K., Odouli, R., & Hendrick, V. (2011). Antidepressant use during pregnancy and childhood autism spectrum disorders. *Archives of General Psychiatry, 68*(11), 1104–12.

Dalton, M. A., Adachi-Meija, A. M., & Longacre, M. R. (2006). Parental rules and monitoring of children's movie viewing associated with children's risk for smoking and drinking. *Pediatrics, 118*(5), 1932–42.

Damasio, A. R. (1998). Emotion in the perspective of an integrated nervous system. *Brain Research Reviews, 26*, 83–86.

Dang-Vu, T. T., Desseilles, M., Peigneux, P., & Maquet, P. (2006). A role for sleep in brain plasticity. *Pediatric Rehabilitation, 9*(2), 98–118.

Dasinger, L. K., Shane, P. A., & Martinovich, Z. (2004). Assessing the effectiveness of community-based substance abuse treatment for adolescents. *Journal of Psychoactive Drugs, 36*(1), 27–33.

Davé, S., Petersen, I., Sherr, L., & Nazareth, I. (2010). Incidence of maternal and paternal depression in primary care: A cohort study using a primary care database. *Archives of Pediatric and Adolescent Medicine, 164*, 1038–44.

Dawson, G., Rogers, S., Munson, J., Smith, M., Winter, J., Greenson, J., . . . Varley, J. (2010). Randomized, controlled trial of an intervention for toddlers with autism: The early start Denver model. *Pediatrics*. Retrieved from http://pediatrics.aappublications.org/content/125/1/e17.full

Deault, L. C. (2010). A systematic review of parenting in relation to the development of comorbidities and functional impairments in children with attention-deficit/hyperactivity disorder (ADHD). *Child Psychiatry and Human Development, 41*(2), 168–92.

Del Angel-Meza, A. R., Davalos-Marin, A. J., Ontiveros-Martinez, L. L., Ortiz, G. G., Beas-Zarate, C., Chaparro-Huerta, V., . . . Bitzer-Quintero, O. K. (2011). Protective effects of tryptophan on neuro-inflammation in rats after administering lipopolysaccharide. *Biomedicine and Pharmacotherapy, 65*(3), 215–19.

de Magistris, L., Familiari, V., Pascotto, A., Sapone, A., Frolli, A., Iardino, P., . . . Bravaccio, C. (2010). Alterations of the intestinal barrier in patients with autism spectrum disorders and in their first-degree relatives. *Journal of Pediatric Gastroenterology and Nutrition, 51*(4), 418–24.

Denton, R. E., & Kampfe, C. M. (1994). The relationship between family variables and adolescent substance abuse: A literature review. *Adolescence, 29*(114), 475–95.

DeStefano, F. (2007). Vaccines and autism: Evidence does not support a causal association. *Clinical Pharmacology and Therapeutics, 82*(6), 756–59.

D'Eufemia, P., Celli, M., Finocchiaro, R., Pacifico, L., Viozzi, L., Zaccagnini, M., . . . Giardini, O. (1996). Abnormal intestinal permeability in children with autism. *Acta Paediatrica, 85*(9), 1076–79.

Dew, R. E., Daniel, S. S., Armstrong, T. D., Goldston, D. B., Triplett, M. F., & Koenig, H. G. (2008). Religion/spirituality and adolescent psychiatric symptoms: A review. *Child Psychiatry and Human Development, 39*(4), 381–98.

Dewald, P. (1976). Toward a general concept of the therapeutic process. *International Journal of Psychoanalytic Psychotherapy, 5,* 283–99.

Dias, A. M., & van Deusen, A. (2011). A new neurofeedback protocol for depression. *Spanish Journal of Psychology, 14*(1), 374–84.

Dietz, P. M., Williams, S. B., Callaghan, W. M., Bachman, D. J., Whitlock, E. P., & Hornbrook, M. C. (2007). Clinically identified maternal depression before, during, and after pregnancies ending in live births. *American Journal of Psychiatry, 164*(10), 1515–20.

Diller, L. (1998). *Running on Ritalin.* New York: Bantam.

Dodge, K. A., & Pettit, G. S. (2003). A biopsychosocial model of the development of chronic conduct problems in adolescence. *Developmental Psychology, 39*(2), 349–71.

Doidge, N. (2007). *The brain that changes itself.* New York: Penguin.

Dolinoy, D. C., Huang, D., & Jirtle, R. L. (2007). Maternal nutrient supplementation counteracts bisphenol a–induced DNA hypomethylation in early development. *Proceedings of the National Academy of Sciences, 104*(32), 13056–61.

Dori, N., & Green, T. (2011). The metabolic syndrome and antipsychotics in children and adolescents [in Hebrew]. *Harefuah, 150*(10), 791–96.

Doshi, J. A., Hodgkins, P., Kahle, J., Sikirica, V., Cangelosi, M. J., Setyawan, J., . . . Neumann, P. J. (2012). Economic impact of childhood and adult attention-deficit/ hyperactivity disorder in the United States. *Journal of the American Academy of Child and Adolescent Psychiatry, 51*(10), 990–1002 e2.

Dossey, L. (1993). *Healing words.* New York: HarperCollins.

Duckworth, A. L., Peterson, C., Matthews, M. D., & Kelly, D. R. (2007). Grit: Perseverance and passion for long-term goals. *Personality Processes and Individual Differences, 92*(6), 1087.

Dumont, I. P., & Olson, A. L. (2012). Primary care, depression, and anxiety: Exploring somatic and emotional predictors of mental health status in adolescents. *Journal of the American Board of Family Medicine, 25*(3), 291–99.

Durbin, C. E., Klein, D. N., Hayden, E. P., Buckley, M. E., & Moerk, K. C. (2005).

Temperamental emotionality in preschoolers and parental mood disorders. *Journal of Abnormal Psychology, 114*, 28–37.

Eaves, L. C., & Ho, H. H. (2008). Young adult outcome of autism spectrum disorders. *Journal of Autism and Developmental Disorders, 38*(4), 739–47.

Eaves, L. J., Prom, E. C., & Silberg, J. L. (2010). The mediating effect of parental neglect on adolescent and young adult anti-sociality: A longitudinal study of twins and their parents. *Behavioral Genetics, 40*(4), 425–37.

Eby, G. A., & Eby, K. L. (2006). Rapid recovery from major depression using magnesium treatment. *Medical Hypotheses, 67*(2), 362–70.

Ecker, J. R., Bickmore, W. A., Barroso, I., Pritchard, J. K., Gilad, Y., & Segal, E. (2012). Genomics: ENCODE explained. *Nature, 489*(7414), 52–55.

Egger, H. L., Costello, E. J., Erkanli, A., & Angold, A. (1999). Somatic complaints and psychopathology in children and adolescents: Stomach aches, musculoskeletal pains, and headaches. *Journal of the American Academy of Child and Adolescent Psychiatry, 28*(7), 852–60.

Egger, J., Carter, C. M., & Graham, P. J. (1985). Controlled trial of oligoantigenic treatment in the hyperkinetic syndrome. *Lancet, 1*(8428), 540–45.

Ehman, J. W., Ott, B. B., Short, T. H., Ciampa, R. C., & Hansen-Flaschen, J. (1999). Do patients want physicians to inquire about their spiritual or religious beliefs if they become gravely ill? *Archives of Internal Medicine, 159*(15), 1803–6.

Ekeland, E., Heian, F., Hagen, K. B., Abbott, J., & Nordheim, L. (2004). Exercise to improve self-esteem in children and young people. *Cochrane Database of Systematic Review, 1*, CD003683.

Eldar, S., Apter, A., Lotan, D., Edgar, K. P., Naim, R., Fox, N. A., . . . Bar-Haim, Y. (2012). Attention bias modification treatment for pediatric anxiety disorders: A randomized controlled trial. *American Journal of Psychiatry, 169*(2), 213–20.

Enoch, M. A. (2012). The influence of gene-environment interactions on the development of alcoholism and drug dependence. *Current Psychiatry Reports, 14*(2), 150–58.

Epkins, C. C., & Heckler, D. R. (2011). Integrating etiological models of social anxiety and depression in youth: Evidence for a cumulative interpersonal risk model. *Clinical Child and Family Psychology Review, 14*(4), 329–76.

Erenberg, G. (2005). The relationship between Tourette syndrome, attention deficit hyperactivity disorder, and stimulant medication: A critical review. *Seminars in Pediatric Neurology, 12*(4), 217–21.

Eriksson, M., & Lindstrom, B. (2007). Antonovsky's sense of coherence scale and its relation with quality of life: A systematic review. *Journal of Epidemiology and Community Health, 61*(11), 938–44.

Erkkila, J., Punkanen, M., Fachner, J., Ala-Ruona, E., Pontio, I., Tervaniemi, M., . . . Gold, C. (2011). Individual music therapy for depression: Randomised controlled trial. *British Journal of Psychiatry, 199*(2), 132–39.

Esposito-Smythers, C., Birmaher, B., Valeri, S., Chiappetta, L., Hunt, J., Ryan, N., . . . Keller, M. (2006). Child comorbidity, maternal mood disorder, and perceptions of family functioning among bipolar youth. *Journal of the American Academy of Child and Adolescent Psychiatry, 45*(8), 955–64.

Evans, S. J., Prossin, A. R., Harrington, G. J., Kamali, M., Ellingrod, V. L., Burant, C. F., & McInnis, M. G. (2012). Fats and factors: Lipid profiles associate with personality factors and suicidal history in bipolar subjects. *PLoS One, 7*(1), e29297.

Evans, S. W., Pelham, W. E., Smith, B. H., Bukstein, O., Gnagy, E. M., Greiner, A. R., . . . Baron-Myak, C. (2001). Dose-response effects of methylphenidate on ecologically valid measures of academic performance and classroom behavior in adolescents with ADHD. *Experimental and Clinical Psychopharmacology, 9*(2), 163–75.

Fair, D. A., Bathula, D., Nikolas, M. A., & Nigg, J. T. (2012). Distinct neuropsychological subgroups in typically developing youth inform heterogeneity in children with ADHD. *Proceedings of the National Academy of Sciences, 109*(17), 6769–74.

Fallone, G., Acebo, C., Seifer, R., & Carskadon, M. A. (2005). Experimental restriction of sleep opportunity in children: Effects on teacher ratings. *Sleep, 28*(12), 1561–67.

Famularo, R., Kinscherff, R., & Fenton, T. (1991). Posttraumatic stress disorder among children clinically diagnosed as borderline personality disorder. *Journal of Nervous and Mental Disease, 179*(7), 428–31.

Fassler, D. (1997). *Help me, I am sad*. New York: Penguin.

Feeny, N. C., Danielson, C. K., Schwartz, L., Youngstrom, E. A., & Findling, R. L. (2006). Cognitive-behavioral therapy for bipolar disorders in adolescents: A pilot study. *Bipolar Disorder, 8*, 508–15.

Felitti, V. J., Anda, R. F., Nordenberg, D., Williamson, D. F., Spitz, A. M., Edwards, V., . . . Marks, J. S. (1998). Relationship of childhood abuse and household dysfunction to many of the leading causes of death in adults. The adverse childhood experiences (ACE) study. *American Journal of Preventive Medicine, 14*(4), 245–58.

Ferguson, J. H. (2000). National Institutes of Health Consensus Development Conference statement: Diagnosis and treatment of attention-deficit/hyperactivity disorder (ADHD). *Journal of the American Academy of Child and Adolescent Psychiatry, 39*(2), 182–93.

Feucht, C., & Patel, D. R. (2011). Herbal medicines in pediatric neuropsychiatry. *Pediatric Clinics of North America, 58*(1), 33–54, x.

Findling, R. L., McNamara, N. K., O'Riordan, M. A., Reed, M. D., Demeter, C. A., Branicky, L. A., & Blumer, J. L. (2003). An open-label pilot study of St. John's wort in juvenile depression. *Journal of the American Academy of Child and Adolescent Psychiatry, 42*(8), 908–14.

Finegold, S. M. (2011). Desulfovibrio species sre potentially important in regressive autism. *Medical Hypotheses, 77*(2), 270–74.

Floch, M. H. (2011). Intestinal microecology in health and wellness. *Journal of Clinical Gastroenterology, 45*(Suppl.), S108–10.

Fontanella, C. A., Bridge, J. A., Marcus, S. C., & Campo, J. V. (2011). Factors associated with antidepressant adherence for Medicaid-enrolled children and adolescents. *Annals of Pharmacotherapy, 46*(7–8), 898–908.

Forbes, E. E., Christopher, M. J., Siegle, G. J., Ladouceur, C. D., Ryan, N. D., Carter, C. S.,... Dahl, R. E. (2006). Reward-related decision making in pediatric major depressive disorder: An fMRI study. *Journal of Child Psychology and Psychiatry, 47*(10), 1031–41.

Fournier, J. C., DeRubeis, R. J., & Hollon, S. D. (2010). Antidepressant drug effects and depression severity: A patient-level meta-analysis. *Journal of the American Medical Association, 303*(1), 47–53.

Fox, N. A., & Davidson, R. J. (1988). Patterns of brain electrical activity during facial signs of emotion in 10-month-old infants. *Developmental Psychology, 24*, 230–36.

Foxcroft, D. R., & Tsertsvadze, A. (2011). Universal family-based prevention programs for alcohol misuse in young people. *Cochrane Database of Systematic Reviews, 9*, CD009308.

Frances, A. (2009). A warning sign on the road to DSM-V: Beware of its unintended consequences. *Psychiatric Times, 26*(8).

Frances, A. (2011, July 22). DSM-5 approves new fad diagnosis for child psychiatry: Antipsychotic use likely to rise. *Psychiatric Times.* Retrieved from http://www.psychiatrictimes.com/display/article/10168/1912195

Frances, A. (2012a, May 2). Wonderful news: DSM 5 finally begins its belated and necessary retreat. *Psychology Today.* Retrieved from http://www.psychologytoday.com/blog/dsm5-in-distress/201205/wonderful-news-dsm-5-finally-begins-its-belated-and-necessary-retreat

Frances, A. (2012b, December 2). DSM 5 is guide not Bible—ignore its ten worst changes: APA approval of DSM-5 is a sad day for psychiatry. *Psychology Today.* Retrieved from http://www.psychologytoday.com/blog/dsm5-in-distress/201212/dsm-5-is-guide-not-bible-ignore-its-ten-worst-changes

Frank, E., Kupfer, D. J., Thase, M. E., Mallinger, A. G., Swartz, H. A., Fagiolini, A. M., . . . Monk, T. (2005). Two-year outcomes for interpersonal and social rhythm therapy in individuals with Bipolar I disorder. *Archives of General Psychiatry, 62*(9), 996–1004.

Frank, J. (1961). *Persuasion and healing: A comparative study of psychotherapy.* Baltimore, MD: Johns Hopkins University Press.

Frank, J. (1971). Therapeutic factors in psychotherapy. *American Journal of Psychotherapy, 25*(3), 350–61.

Frank, J. D., Hoehn-Saric, R., Imber, S. D., et al. (1978). *Effective ingredients of successful psychotherapy.* New York: Brunner/Mazel.

Frankl, V. (1997). *Man's search for meaning.* New York: Pocket Books.

Franklin, M. E., Sapyta, J., Freeman, J. B., Khanna, M., Compton, S., Almirall, D., . . . March, J. S. (2011). Cognitive behavior therapy augmentation of pharmacotherapy in pediatric obsessive-compulsive disorder: The pediatric OCD treatment study II (POTS II) randomized controlled trial. *Journal of the American Medical Association, 306*(11), 1224–32.

Frazier, E. A., Fristad, M., & Arnold, L. E. (2009). Multinutrient supplement as treatment: Literature review and case report of a 12-year-old boy with bipolar disorder. *Journal of Child and Adolescent Psychopharmacology, 19*, 453–60.

Frazier, E. A., Fristad, M. A., & Arnold, L. E. (2012). Feasibility of a nutritional supplement as treatment for pediatric bipolar spectrum disorders. *Journal of Alternative and Complementary Medicine, 18*(7), 678–85.

Freed, J., & Parsons, L. (1998). *Right-brained children in a left-brained world: Unlocking the potential of your ADHD child.* New York: Fireside.

Fristad, M. A. (2006). Psychoeducational treatment for school-aged children with bipolar disorder. *Developmental Psychopathology, 18*(4), 1289–1306.

Furlong, M., McGilloway, S., Bywater, T., Hutchings, J., Smith, S. M., & Donnelly, M. (2012). Behavioural and cognitive-behavioural group-based parenting programmes for early-onset conduct problems in children aged 3 to 12 years. *Cochrane Database of Systematic Reviews, 2*, CD008225.

Fux, M., Benjamin, J., & Belmaker, R. H. (1999). Inositol versus placebo augmentation of serotonin reuptake inhibitors in the treatment of obsessive-compulsive disorder: A double-blind cross-over study. *International Journal of Neuropsychopharmacology, 2*(3), 193–95.

Galiatsatos, P., Gologan, A., & Lamoureux, E. (2009). Autistic enterocolitis: Fact or fiction? *Canadian Journal of Gastroenterology, 23*(2), 95–98.

Gallup, G., Jr. (2000). *The next American spirituality.* Colorado Springs, CO: Cook Communications.

Ganz, M. L. (2007). The lifetime distribution of the incremental societal costs of autism. *Archives of Pediatric and Adolescent Medicine, 161*, 343–49.

Gardner, H. (1993*). Multiple intelligences: The theory in practice.* New York: Basic Books.

Garnier-Dykstra, L. M., Caldeira, K. M., Vincent, K. B., O'Grady, K. E., & Arria, A. M. (2012). Nonmedical use of prescription stimulants during college: Four-year trends in exposure opportunity, use, motives, and sources. *Journal of American College Health, 60*(3), 226–34.

Gaskins, H. R., Croix, J. A., Nakamura, N., & Nava, G. M. (2008). Impact of the intestinal microbiota on the development of mucosal defense. *Clinical Infectious Diseases, 46*(Suppl 2), S80–S86.

Gaylor, E. E. (2011, June 14)."Sleep efficacy and working memory" presented at the meeting of the Association for Sleep Societies, APSS, Minneapolis, MN.

Gaylor, E. E., Burnham, M. M., Goodlin-Jones, B. L., & Anders, T. F. (2005). A longitudinal follow-up study of young children's sleep patterns using a developmental classification system. *Behavioral Sleep Medicine, 3*, 44–61.

Geller, B., Craney, J. L., Bolhofner, K., Nickelsburg, M. J., Williams, M., & Zimerman, B. (2002). Two-year prospective follow-up of children with a prepubertal and early adolescent bipolar disorder phenotype. *American Journal of Psychiatry, 159*(6), 927–33.

Ghazavi, Z., Namnabati, M., Faghihinia, J., Mirbod, M., Ghalriz, P., Nekuie, A., & Fanian, N. (2010). Effects of massage therapy of asthmatic children on the anxiety level of mothers. *Iranian Journal of Nursing and Midwifery Research, 15*(3), 130–34.

Giannini, A. J., Nakoneczie, A. M., Melemis, S. M., Ventresco, J., & Condon, M. (2000). Magnesium oxide augmentation of verapamil maintenance therapy in mania. *Psychiatry Research, 93*(1), 83–7.

Giles, L. C., Davies, M. J., Whitrow, M. J., Warin, M. J., & Moore, V. (2011). Maternal depressive symptoms and child care during toddlerhood relate to child behavior at age 5 years. *Pediatrics, 128*(1), e78–e84.

Ginsburg, G. S., Riddle, M. A., & Davies, M. (2006). Somatic symptoms in children and adolescents with anxiety disorders. *Journal of the American Academy of Child and Adolescent Psychiatry, 45*(10), 1179–87.

Glasser, H. E., & Easley, J. (1998*). Transforming the difficult child: The nurtured heart approach.* Tucson, AZ: Center for the Difficult Child Publications.

Goldenberg, H., & Goldenberg, I. (2008). *Family therapy: An overview.* Belmont, CA: Thomson.

Golding, J., Steer, C., Emmett, P., Davis, J. M., & Hibbeln, J. R. (2009). High levels of depressive symptoms in pregnancy with low omega-3 fatty acid intake from fish. *Epidemiology, 20*(4), 598–603.

Goldstein, B. I., & Birmaher, B. (2012). Prevalence, clinical presentation and differential diagnosis of pediatric bipolar disorder. *Israel Journal of Psychiatry and Related Sciences, 49*(1), 3–14.

Goldstein, T. R., Axelson, D. A., Birmaher, B., & Brent, D. A. (2007). Dialectical behavior therapy for adolescents with bipolar disorder: A 1-year open trial. *Journal of the American Academy of Child Adolescent Psychiatry, 46*, 820–30.

Gomez-Pinilla, F. (2011). Collaborative effects of diet and exercise on cognitive enhancement. *Nutrition and Health, 20*(3–4), 165–69.

Goraya, J. S., Cruz, M., Valencia, I., Kaleyias, J., Khurana, D. S., Hardison, H. H., . . . Kothare, S. V. (2009). Sleep study abnormalities in children with attention deficit hyperactivity disorder. *Pediatric Neurology, 40*(1), 42–46.

Gordon, J. S., Staples, J. K., Blyta, A., Bytyqi, M., & Wilson, A. T. (2008). Treatment of posttraumatic stress disorder in postwar Kosovar adolescents using mind-body skills groups: A randomized controlled trial. *Journal of Clinical Psychiatry, 69*(9), 1469–76.

Gracious, B. L., Chirieac, M. C., Costescu, S., Finucane, T. L., Youngstrom, E. A., & Hibbeln, J. R. (2010). Randomized, placebo-controlled trial of flax oil in pediatric bipolar disorder. *Bipolar Disorders, 12*(2), 142–54.

"Grade-schoolers grow into sleep loss." (2000, May 1). *Science News, 157*(21), 324.

Grandin, L. D., Alloy, L. B., & Abramson, L. Y. (2006). The social Zeitgeber theory, circadian rhythms, and mood disorders: Review and evaluation. *Clinical Psychology Review, 26*(6), 679–94.

Grant, L. P., Haughton, B., & Sachan, D. S. (2004). Nutrition education is positively associated with substance abuse treatment program outcomes. *Journal of the American Dietetic Association, 104*(4), 604–10.

Greiner, C., Enss, E., & Haen, E. (2009). Drug-induced psychosis after intake of a modified-release formulation of methylphenidate. *Psychiatrische Praxis, 36*(2), 89–91.

Grissom, J. B. (2005). Physical fitness and academic achievement. *Journal of Exercise Physiology, 8*(1), 11–25.

Guzder, J., Bond, S., Rabiau, M., Zelkowitz, P., & Rohar, S. (2011). The relationship between alliance, attachment and outcome in a child multi-modal treatment population: Pilot study. *Journal of the Canadian Academy of Child and Adolescent Psychiatry, 20*(3), 196–202.

Hagerman, R. J., & Falkenstein, A. R. (1987). An association between recurrent otitis media in infancy and later hyperactivity. *Clinical Pediatrics, 26*(5), 253–57.

Haley, J. (1993). *Uncommon therapy.* New York: Norton.

Hallmayer, J., Cleveland, S., Torres, A., Phillips, J., Cohen, B., Torigoe, T., Miller, J., . . . Risch, N. (2011). Genetic heritability and shared environmental factors among twin pairs with autism. *Archives of General Psychiatry, 68*(11):1095–102.

Hammen, C., & Brennan, P. A. (2003). Severity, chronicity, and timing of maternal depression and risk for adolescent offspring diagnoses in a community sample. *Archives of General Psychiatry, 60*(3), 253–58.

Hammen, C., Shih, J., Altman, T., & Brennan, P. A. (2003). Interpersonal impairment and the prediction of depressive symptoms in adolescent children of depressed and nondepressed mothers. *Journal of American Academy of Child and Adolescent Psychiatry, 42*(5), 571–77.

Hanson, E., Kalish, L. A., Bunce, E., Curtis, C., McDaniel, S., Ware, J., & Petry, J. (2007). Use of complementary and alternative medicine among children diagnosed with autism spectrum disorder. *Journal of Autism and Developmental Disorders, 37*(4), 628–36.

Harnish, J. D., Dodge, K. A., & Valente, E. (1995). Mother-child interaction quality as a partial mediator of the roles of maternal depressive symptomatology and socioeconomic status in the development of child behavior problems. Conduct Problems Prevention Research Group. *Child Development, 66*(3), 739–53.

Harris, G. (2006, March 23). Panel advises disclosure of drugs' psychotic effects. *New York Times.*

Harvey, E. A., Metcalfe, L. A., Herbert, S. D., & Fanton, J. H. (2011). The role of family experiences and ADHD in the early development of oppositional defiant disorder. *Journal of Consulting and Clinical Psychology, 79*(6), 784–95.

Heiden, A., Frey, R., Presslich, O., Blasbichler, T., Smetana, R., & Kasper, S. (1999). Treatment of severe mania with intravenous magnesium sulphate as a supplementary therapy. *Psychiatry Research, 89*(3), 239–46.

Heijtz, R. D., Wang, S., Anuar, F., Qian, Y., Bjorkholm, B., Samuelsson, A., . . . Pettersson, S. (2011). Normal gut microbiota modulates brain development and behavior. *Proceedings of the National Academy of Sciences, 108*(7), 3047–52.

Herpertz, S. C., Mueller, B., Wenning, B., Qunaibi, M., Lichterfeld, C., & Herpertz-Dahlmann, B. (2003). Autonomic responses in boys with externalizing disorders. *Journal of Neural Transmission, 110*(10), 1181–95.

Hetrick, S., Merry, S., McKenzie, J., Sindahl, P., & Proctor, M. (2007). Selective serotonin reuptake inhibitors (SSRIs) for depressive disorders in children and adolescents. *Cochrane Database Systematic Reviews, 18*(3), CD004851.

Hill, J. (2002). Biological, psychological and social processes in the conduct disorders. *Journal of Child Psychology and Psychiatry, 43*(1), 133–64.

Hinshaw, S. P., Owens, E. B., Wells, K. C., Kraemer, H. C., Abikoff, H. B., Arnold, L. E., . . . Wigal, T. (2000). Family processes and treatment outcome in the MTA: Negative/ineffective parenting practices in relation to multimodal treatment. *Journal of Abnormal Child Psychology, 28*(6), 555–68.

Hofer, M. A. (1994). Hidden regulators in attachment, separation, and loss. *Monographs of the Society for Research in Child Development, 59*(2–3), 192–207.

Hogan, D. B. (1979). *The regulation of psychotherapists (Vol. 1)*. Cambridge, MA: Ballinger.

Honos-Webb, L. (2010). *The gift of ADHD*. Oakland, CA: New Harbinger.

Hossain, K. J., Kamal, M. M., Ahsan, M., & Islam, S. N. (2007). Serum antioxidant micromineral (Cu, Zn, Fe) status of drug dependent subjects: Influence of illicit drugs and lifestyle. *Substance Abuse, Treatment and Prevention Policy, 2*(1), 12.

Howard, M. O., Perron, B. E., Sacco, P., Ilgen, M., Vaughn, M. G., Garland, E., & Freedentahl, S. (2010). Suicide ideation and attempts among inhalant users: Results from the national epidemiologic survey on alcohol and related conditions. *Suicide and Life-Threatening Behavior, 40*(3), 276–86.

Howard, M. O., Perron, B. E., Vaughn, M. G., Bender, K. A., & Garland, E. (2010). Inhalant use, inhalant-use disorders, and antisocial behavior: Findings from the National Epidemiologic Survey on Alcohol and Related Conditions (NESARC). *Journal of Studies on Alcohol and Drugs, 71*(2), 201–9.

Hoza, B. (2007). Peer functioning in children with ADHD. *Journal of Pediatric Psychology, 32*(2), 655–63.

Hoza, B., Mrug, S., Gerdes, A. C., Hinshaw, S. P., Bukowski, W. M., Gold, J. A., Kraemer, H. C., . . . Arnold, L. E. (2005). What aspects of peer relationships are impaired in children with attention-deficit/hyperactivity disorder? *Journal of Consulting and Clinical Psychology, 73*(3), 411–23.

Hsu, C. L., Lin, C. Y., Chen, C. L., Wang, C. M., & Wong, M. K. (2009). The effects of a gluten and casein-free diet in children with autism: A case report. *Chang Gung Medical Journal, 32*(4), 459–65.

Hubner, W. D., & Kirste, T. (2001). Experience with St John's wort (hypericum perforatum) in children under 12 years with symptoms of depression and psychovegetative disturbances. *Phytotherapy Research: PTR, 15*(4), 367–70.

Hughes, A. A., Lourea-Waddell, B., & Kendall, P. C. (2008). Somatic complaints in children with anxiety disorders and their unique prediction of poorer academic performance. *Child Psychiatry and Human Development, 29*(2), 211–20.

Hurst, E., Lofthouse, N., & Arnold, E. (2010). Non-ingestible alternative and complementary treatments for ADHD. In B. Hoza & S. Evans (Eds.), *Treating attention-deficit disorder*. Kingston, NJ: Civic Research Institute.

Insel, B. J., Schaefer, C. A., McKeague, I. W., Susser, E. S., & Brown, A. S. (2008). Maternal iron deficiency and the risk of schizophrenia in offspring. *Archives of General Psychiatry, 65*(10), 1136–44.

Jacka, F. N., Kremer, P. J., Berk, M., de Silva-Sanigorki, A. M., Moodie, M., Leslie, E. R., . . . Swinburn, B. A. (2011). A prospective study of diet quality and mental health in adolescents. *PLoS, 6*(9), e24805.

Jacka, F. N., Mykletun, A., Berk, M., Bjelland, I., & Tell, G. S. (2011). The association between habitual diet quality and the common mental disorders in community-dwelling adults: The Hordaland health study. *Psychosomatic Medicine, 73*(6), 483–90.

Jacka, F. N., Overland, S., Stewart, R., Tell, G. S., Bjelland, I., & Mykletun, A. (2009). Association between magnesium intake and depression and anxiety in community-dwelling adults: The Hordaland health study. *Australian and New Zealand Journal of Psychiatry, 43*(1), 45–52.

Jacka, F. N., Pasco, J. A., Mykletun, A., Williams, L. J., Hodge, A. M., O'Reilly, S. L., . . . Berk, M. (2010). Association of Western and traditional diets with depression and anxiety in women. *American Journal of Psychiatry, 167*(3), 305–11.

Jacka, F. N., Pasco, J. A., Mykletun, A., Williams, L. J., Nicholson, G. C., Kotowicz, M. A., & Berk, M. J. (2011). Diet quality in bipolar disorder in a population-based sample of women. *Affective Disorders, 129*(1–3), 332–37.

James, A., Soler, A., & Weatherall, R. (2005). Cognitive behavioural therapy for anxiety disorders in children and adolescents. *Cochrane Database of Systematic Reviews, 4,* CD004690.

Janssen, P. A., Demorest, L. C., & Whynot, E. M. (2005). Acupuncture for substance abuse treatment in the downtown eastside of Vancouver. *Journal of Urban Health, 82*(2), 285–95.

Jensen, P. S., Arnold, L. E., Swanson, J. M., Vitiello, B., Abikoff, H. B., Greenhill, L. L., . . . Hur, K. (2007). 3-year follow-up of the NIMH MTA study. *Journal of the American Academy of Child and Adolescent Psychiatry, 46*(8), 989–1002.

Jensen, P. S., Kettle, L., Roper, M. T., Sloan, M. T., Dulcan, M. K., Hoven, C., . . . Payne, J. D. (1999). Are stimulants overprescribed? Treatment of ADHD in four

U.S. communities. *Journal of the American Academy of Child and Adolescent Psychiatry, 38*(7), 797–804.

Jones, N. A., Field, T., & Almeida, A. (2009). Right frontal EEG asymmetry and behavioral inhibition in infants of depressed mothers. *Infant Behavior and Development, 32,* 298–304.

Jones, V., & Prior, M. (1985). Motor imitation abilities and neurological signs in autistic children. *Journal of Autism and Developmental Disorders, 15*(1), 37–46.

Jorde, R., Sneve, M., Figenschau, Y., Svartberg, J., & Waterloo, K. (2008). Effects of Vitamin D supplementation on symptoms of depression in overweight and obese subjects: Randomized double blind trial. *Journal of Internal Medicine, 264*(6), 599–609.

Joseph, J. (2003). *The gene illusion: Genetic research in psychiatry and psychology under the microscope.* Herefordshire: PCCS Books.

Jung, C. (1933). *Modern man in search of a soul.* New York: Harcourt.

Jung, C. (1939). *The integration of the personality.* New York: Farrar and Rinehart.

Jung, C. (1971). *Psychological types.* Princeton, NJ: Princeton University Press. (Original work published 1921)

Kaati, G., Bygren, L. O., Pembrey, M., & Sjostrom, M. (2007). Transgenerational response to nutrition, early life circumstances and longevity. *European Journal of Human Genetics, 15*(7), 784–90.

Kahn, E. & Cohen, L. H. (1934). Organic drivenness: A brain stem syndrome and an experience with case reports. *New England Journal of Medicine, 210,* 748–756.

Kaplan, B. J., Crawford, S. G., Field, C. J., & Simpson, J. S. (2007). Vitamins, minerals, and mood. *Psychological Bulletin, 133*(5), 747–60.

Kaplan, G. A., Wilson, T. W., Cohen, R. D., Kauhanen, J., Wu, M., & Salonen, J. T. (1994). Social functioning and overall mortality: Prospective evidence from the Kuopio Ischemic heart disease risk factor study. *Epidemiology, 5*(5), 495–500.

Kaplan, H., & Sadock, B. (1985). *Comprehensive textbook of psychiatry.* Baltimore, MD: Williams and Wilkins.

Karasu, T. B. (1977). Psychotherapies: An overview. *American Journal of Psychiatry, 134*(8), 851–63.

Karasu, T. B. (1979). Toward unification of psychotherapies: A complementary model. *American Journal of Psychotherapy, 33*(4), 555–63.

Karasu, T. B. (1982). *APA Commission on psychotherapies: Psychotherapy research, methodological, and efficacy issues.* Washington, DC: APA Press.

Karasu, T. B. (1999). Spiritual psychotherapy. *American Journal of Psychotherapy, 53*(2), 145.

Karlsson, H., Blomstrom, A., Wicks, S., Yang, S., Yolken, R. H., & Dalman, C. (2012). Maternal antibodies to dietary antigens and risk for nonaffective psychosis in offspring. *American Journal of Psychiatry, 169*(6), 625–32.

Kasper, S., Volz, H. P., Moller, H. J., Dienel, A., & Kieser, M. (2008). Continuation and long-term maintenance treatment with hypericum extract WS 5570 after recovery from an acute episode of moderate depression—a double-blind, randomized, placebo-controlled long-term trial. *European Neuropsychopharmacology, 18*(11), 803–13.

Katz, M., Levine, A. A., Kol-Degani, H., & Kav-Venaki, L. (2010). A compound herbal preparation (CHP) in the treatment of children with ADHD: A randomized controlled trial. *Journal of Attention Disorders, 14*(3), 281–91.

Kaufman, S. (1995). *At home in the universe: The search for the laws of self-organization and complexity.* New York: Oxford University Press.

Kendall, P. C., Safford, S., Flannery-Schroeder, E., & Webb, A. (2004). Child anxiety treatment: Outcomes in adolescence and impact on substance use and depression at 7.4-year follow-up. *Journal of Consulting and Clinical Psychology, 72*(2), 276–87.

Kessler, R. C., Aguilar-Gaxiola, S., Alonso, J., Chatterji, S., Lee, S., Ormel, J., . . . Wang, P. S. (2009). The global burden of mental disorders: An update from the WHO world mental health (WMH) surveys. *Epidemiologia e Psichiatria Sociale, 18*(1), 23–33.

Kessler, R. C., & Walters, E. E. (1998). Epidemiology of DSM-III-R major depression and minor depression among adolescents and young adults in the national Comorbidity Survey. *Depression and Anxiety, 7*(1), 3–14.

Khan, A., Faucett, J., Lichtenberg, P., Kirsch, I., & Brown, W. A. (2012). A systematic review of comparative efficacy of treatments and controls for depression. *PLoS One, 7*(7), e41778.

Kirsch, I. (2009). *The emperor's new drugs: Exploding the antidepressant myth.* New York: Basic Books.

Kirsch, I., Deacon, B. J., Huedo-Medina, T. B., Scoboria, A., Moore, T. J., & Johnson, B. T. (2008). Initial severity and antidepressant benefits: A meta-analysis of data submitted to the Food and Drug Administration. *PLoS Medicine, 5*(2), e45.

Klingberg, T. (2010). Training and plasticity of working memory. *Trends in Cognitive Science, 14*(7), 317–24.

Klingberg, T., Fernell, E., Olesen, P. J., Johnson, M., Gustafsson, P., Dahlstrom, K., . . . Westerberg, H. (2005). Computerized training of working memory in children with ADHD—a randomized, controlled trial. *Journal of the American Academy of Child and Adolescent Psychiatry, 44*(2), 177–86.

Kobasa, S. C., Maddi, S. R., & Courington, S. (1981). Personality and constitution as mediators in the stress-illness relationship. *Journal of Health and Social Behavior, 22*(4), 368–378.

Kochupillai, V., Kumar, P., & Singh, D. (2005). Effect of rhythmic breathing (Sudarshan Kriya and Pranayam) on immune functions and tobacco addiction. *Annals of the New York Academy of Sciences, 1056,* 242–52.

Koenig, H. (2012). *Handbook of religion and health.* New York: Oxford University Press.

Konichezky, A., & Gothelf, D. (2011). Somatoform disorders in children and adolescents. *Harefuah, 150*(2), 180–84, 203.

Kopas, A. (2010). SSRI prescription rates for young people in Australia. S. Hetrick (Ed.), Pharmaceutical Benefits Division, Department of Health and Ageing. Canberra, Australia.

Koran, L. M., Aboujaoude, E., & Gamel, N. N. (2009). Double-blind study of dextro-amphetamine versus caffeine augmentation for treatment-resistant obsessive-compulsive disorder. *Journal of Clinical Psychiatry, 70*(11), 1530–35.

Korte, S. M. (2001). Corticosteroids in relation to fear, anxiety and psychopathology. *Neuroscience and Biobehavioral Reviews, 25*(2), 117–42.

Kovacs, M., & Lopez-Duran, N. L. (2010). Prodromal symptoms and atypical affectivity as predictors of major depression in juveniles: Implications for prevention. *Journal of Child Psychology and Psychiatry, 51*(4), 472–96.

Kraemer, M., Uekermann, J., Wiltfang, J., & Kis, B. (2010). Methylphenidate-induced psychosis in adult attention-deficit/hyperactivity disorder: Report of 3 new cases and review of the literature. *Clinical Neuropharmacology, 33*(4), 204–6.

Kripke, D. F., Langer, R. D., & Kline, L. E. (2012). Hypnotics' association with mortality or cancer: A matched cohort study. *BMJ Open*, 2:e000850.

Kruisdijk, F. R., Hendriksen, I. J., Tak, E. C., Beekman, A. T., & Hopman-Rock, M. (2012). Effect of running therapy on depression (EFFORT-D). Design of randomised controlled trial in adult patients [ISRCTN 1894]. *BMC Public Health, 12*, 50.

Kuo, F. E., & Taylor, A. F. (2004). A potential natural treatment for attention-deficit/hyperactivity disorder: Evidence from a national study. *American Journal of Public Health, 94*(9), 1580–86.

Kupfer, D. J. (1998). Stressful life events and social rhythm disruption in the onset of manic and depressive bipolar episodes: A preliminary investigation. *Archives of General Psychiatry, 55*(8), 702–7.

Lahey, B. B. (1990). Comparison of DSM-III and DSM-IIIR diagnosis for prepubertal children. *Journal of the American Academy of Child and Adolescent Psychiatry, 29*(4), 620–26.

Laible, D., Panfile, T., & Makariev, D. (2008). The quality and frequency of mother-toddler conflict: Links with attachment and temperament. *Child Development, 79*(2), 426–43.

Laplante, D. P., Barr, R. G., Brunet, A., Galbaud du Fort, G., Meaney, M. L., Saucier, J. F., . . . King, S. (2004). Stress during pregnancy affects general intellectual and language functioning in human toddlers. *Pediatric Research, 56*(3), 400–10.

Larson, J. M. (1992). *Seven weeks to sobriety*. New York: Random House.

Lawlor, D. A., Ronalds, G., Clark, H., Smith, G. D., & Leon, D. A. (2005). Birth weight is inversely associated with incident coronary heart disease and stroke among individuals born in the 1950s: Findings from the Aberdeen children of the 1950s prospective cohort study. *Circulation, 112*(10), 1414–18.

Lazarus, R. (1966). *Psychological stress and the coping process*. New York: Mc-Graw-Hill.

Lebowitz, E. R., Panza, K. E., Su, J., & Bloch, M. H. (2012). Family accommodation in obsessive-compulsive disorder. *Expert Review of Neurotherapeutics, 12*(2), 229–38.

Leboyer, M., Soreca, I., Scott, J., Frye, M., Henry, C., Tamouza, R., & Kupfer, D. J. (2012). Can bipolar disorder be viewed as a multi-system inflammatory disease? *Journal of Affective Disorders, 141*(1), 1–10.

Lee, E., Teschemaker, A. R., Johann-Liang, R., Bazemore, G., Yoon, M., Shim, K. S., . . . Wutoh, A. K. (2012). Off-label prescribing patterns of antidepressants in children and adolescents. *Pharmacoepidemiology and Drug Safety, 21*(2), 137–44.

Lerner, R. M. (1986). *Concepts and theories of human development* (2nd ed.). New York: Random House.

Leslie, D. L., & Rosenheck, R. (2012). Off-label use of antipsychotic medications in Medicaid. *American Journal of Managed Care, 18*(3), e109–17.

Leveille, S. G., Guralnik, J. M., Ferrucci, L., & Langlois, J. A. (1999). Aging successfully until death in old age: Opportunities for increasing active life expectancy. *American Journal of Epidemiology, 149*(7), 654–64.

Levine, M. (2006). *The price of privilege: How parental pressure and material advantage are creating a generation of disconnected and unhappy kids*. New York: HarperCollins.

Linde, K., Berner, M. M., & Kriston, L. (2008). St John's wort for major depression. *Cochrane Database of Systematic Reviews*, (4), CD000448.

Lionetti, E., Francavilla, R., Maiuri, L., Ruggieri, M., Spina, M., Pavone, P., . . . Pavone, L. (2009). Headache in pediatric patients with celiac disease and its prevalence as a diagnostic clue. *Journal of Pediatric Gastroenterology and Nutrition, 49*(2), 202–7.

Liu, Z., Li, N., & Neu, J. (2005). Tight junctions, leaky intestines, and pediatric diseases. *Acta Paediatrica, 94*(4), 386–93.

Llinás, R. (2001). *I of the vortex: From neurons to self*. Boston: MIT Press.

Loe, I. M., Balestrino, M. D., Phelps, R. A., Kurs-Lasky, M., Chaves-Gnecco, D., Paradise, J. L., & Feldman, H. M. (2008). Early histories of school-aged children with attention-deficit/hyperactivity disorder. *Child Development, 79*(6), 1853–68.

Lofthouse, N., Arnold, L. E., Hersch, S., Hurt, E., & Debeus, R. (2012). A review of neurofeedback treatment for pediatric ADHD. *Journal of Attention Issues, 16*(5), 351–72.

Lopez-Duran, N. L., Kovacs, M., & George, C. J. (2009). Hypothalamic-pituitary-adrenal axis dysregulation in depressed children and adolescents: A meta-analysis. *Psychoneuroendocrinology, 34*(9), 1272–83.

Lord, S., & Marsch, L. (2011). Emerging trends and innovations in the identification and management of drug use among adolescents and young adults. *Adolescent Medicine: State of the Art Reviews, 22*(3), 649–69, xiv.

Lu, C., Toepel, K., Irish, R., Fenske, R. A., Barr, D. B., & Bravo, R. (2006). Organic diets significantly lower children's dietary exposure to organophosphorus pesticides. *Environmental Health Perspectives, 114*(2), 260–3.

Lutz, A., Slagter, H. A., Rawlings, N. B., Francis, A. D., Greischar, L. L., & Davidson, R. J. (2009). Mental training enhances attentional stability: Neural and behavioral evidence. *Journal of Neuroscience, 29*(42), 13418–27.

Luxton, D. D., Greenburg, D., Ryan, J., Niven, A., Wheeler, G., & Mysliwiec, V. (2011). Prevalence and impact of short sleep duration in redeployed OIF soldiers. *Sleep, 34*(9), 1189–95.

Mabe, P. A., & Josephson, A. M. (2004). Child and adolescent psychopathology: Spiritual and religious perspectives. *Child and Adolescent Psychiatric Clinics of North America, 13*(1), 111–25, vii–viii.

Mahoney, D. (2011). Sleep debt takes toll on health, relationships: Insufficient shut-eye linked to ADHD symptoms, genetic risk of obesity, and marital discontent. *Clinical Psychiatry News, 40*(1).

Main, M., & Goldwyn, R. (1994). *Adult attachment rating and classification system, manual in draft: Version 6.0.* [Unpublished manuscript.] University of California at Berkeley.

Malina, R. M. (1996). Tracking of physical activity and physical fitness across the lifespan. *Research Quarterly for Exercise and Sport, 67*(3 Suppl), S48–S57.

Malkoff-Schwartz, S., Frank, E., Anderson, B., Sherrill, J. T., Siegel, L., Patterson, D., & Murck, H. (2002). Magnesium and affective disorders. *Nutritional Neuroscience, 5*(6), 375–89.

Mancebo, M. C., Garcia, A. M., Pinto, A., Freeman, J. B., Przeworski, A., Stout, R., ... Rasmussen, S. A. (2008). Juvenile-onset OCD: Clinical features in children, adolescents and adults. *Acta Psychiatrica Scandinavica, 118*(2), 149–59.

March, J., Silva, S., Petrycki, S., Curry, J., Wells, K., Fairbank, J., ... Severe, J. (2004). Fluoxetine, cognitive-behavioral therapy, and their combination for adolescents with depression: Treatment for adolescents with depression study (TADS) randomized controlled trial. *Journal of the American Medical Association, 292*(7), 807–20.

March, J. S., Silva, S., Petrycki, S., Curry, J., Wells, K., Fairbank, J., ... Severe, J. (2007). The treatment for adolescents with depression study (TADS): Long-term effectiveness and safety outcomes. *Archives of General Psychiatry, 64*(10), 1132–43.

Marco, E. M., Adriani, W., Ruocco, L. A., Canese, R., Sadile, A. G., & Laviola, G. (2011). Neurobehavioral adaptations to methylphenidate: The issue of early adolescent exposure. *Neuroscience and Biobehavioral Reviews, 35*(8), 1722–39.

Margolin, A., Kleber, H. D., & Avants, S. K. (2002). Acupuncture for the treatment of cocaine addiction: A randomized controlled trial. *Journal of the American Medical Association, 287*(1), 55–63.

Marshall, R. D., Olfson, M., Hellman, F., Blanco, C., Guardino, M., & Struening, E. L. (2001). Comorbidity, impairment, and suicidality in subthreshold PTSD. *American Journal of Psychiatry 158*(9), 1467–73.

Martin, Andres, & Volkmar, Fred R. (Eds.). (2007). *Lewis's child and adolescent psychiatry: A comprehensive textbook* (4th ed.). New York: Lippincott Williams & Wilkins.

Martinez, W., Carter, J. S., & Legato, L. J. (2011). Social competence in children with chronic illness: A meta-analytic review. *Journal of Pediatric Psychology, 36*(8), 878–90.

Maslow, A. (1993). *The farther reaches of human nature.* New York: Penguin/ Arkana.

Massat, I., & Victoor, L. (2008). Early bipolar disorder and ADHD: Differences and similarities in pre-pubertal and early adolescence. *Clinical Approaches to Bipolar Disorder, 6,* 20–28.

Mataix-Cols, D., Nakatani, E., Micali, N., & Heyman, I. (2008). Structure of obsessive-compulsive symptoms in pediatric OCD. *Journal of the American Academy of Child and Adolescent Psychiatry, 47*(7), 773–78.

May, R. (1958). *Man's search for himself.* New York: Norton.

Mayberg, H. S., Silva, J. A., Brannan, S. K., Tekell, J. L., Mahurin, R. K., McGinnis, S., . . . & Jerabek, P. A. (2002). The functional neuroanatomy of the placebo effect. *American Journal of Psychiatry, 159*(5), 728–37.

McCabe, S. E., West, B. T., Teter, C. J., Cranford, J. A., Ross-Durow, P. L., & Boyd, C. J. (2012). Adolescent nonmedical users of prescription opioids: Brief screening and substance use disorders. *Addictive Behaviors, 37*(5), 651–56.

McCann, D., Barrett, A., Cooper, A., Crumpler, D., Dalen, L., Grimshaw, K., . . . Stevenson, J. (2007). Food additives and hyperactive behaviour in 3-year-old and 8/9-year-old children in the community: A randomised, double-blinded, placebo-controlled trial. *Lancet, 370*(9598), 1560–67.

McCarty, D. (2007, May 5). Substance abuse treatment benefits and costs. Substance Abuse Policy Research Program. Retrieved from http://www.rwjf.org/en/ research-publications/find-rwjf-research/2007/05/substance-abuse-treatment-benefits-and-costs.html

McCrory, E., De Brito, S. A., & Viding, E. (2011). The impact of childhood maltreatment: A review of neurobiological and genetic factors. *Frontiers in Psychiatry/Frontiers Research Foundation, 2,* 48.

McCrory, E., De Brito, S. A., & Viding, E. (2012). The link between child abuse and psychopathology: A review of neurobiological and genetic research. *Journal of the Royal Society of Medicine, 105*(4), 151–56.

McDonagh, M. S., Christensen, V., Peterson, K., & Thakurta, S. (2007). Drug class review on pharmacologic treatments for ADHD. Portland, OR: Oregon Health and Science University. Retrieved from http://www.rx.wa.gov/documents/adhd_final_report_update3_1009.pdf

McGowan, P. O., Sasaki, A., D'Alessio, A. C., Dymov, S., Labonte, B., Szyf, M., . . . Meaney, M. J. (2009). Epigenetic regulation of the glucocorticoid receptor in human brain associates with childhood abuse. *Nature Neuroscience, 12*(3), 342–48.

McHenry, L. (2006). Ethical issues in psychopharmacology. *Journal of Medical Ethics, 32*(7), 405–10.

McNamara, R. K., Nandagopal, J. J., Strakowski, S. M., DelBello, M. P. (2010). Preventative strategies for early-onset bipolar disorder: Towards a clinical staging model. *CNS Drugs, 24*(12), 983–96.

McNeill, C. (2012, July 7). CMS survey finds suicidal thoughts, bullying, binge drinking on the rise. *Charlotte Observer.* Retrieved from charlotteobserver.com/2012/07/05/3368849/cms-survey-finds-suicidal-thoughts.html

McPheeters, M. L., Warren, Z., Sathe, N., Bruzek, J. L., Krishnaswami, S., Jerome, R. N., & Veenstra-Vanderweele, J. (2011). A systematic review of medical treatments for children with autism spectrum disorders. *Pediatrics, 127*(5), e1312–21.

Mead, G. E., Morley, W., Campbell, P., Greig, C. A., McMurdo, M., & Lawlor, D. A. (2009). Exercise for depression. *Cochrane Database of Systematic Reviews, 3,* CD004366.

Mehl-Madrona, L., Leung, B., Kennedy, C., Paul, S., & Kaplan, B. J. (2010). Micronutrients versus standard medication management in autism: A naturalistic case-control study. *Journal of Child and Adolescent Psychopharmacology, 20*(2), 95–103.

Meier, M. H., Caspi, A., Ambler, A., Harrington, H., Houts, R., Keefe, R. S., . . . Moffitt, T. E. (2012). Persistent cannabis users show neuropsychological decline from childhood to midlife. *Proceedings of the National Academy of Sciences, 109*(40), 32657–64.

Merikangas, K. R., He, J. P., Burstein, M., Swanson, S. A., Avenevoli, S., Cui, L., . . . Swendsen, J. (2010). Lifetime prevalence of mental disorders in U.S. adolescents: Results from the national comorbidity survey replication—adolescent supplement (NCS-A). *Journal of the American Academy of Child and Adolescent Psychiatry, 49*(10), 980–89.

Meyer, T. D., Koßmann-Böhm, S., & Schlottke, P. F. (2004). Do child psychiatrists in Germany diagnose bipolar disorders in children and adolescents? Results from a survey. *Bipolar Disorders, 6*(5), 426–31.

Micheva, K. D., Busse, B., Weiler, N. C., O'Rourke, N., & Smith, S. J. (2010). Single synapse analysis of a diverse synapse population: Proteomic imaging methods and markers. *Neuron, 68*(4), 639–53.

Mignot, E. (2012). Message from the director. Stanford Center for Sleep Sciences and Medicine. Retrieved from http://sleep.stanford.edu/

Miklowitz, D. J., George, E. L., Axelson, D. A., Kim, E. Y., Birmaher, B., Schneck,

C., . . . Brent, D. A. (2004). Family-focused treatment for adolescents with bipolar disorder. *Journal of Affective Disorders, 82*(suppl), S113–28.

Miller, P. (2012, January). A thing or two about twins. *National Geographic.* Retrieved from http://ngm.nationalgeographic.com/2012/01/twins/miller-text

Miller, W., & Thoresen, C. E. (2003). Spirituality, religion and health. *American Psychologist, 58*(1), 24–35.

Milne, D. B. (2000). *Lab assessment of trace elements and minerals.* Totowa, NJ: Humana Press.

Miodownik, C., Maayan, R., Ratner, Y., Lerner, V., Pintov, L., Mar, M., . . . Ritsner, M. S. (2011). Serum levels of brain-derived neurotrophic factor and cortisol to sulfate of dehydroepiandrosterone molar ratio associated with clinical response to L-theanine as augmentation of antipsychotic therapy in schizophrenia and schizoaffective disorder patients. *Clinical Neuropharmacology, 34*(4), 155–60.

Miranda, J. K., de la Osa, N., Granero, R., & Ezpeleta, L. (2011). Maternal experiences of childhood abuse and intimate partner violence: Psychopathology and functional impairment in clinical children and adolescents. *Child Abuse and Neglect, 35*(9), 700–11.

Mischel, W., Ayduk, O., Berman, M. G., Casey, B. J., Gotlib, I. H., Jonides, J., . . . Shoda, Y. (2011). "Willpower" over the life span: Decomposing self-regulation. *Social Cognitive and Affective Neuroscience, 6*(2), 252–56.

Mischel, W., Ebbesen, E. B., & Zeiss, A. R. (1972). Cognitive and attentional mechanisms in delay of gratification. *Journal of Personality and Social Psychology, 21*(2), 204–18.

Mojtabai, R., & Olfson, M. (2011). Proportion of antidepressants prescribed without a psychiatric diagnosis is growing. *Health Affairs, 30*(8), 1434–42.

Molina, B. S., Hinshaw, S. P., Swanson, J. M., Arnold, L. E., Vitiello, B., Jensen, P. S . . . . Houck, P. R. (2009). The MTA at 8 years: Prospective follow-up of children treated for combined-type ADHD in a multisite study. *Journal of the American Academy of Child and Adolescent Psychiatry, 48*(5), 484–500.

Moll, G. H., Hause, S., Ruther, E., Rothenberger, A., & Huether, G. (2001). Early methylphenidate administration to young rats causes a persistent reduction in the density of striatal dopamine transporters. *Journal of Child and Adolescent Psychopharmacology, 11*(1), 15–24.

Monteggia, L. M., Barrot, M., Powell, C. M., Berton, O., Galanis, V., Gemelli, T., . . . Nestler, E. J. (2004). Essential role of brain-derived neurotrophic factor in adult hippocampal function. *Proceedings of the National Academy of Sciences, 101*(29), 10827–32.

Montes, G., & Halterman, J. S. (2008). Association of childhood autism spectrum disorders and loss of family income. *Pediatrics, 121*(4), e821–26.

Moreno, C., Laje, G., Blanco, C., Jiang, H., Schmidt, A. B., & Olfson, M. (2007). National trends in the outpatient diagnosis and treatment of bipolar disorder in youth. *Archives of General Psychiatry, 64*, 1032–39.

Moretti, G., Pasquini, M., Mandarelli, G., Tarsitani, L., & Biondi, M. (2008). What every psychiatrist should know about PANDAS: A review. *Clinical Practice and Epidemiology in Mental Health, 4*, 13.

Morrissey, M. J., Duntley, S. P., Anch, A. M., & Nonneman, R. (2004). Active sleep and its role in the prevention of apoptosis in the developing brain. *Medical Hypotheses, 62*(6), 876–79.

M'Rabet, L., Vos, A. P., Boehm, G., & Garssen, J. (2008). Breast-feeding and its role in early development of the immune system in infants: Consequences for health later in life. *Journal of Nutrition, 138*(9), 1782S–90S.

MTA Cooperative Group. (1999). The multimodal treatment study of children with ADHD (MTA). *Archives of General Psychiatry, 56*(12), 1073–86.

Muller, S. F., & Klement, S. (2006). A combination of valerian and lemon balm is effective in the treatment of restlessness and dyssomnia in children. *Phytomedicine, 13*(6), 383–87.

Murck, H. (2002). Magnesium and affective disorders. *Nutritional Neuroscience, 5*(6), 375–89.

Murphy, P. K., & Wagner, C. L. (2008). Vitamin D and mood disorders among women: An integrative review. *Journal of Midwifery and Women's Health, 53*(5), 440–46.

National Institute on Drug Abuse. (2011). Monitoring the future survey, Overview of Findings 2011. Retrieved from http://www.drugabuse.gov/related-topics/trends-statistics/monitoring-future/overview-findings-2011

National Sleep Foundation. (2004). Survey Data. Retrieved from sleepfoundation.org/sites/default/files/FINAL%20SOF%202004.pdf

Nazrul Islam, S. K., Jahangir Hossain, K., & Ahsan, M. (2001). Serum Vitamin E, C and a status of the drug addicts undergoing detoxification: Influence of drug habit, sexual practice and lifestyle factors. *European Journal of Clinical Nutrition, 55*(11), 1022–27.

Neki, J. S. (1973). Guru-Chela Relationship: The possibility of a therapeutic paradigm. *American Journal of Orthopsychiatry, 43*(5), 755–66.

Nestadt, G., Lan, T., Samuels, J., Riddle, M., Bienvenu, O. J., 3rd, Liang, K. Y., . . . Shugart, Y. Y. (2000). Complex segregation analysis provides compelling evidence for a major gene underlying obsessive-compulsive disorder and for heterogeneity by sex. *American Journal of Human Genetics, 67*(6), 1611–16.

Niederhofer, H., & Pittschieler, K. (2006). A preliminary investigation of ADHD symptoms in persons with celiac disease. *Attention Disorders, 10*(2), 200–4.

Nierenberg, A. A., Ostacher, M. J., Calabrese, J. R., Ketter, T. A., Marangell, L. B., Miklowitz, D. J., . . . Sachs, G. S. (2006). Treatment-resistant bipolar depression: A STEP-BD equipoise randomized effectiveness trial of antidepressant augmentation with Lamotrigine, Inositol, or Risperidone. *American Journal of Psychiatry, 163*(2), 210–16.

Nierenberg, A. A., Kansky, C., Brennan, B. P., Shelton, R. C., Perlis, R., & Iosifescu, D. V. (2013, January). Mitochondrial modulators for bipolar disorder: A pathophysiologically informed paradigm for new drug development. *Australian and New Zealand Journal of Psychiatry, 47*(1), 26–42.

Nugent, N. R., Tyrka, A. R., Carpenter, L. L., & Price, L. H. (2011). Gene-environment interactions: Early life stress and risk for depressive and anxiety disorders. *Psychopharmacology, 214*(1), 175–96.

Ogata, S. N., Silk, K. R., Goodrich, S., Lohr, N. E., Westen, D., & Hill, E. M. (1990). Childhood sexual and physical abuse in adult patients with borderline personality disorder. *American Journal of Psychiatry, 147*(8), 1008–13.

Okun, M. A., August, K. J., Rook, K. S., & Newsom, J. T. (2010). Does volunteering moderate the relation between functional limitations and mortality? *Social Science and Medicine, 71*(9), 1662–68.

Olino, T. M., Lopez-Duran, N. L., Kovacs, M., George, C. J., Gentzler, A. L., & Shaw, D. S. (2009). Developmental trajectories of positive and negative affect in children at high and low familial risk for depression. *Journal of Child Psychology and Psychiatry, 52*(7), 792–99.

Olson, S. L., Bates, J. E., Sandy, J. M., & Lanthier, R. (2000). Early developmental precursors of externalizing behavior in middle childhood and adolescence. *Journal of Abnormal Child Psychology, 28*(2), 199–233.

Ornish, D. (1998). *Love and survival.* New York: Harper Collins.

Ortega, F. B., Ruiz, J. R., Castillo, M. J., & Sjostrom, M. (2007). Physical fitness in childhood and adolescence: A powerful marker of health. *International Journal of Obesity, 32*(1), 1–11.

Osler, W. (1902, September 17). Address to the Canadian Medical Association, Montreal. *Montreal Medical Journal, XXXI,* 132.

Ospina, M. B., Krebs Seida, J., Clark, B., Karkhaneh, M., Hartling, L., Tjosvold, L., . . . Smith, V. (2008). Behavioural and developmental interventions for autism spectrum disorder: A clinical systematic review. *PLoS One, 3*(11), e3755.

Page, A. N., Swannell, S., Martin, G., Hollingworth, S., Hickie, I. B., & Hall, W. D. (2009). Sociodemographic correlates of antidepressant utilization in Australia. *Medical Journal of Australia, 190*(9), 479–83.

Palatnik, A., Frolov, K., Fux, M., & Benjamin, J. (2001). Double-blind, controlled, crossover trial of inositol versus fluvoxamine for the treatment of panic disorder. *Journal of Clinical Psychopharmacology, 21*(3), 335–39.

Parfitt, G., Pavey, T., & Rowlands, A. V. (2009). Children's physical activity and psychological health: The relevance of intensity. *Acta Paediatrica, 98*(6), 1037–43.

Pargament, K. (1997). *The psychology of religion and coping: Theory, research, practice.* New York: Guilford.

Parker-Pope, T. (2012, April 22). Well, it ain't me. *New York Times Magazine.*

Parlak Gurol, A., Polat, S., & Akcay, M. N. (2010). Itching, pain, and anxiety levels are reduced with massage therapy in burned adolescents. *Journal of Burn Care and Research, 13*(3), 420–32.

Parloff, M. B., Waskow, I. E., & Wolfe, B. E. (1978). Research on therapist variables in relation to process and outcome. In S. L. Garfield and A. E. Bergin (Eds.),

Handbook of psychotherapy and behavior change: An empirical analysis (2nd ed.). New York: Wiley.

Parracho, H. M., Bingham, M. O., Gibson, G. R., & McCartney, A. L. (2005). Differences between the gut microflora of children with autistic spectrum disorders and that of healthy children. *Journal of Medical Microbiology, 54*(pt.10), 987–91.

Parry, P., & Allison, S. (2008). Paediatric bipolar disorder. *Australasian Psychiatry: Bulletin of Royal Australian and New Zealand College of Psychiatrists, 16*(4), 293.

Parry, P., Furbe, G., & Allison, S. (2009). The pediatric bipolar hypothesis: The view from Australia and New Zealand. *Child and Adolescent Mental Health 14*(3), 140–47.

Pasco, J. A., Nicholson, G. C., Williams, L. J., Jacka, F. N., Henry, M. J., Kotowicz, M. A., . . . Berk, M. (2010). Association of high-sensitivity C-reactive protein with de Novo major depression. *British Journal of Psychiatry, 197*(5), 372–77.

Paul, G. L. (1967). Strategy of outcome research in psychotherapy. *Journal of Consulting Psychology, 31*(2), 109–19.

Paulson, J. F., & Bazemore, S. D. (2010). Prenatal and postpartum depression in fathers and its association with maternal depression: A meta-analysis. *Journal of the American Medical Association, 303*, 1961–69.

Pavuluri, M. N., Birmaher, B., & Naylor, M. W. (2005). Pediatric bipolar disorder: A review of the past 10 years. *Journal of the American Academy of Child and Adolescent Psychiatry, 44*(9), 846–71.

Pediatric OCD Treatment Study (POTS) Team. (2004). Cognitive-behavior therapy, sertraline, and their combination for children and adolescents with obsessive-compulsive disorder: The pediatric OCD treatment study (POTS) randomized controlled trial. *Journal of the American Medical Association, 292*(16), 1969–76.

Peeke, S., Halliday, R., Callaway, E., Prael, R., & Reus, V. (1984). Effects of two doses of methylphenidate on verbal information processing in hyperactive children. *Journal of Clinical Psychopharmacology, 4*(2), 82–88.

Pelham, W. (2008, August). Beyond the MTA: Multimodal treatment of ADHD. Presentation at the meeting of the American Psychological Association in Boston, MA. Retrieved from http://ccf.buffalo.edu/pdf/Pelham_APA2008.pdf

Pelsser, L. M., Frankena, K., Toorman, J., Savelkoul, H. F., Dubois, A. E., Pereira, R. R., . . . Buitelaar, J. K. (2011). Effects of a restricted elimination diet on the behaviour of children with attention-deficit hyperactivity disorder (INCA Study): A randomised controlled trial. *Lancet, 377*(9764), 494–503.

Pennesi, C. M., & Klein, L. C. (2012). Effectiveness of the gluten-free, casein-free diet for children diagnosed with autism spectrum disorder: Based on parental report. *Nutritional Neuroscience, 15*(2), 85–91.

Perlis, R. H., Miyahara, S., Marangell, L. B., Wisniewski, S. R., Ostacher, M., Del-Bello, M. P., . . . Nierenberg, A. A. (2004). Long-term implications of early onset in bipolar disorder: Data from the first 1000 participants in the systematic treatment enhancement program for bipolar disorder (STEP-BD). *Biological Psychiatry, 55*(9), 875–81.

Perlmutter, S. J., Leitman, S. F., Garvey, M. A., Hamburger, S., Feldman, E., Leonard, H. L., & Swedo, S. E. (1999). Therapeutic plasma exchange and intravenous immunoglobulin for obsessive-compulsive disorder and tic disorders in childhood. *Lancet, 354*(9185), 1153–58.

Perry, B. (2006). Applying principles of neurodevelopment to clinical work and maltreated and traumatized children: The neurosequential model of therapeutics. In N. B. Webb (Ed.), *Working with traumatized youth in child welfare* (pp. 27–52). New York: Guilford.

Perry, B. D., & Pollard, R. (1998). Homeostasis, stress, trauma, and adaptation: A neurodevelopmental view of childhood trauma. *Child and Adolescent Psychiatric Clinics of North America, 7*(1), 33–51, viii.

Peterson, C., & Seligman, M. (2004). *Character strength and virtues.* New York: Oxford University Press.

Pettigrew, J. D., & Miller, S. M. (1998). A "sticky" interhemispheric switch in bipolar disorder? *Proceedings of the Royal Society of Biological Sciences, 265*(1411), 2141–48.

Pezet, A. W. (1967). *Body, mind and sugar.* New York: Holt, Rinehart and Winston.

Pfefferbaum, B., Seale, T. W., McDonald, N. B., Brandt, E. N., Jr., Rainwater, S. M., Maynard, B. T., . . . & Miller, P. D. (2000). Posttraumatic stress two years after the Oklahoma City bombing in youths geographically distant from the explosion. *Psychiatry, 63*(4), 358–70.

Pittler, M. H., & Ernst, E. (2002). Kava extract for treating anxiety. *Cochrane Database of Systematic Reviews, 2,* CD003383.

Popper, C. W. (2001). Do vitamins or minerals (apart from lithium) have mood-stabilizing effects? *Journal of Clinical Psychiatry, 62*(12), 933–35.

Porges, S. W. (1997). Emotion: An evolutionary by-product of the neural regulation of the autonomic nervous system. *Annals of the New York Academy of Sciences, 15*(807), 62–77.

Prince, R. (1972). Fundamental differences of psychoanalysis and faith healing. *Journal of American Psychoanalytic Association, 27*(Suppl.), 41–69.

PRNewswire. (2008, August 5). Raising happy kids: Survey highlights the importance of teaching children good social skills. Retrieved from http://multivu. prnewswire.com/mnr/hasbro/31656/

Prohaska, J. R. (1987). Functions of trace elements in brain metabolism. *Physiological Review, 67*(3), 858–901.

Pryor, J. H., DeAngelo, L., Palucki Blake, L., Hurtado, S., & Tran, S. (2011). The American freshman: National Norms Fall 2011. Los Angeles: Higher Education Research Institute, UCLA.

Pynnönen, P., Isometsä, E., Aronen, E., Verkasalo, M. A., Savilahti, E., & Aalberg,

V. A. (2004). Mental disorders in adolescents with celiac disease. *Psychosomatics, 45*(4), 325–35.

Pynnönen, P. A., Isometsä, E. T., Verkasalo, M. A., Kähkönen, S. A., Sipilä, I., Savilahti, E., & Aalberg, V. A. (2005). Gluten-free diet may alleviate depressive and behavioural symptoms in adolescents with celiac disease: A prospective follow-up case-series study. *BMC Psychiatry, 5*(14).

Rabkin, J. G., McElhiney, M. C., Rabkin, R., McGrath, P. J., & Ferrando, S. J. (2006). Placebo-controlled trial of dehydroepiandrosterone (DHEA) for treatment of nonmajor depression in patients with HIV/AIDS. *American Journal of Psychiatry, 163*(1), 59–66.

Radley, D. C., Finkelstein, S. N., & Stafford, R. S. (2006). Off-label prescribing among office-based physicians. *Archives of Internal Medicine, 166*(9), 1021–26.

Ramchand, R., Griffin, B. A., Harris, K. M., McCaffrey, D. F., & Morral, A. R. (2008). A prospective investigation of suicide ideation, attempts, and use of mental health service among adolescents in substance abuse treatment. *Psychology of Addictive Behaviors, 22*(4), 524–32.

Ramsawh, H. J., Chavira, D. A., & Stein, M. B. (2010). Burden of anxiety disorders in pediatric medical settings: Prevalence, phenomenology, and a research agenda. *Archives of Pediatrics and Adolescent Medicine, 164*(10), 965–72.

Rapport, M. D., Quinn, S. O., DuPaul, G. J., Quinn, E. P., & Kelly, K. L. (1989). Attention deficit disorder with hyperactivity and methylphenidate: The effects of dose and mastery level on children's learning performance. *Journal of Abnormal Child Psychology, 17*(6), 669–89.

Resnick, M. D., Bearman, P. S., Blum, R. W., Bauman, K. E., Harris, K. M., Jones, J., . . . Udry, J. R. (1997). Protecting adolescents from harm: Findings from the National Longitudinal Study on Adolescent Health. *Journal of the American Medical Association, 278*(10), 823–32.

Rethorst, C. D., Wipfli, B. M., & Landers, D. M. (2009). The antidepressive effects of exercise: A meta-analysis of randomized trials. *Sports Medicine, 39*(6), 491–511.

Rettew, D. C., Lynch, A. D., Achenbach, T. M., Dumenci, L., & Ivanova, M. Y. (2009). Meta-analyses of agreement between diagnoses made from clinical evaluations and standardized diagnostic interviews. *International Journal of Methods in Psychiatric Research, 18(*3), 169–84.

Reynolds, P., Boyd, P. T., Blacklow, R. S., Jackson, J. S., Greenberg, R. S., Austin, D. F., . . . Edwards, B. K. (1994). The relationship between social ties and survival among black and white breast cancer patients. National Cancer Institute Black/White Cancer Survival Study Group. *Cancer Epidemiology, Biomarkers and Prevention, 3*(3), 253–59.

Rice, F., Harold, G., & Thapar, A. (2002).The genetic aetiology of childhood depression: A review. *Journal of Child Psychology and Psychiatry, 43*(1), 65–79.

Rich, B. A., Brotman, M. A., Dickstein, D. P., Mitchell, D. G., Blair, R. J., & Leibenluft, E. (2010). Deficits in attention to emotional stimuli distinguish youth with severe mood dysregulation from youth with bipolar disorder. *Journal of Abnormal Child Psychology, 38*(5), 695–706.

Rich, B. A., Carver, F. W., Holroyd, T., Rosen, H. R., Mendoza, J. K., Cornwell, B. R., . . . Leibenluft, E. (2011). Different neural pathways to negative affect in youth with pediatric bipolar disorder and severe mood dysregulation. *Journal of Psychiatric Research, 45*(10), 1283–94.

Rich, B. A., Schmajuk, M., Perez-Edgar, K. E., Fox, N. A., Pine, D. S., & Leibenluft, E. (2007). Different psychophysiological and behavioral responses elicited by frustration in pediatric bipolar disorder and severe mood dysregulation. *American Journal of Psychiatry, 164*(2), 309–17.

Riggs, P. (2008). Non-medical use and abuse of commonly prescribed medications. *Current Medical Research and Opinion, 24*(3), 869–77.

Rogers, S. J., & Vismara, L. A. (2008). Evidence-based comprehensive treatments for early autism. *Journal of Clinical Child and Adolescent Psychology, 37*(1), 8–38.

Roseboom, T. J., Painter, R. C., van Abeelen, A. F., Veenendaal, M. V., & de Rooij, S. R. (2011). Hungry in the womb: What are the consequences? Lessons from the Dutch Famine. *Maturitas, 70*(2), 141–45.

Rosenhan, D. L. (1973). On being sane in insane places. *Science, 179*(70), 250–58.

Rossignol, D. A. (2009). Novel and emerging treatments for autism spectrum disorders: A systematic review. *Annals of Clinical Psychiatry, 21*(4), 213–36.

Rossignol, D. A., & Frye, R. E. (2012). A review of research trends in physiological abnormalities in autism spectrum disorders: Immune dysregulation, inflammation, oxidative stress, mitochondrial dysfunction and environmental toxicant exposures. *Molecular Psychiatry, 17*(4), 398–401.

Rothbaum, F., & Weisz, J. R. (1994). Parental caregiving and child externalizing behavior in nonclinical samples: A meta-analysis. *Psychological Bulletin, 116*(1), 55–74.

Roy-Byrne, P. P., Davidson, K. W., Kessler, R. C., Asmundson, G. J., Goodwin, R. D., Kubzansky, L., . . . Stein, M. B. (2008). Anxiety disorders and comorbid medical illness. *General Hospital Psychiatry, 30*(3), 208–25.

Rucklidge, J. J., Gately, D., & Kaplan, B. J. (2010). Database analysis of children and adolescents with bipolar disorder consuming a micronutrient formula. *BMC Psychiatry, 10,* 74.

Ruff, M., Schiffmann, E., Terranova, V., & Pert, C.B. (1985). Neuropeptides are chemoattractants for human tumor cells and monocytes: A possible mechanism for metastasis. *Clinical Immunology Immunopathology, 37*(3), 387–96.

Rush, J. (2006). STAR*D: What have we learned? *American Journal of Psychiatry, 164*(2), 201–4.

Russek, L. G., & Schwartz, G. E. (1997). Perceptions of parental caring predict health status in midlife: A 35-year follow-up of the Harvard Mastery of Stress Study. *Psychosomatic Medicine, 59*(2), 144–49.

Russek, L. G., Schwartz, G. E., Bell, I. R., & Baldwin, C. M. (1998). Positive perceptions of parental caring are associated with reduced psychiatric and somatic symptoms. *Psychosomatic Medicine, 60*(5), 654–57.

Ruttle, P. L., Shirtcliff, E. A., Serbin, L. A., Fisher, D. B., Stack, D. M., & Schwartzman, A. E. (2011). Disentangling psychobiological mechanisms underlying internalizing and externalizing behaviors in youth: Longitudinal and concurrent associations with cortisol. *Hormones and Behavior, 59*(1), 123–32.

Sacks, O. (1995). *An anthropologist on Mars.* New York: Vintage Books.

Sanchez-Villegas, A., Delgado-Rodriguez, M., Alonso, A., Schlatter, J., Lahortiga, F., Serra Majem, L., & Martinez-Gonzalez, M. A. (2009). Association of the Mediterranean dietary pattern with the incidence of depression: The Seguimiento Universidad de Navarra/University of Navarra follow-up (SUN) Cohort. *Archives of General Psychiatry, 66*(10), 1090–98.

Sandler, R. H., Finegold, S. M., Bolte, E. R., Buchanan, C. P., Maxwell, A. P., Vaisanen, M. L., . . . Wexler, H. M. (2000). Short-term benefit from oral Vancomycin treatment of regressive-onset autism. *Journal of Child Neurology, 15*(7), 429–35.

Sargent, J., Gibson, J., & Heatherton, T. (2009). Comparing the effects of entertainment media and tobacco marketing on youth smoking. *Tobacco Control, 18*(1), 47–53.

Sarris, J., Camfield, D., & Berk, M. (2012). Complementary medicine, self-help, and lifestyle interventions for obsessive compulsive disorder (OCD) and the OCD spectrum: A systematic review. *Journal of Affective Disorders, 138*(3), 213–21.

Sarris, J., LaPorte, E., & Schweitzer, I. (2011). Kava: A comprehensive review of efficacy, safety, and psychopharmacology. *Australian and New Zealand Journal of Psychiatry, 45*(1), 27–35.

Schatz, D. B., & Rostain, A. L. (2006). ADHD with comorbid anxiety: A review of the current literature. *Journal of Attentional Disorders, 10*(2), 141–49.

Schildkraut, J. J., Gordon, E. K., & Durell, J. (1965). Catecholamine metabolism in affective disorders. I. Normetanephrine and VMA excretion in depressed patients treated with Imipramine. *Journal of Psychiatric Research, 3*(4), 213–28.

Schmidt, H. D., & Duman R. S. (2010). Peripheral BDNF produces antidepressant-like effects in cellular and behavioral models. *Neuropsychopharmacology, 35*(12), 2378–91.

Schore, A. (1994). *Affect regulation and the origin of the self.* Oxford: Psychology Press.

Schultz, S. T. (2010). Does Thimerosal or other mercury exposure increase the risk for autism? A review of current literature. *Acta Neurobiologiae Experimentalis, 70*(2), 187–95.

Schwarz, A. (2012, June 9). Risky rise of the good-grade pill. *New York Times.* Retrieved from http://www.nytimes.com/2012/06/10/education/seeking-academic-edge-teenagers-abuse-stimulants.html?pagewanted=all

Scott, W. C., Kaiser, D., Othmer, S., & Sideroff, S. I. (2005). Effects of an EEG biofeedback protocol on a mixed substance abusing population. *American Journal of Drug and Alcohol Abuse, 31*(3), 455–69.

Scull, T. M., Kupersmidt, J. B., Parker, A. E., Elmore, K. C., & Benson, J. W. (2010). Adolescents' media-related cognitions and substance use in the context of parental and peer influences. *Journal of Youth and Adolescence, 39*(9), 981–98.

Seligman, M. (2007). *The optimistic child.* New York: Mariner Books.

Selye, H. (1956). *The stress of life.* New York: McGraw-Hill.

Shaffer, H. J., LaSalvia, T. A., & Stein, J. P. (1997). Comparing Hatha yoga with dynamic group psychotherapy for enhancing methadone maintenance treatment: A randomized clinical trial. *Alternative Therapies in Health and Medicine, 3*(4), 57–66.

Shannon, S. (2007). *Please don't label my child: Break the doctor-diagnosis-drug cycle and discover safe, effective choices for your child's emotional health.* New York: Rodale.

Shannon, S., Weil, A., & Kaplan, B. J. (2011). Medical decision making in integrative medicine: Safety, efficacy, and patient preference. *Alternative and Complementary Therapies, 17*(2), 84–91.

Shapiro, A. K., & Morris, L. A. (1978). The placebo effect in medical and psychological therapies. In S. L. Garfield and A. E. Bergin (Eds.), *Handbook of psychotherapy and behavior change: An empirical analysis* (2nd ed.). New York: Wiley.

Shattock, P. (2010). The ScanBrit Randomised, controlled, single-blind study of a gluten- and casein-free dietary intervention for children with autism spectrum disorders. *Nutritional Neuroscience, 13*(2), 87–100.

Shaver, P. R., & Mikulincer, M. (2002). Attachment and related psychodynamics. *Attachment and Human Development, 4*(20), 133–61.

Shaw, D. S., Owens, E. B., Giovannelli, J., & Winslow, E. B. (2001). Infant and toddler pathways leading to early externalizing disorders. *Journal of the American Academy of Child and Adolescent Psychiatry, 40*(1), 36–43.

Shaw, P., Eckstrand, K., & Sharp, W. (2007). Attention-deficit/hyperactivity disorder is characterized by a delay in cortical maturation. *Proceedings of the National Academy Sciences, 104*(49), 19649–54.

Siegel, D. J. (1999). *The developing mind: How relationships and the brain interact to shape who we are.* New York: Guilford.

Siegel, D. J., & Hartzell, M. (2003). *Parenting from the inside out.* New York: Tarcher.

Silver, R. B., Measelle, J. R., Armstrong, J. M., & Essex, M. J. (2010). The impact of parents, child care providers, teachers, and peers on early externalizing trajectories. *Journal of School Psychology, 48*(6), 555–83.

Simeon, J., Nixon, M. K., Milin, R., Jovanovic, R., & Walker, S. (2005). Open-label pilot study of St. John's wort in adolescent depression. *Journal of Child and Adolescent Psychopharmacology, 15*(2), 293–301.

Singh, M. K., DelBello, M. P., Kowatch, R. A., & Strakowski, S. M. (2008). Co-occurrence of bipolar and attention-deficit hyperactivity disorders in children. *Bipolar Disorder, 8*(7), 710–20.

Sinn, N., Milte, C., & Howe, P. R. (2010). Oiling the brain: A review of randomized controlled trials of omega-3 fatty acids in psychopathology across the lifespan. *Nutrients, 2*(2), 128–70.

Slagter, H. A., Lutz, A., Greischar, L. L., Francis, A. D., Nieuwenhuis, S., Davis, J. M., & Davidson, R. J. (2007). Mental training affects distribution of limited brain resources. *PLoS Biology, 5*(6), 138.

Slopen, N., Kubzansky, L. D., McLaughlin, K. A., & Koenen, K. C. (2012, June 21). Childhood adversity and inflammatory processes in youth: A prospective study. *Psychoneuroendocrinology* [Epub ahead of print.]

Smith, G., Jongeling, B., Hartmann, P., Russell, C., & Landau, L. (2010). Raine ADHD study: Long-term outcomes associated with stimulant medication in the treatment of ADHD in children. Government of Western Australia, Department of Health. Retrieved from http://www.health.wa.gov.au/publications/documents/MICADHD_Raine_ADHD_Study_report_022010.pdf

Smith, J. E., Lawrence, A. D., Diukova, A., Wise, R. G., & Rogers, P. J. (2011). Storm in a coffee cup: Caffeine modifies brain activation to social signals of threat. *Social Cognitive and Affective Neuroscience 7*(7), 831–840. [Epub ahead of print.]

Smith, M. D., Glass, G. V., & Miller, T. I. (1980). *The benefits of psychotherapy.* Baltimore, MD: Johns Hopkins University Press.

Snyder, H. N. (2000). Sexual assault of young children as reported to law enforcement: Victim, incident, and offender characteristics. National Center for Juvenile Justice, U.S. Department of Justice. Retrieved from http://www.bjs.ojp.usdoj.gov/content/pub/pdf/saycrle.pdf

Sorensen, H. J., Nielsen, P. R., Pedersen, C. B., & Mortensen, P. B. (2011). Association between prepartum maternal iron deficiency and offspring risk of schizophrenia: Population-based cohort study with linkage of Danish national registers. *Schizophrenia Bulletin, 37*(5), 982–87.

Spady, D. W., Schopflocher, D. P., Svenson, L. W., & Thompson, A. H. (2005). Medical and psychiatric comorbidity and health care use among children 6 to 17 years old. *Archives of Pediatrics and Adolescent Medicine, 159*(3), 231–37.

Spasov, A. A., Iezhitsa, I. N., Kharitonova, M. V., & Kravchenko, M. S. (2008). Depression-like and anxiety-related behaviour of rats fed with magnesium-deficient diet. *Zh Vyssh Nerv Deiat Im I P Pavlova, 58*(4), 476–85.

Spence, S. H., Donovan, C. L., March, S., Gamble, A., Anderson, R. E., Prosser, S., & Kenardy, J. (2011). A randomized controlled trial of online versus clinic-based cbt for adolescent anxiety. *Journal of Consulting and Clinical Psychology, 79*(5), 629–42.

Spencer, T., Biederman, J., & Wilens, T. (1999). Attention-deficit/hyperactivity disorder and comorbidity. *Pediatric Clinics of North America, 46*(5), 915–27.

Spencer, T. J., Faraone, S. V., Biederman, J., Lerner, M., Cooper, K. M., & Zimmerman, B. (2006). Does prolonged therapy with a long-acting stimulant suppress growth in children with ADHD? *Journal of the American Academy of Child and Adolescent Psychiatry, 45*(5), 527–37.

Splete, H. (2011). Low vitamin D levels tied to psychotic symptoms in teens. *Clinical Psychiatry News, 40*(4), 20.

Sroufe, L. A. (1996). *Emotional development.* New York: Cambridge University Press.

Sroufe, L. A. (2005a). Attachment and development: A prospective, longitudinal study from birth to adulthood. *Attachment and Human Development, 7*(4), 349–67.

Sroufe, L. A. (2005b). *The development of the person: The Minnesota study of risk and adaption.* New York: Guilford.

Steenari, M. R., Vuontela, V., Paavonen, E. J., Carlson, S., Fjallberg, M., & Aronen, E. (2003). Working memory and sleep in 6- to 13-year-old schoolchildren. *Journal of the American Academy of Child and Adolescent Psychiatry, 42*(1), 85–92.

Stefanatos, G. A. (2008). Regression in autistic spectrum disorders. *Neuropsychology Review, 18*(4), 305–19.

Stefansson, H., Ophoff, R. A., Steinberg, S., Andreassen, O. A., Cichon, S., Rujescu, D., ... Collier, D. A. (2009). Common variants conferring risk of schizophrenia. *Nature, 260*(7256), 744–47.

Stewart, J. C., Rand, K. L., Muldoon, M. F., & Kamarck, T. W. (2009). A prospective evaluation of the directionality of the depression-inflammation relationship. *Brain, Behavior, and Immunity, 23*(7), 936–44.

Stoll, A. L., Locke, C. A., Marangell, L. B., & Severus, W. E. (1999). Omega-3 fatty acids and bipolar disorder: A review. *Prostaglandins, Leukotrienes, and Essential Fatty Acids, 60*(5–6), 329–37.

Stoolmiller, M., Patterson, G. R., & Snyder, J. (1997). Parental discipline and child antisocial behavior: A contingency-based theory and some methodological refinements. *Psychological Inquiry, 8*(3), 223–29.

Storch, E. A., Bjorgvinsson, T., Riemann, B., Lewin, A. B., Morales, M. J., & Murphy, T. K. (2010). Factors associated with poor response in cognitive-behavioral therapy for pediatric obsessive-compulsive disorder. *Bulletin of the Menninger Clinic, 74*(2), 167–85.

Storch, E. A., Larson, M. J., Muroff, J., Caporino, N., Geller, D., Reid, J. M., . . . Murphy, T. K. (2010). Predictors of functional impairment in pediatric obsessive-compulsive disorder. *Journal of Anxiety Disorders, 24*(2), 275–83.

Storch, E. A., Lewin, A. B., Larson, M. J., Geffken, G. R., Murphy, T. K., & Geller, D. A. (2012). Depression in youth with obsessive-compulsive disorder: Clinical phenomenology and correlates. *Psychiatry Research, 196*(1), 83–89.

Strupp, H. (1970). Specific versus nonspecific factors in psychotherapy and the problem of control. *Archives of General Psychiatry, 23*(5), 393–401.

Strupp, H. (1974). On the basic ingredients of psychotherapy. *Psychotherapy and Psychosomatics, 24*(4–6), 249–60.

Strupp, H. (1975). Psychoanalysis, "focal psychotherapy," and the nature of the therapeutic influence. *Archives of General Psychiatry, 32*(1), 127–35.

Strupp, H. H. (1977). A reformulation of the dynamics of the therapist's contribution. In A. S. Gurman and A. M. Razin (Eds.), *Effective psychotherapy: A handbook of research.* New York: Pergamon.

Strupp, H. H., & Hadley, S. W. (1979). Specific vs. nonspecific factors in psychotherapy. *Archives of General Psychiatry, 36*(10), 1125–36.

Styron, W. (1992). *Darkness visible: A memoir of madness.* New York: Vintage.

Substance Abuse and Mental Health Services Administration. (2006). Results from the 2006 National Survey on Drug Use and Health: National Findings. Department of Health and Human Services: Substance Abuse and Mental Health Services Administration, Office of Applied Studies. Retrieved from http://oas.samhsa.gov/nsduh/2k6nsduh/2k6results.pdf

Substance Abuse and Mental Health Services Administration. (2008). Results from the 2008 National Survey on Drug Use and Health: National Findings. Department of Health and Human Services: Substance Abuse and Mental Health Services Administration, Office of Applied Studies. Retrieved from http://oas.samhsa.gov/nsduh/2k6nsduh/2k6results.pdf

Sung, V., Hiscock, H., Sciberras, E., & Efron, D. (2008). Sleep problems in children with attention-deficit/hyperactivity disorder: Prevalence and the effect on the child and family. *Archive of Pediatric and Adolescent Medicine, 168,* 336–42.

Surles, L. K., May, H. J., & Garry, J. P. (2002). Adderall-induced psychosis in an adolescent. *Journal of the American Board of Family Practice, 15*(6), 498–500.

Swartz, H. A., Shear, M. K., Wren, F. J., Greeno, C. G., Sales, E., Sullivan, B. K., & Ludewig, D. P. (2005). Depression and anxiety among mothers who bring their children to a pediatric mental health clinic. *Psychiatric Services, 56*(9), 1077–83.

Swedo, S. E. (1994). Sydenham's chorea: A model for childhood autoimmune neuropsychiatric disorders. *Journal of the American Medical Association, 272*(22), 1788–91.

Swedo, S. E., & Grant, P. J. (2005). Annotation: PANDAS: a model for human autoimmune disease. *Journal of Child Psychology and Psychiatry, and Allied Disciplines, 46*(3), 227–34.

Swedo, S. E., Leonard, H. L., Garvey, M., Mittleman, B., Allen, A. J., Perlmutter, S., . . . Dubbert, B. K. (1998). Pediatric autoimmune neuropsychiatric disorders associated with streptococcal infections: Clinical description of the first 50 cases. *American Journal of Psychiatry, 155*(2), 264–71.

Swek, M. (2005). The role of copper and magnesium in affective disorders. *Psychiatria Polska, 239*(5), 911–20.

Szaz, T. (1984). *The myth of mental illness*. New York: HarperCollins.

Tanner-Smith, E. E., Wilson, S. J., & Lipsey, M. W. (2012). The comparative effectiveness of outpatient treatment for adolescent substance abuse: A meta-analysis. *Journal of Substance Abuse Treatment*, doi: 10.1016/j.jsat.2012.05.006

Tasali, E., Leproult, R., Ehrmann, D. A., & Van Cauter, E. (2008). Slow-wave sleep and the risk of type 2 diabetes in humans. *Proceedings of the National Academy of Sciences of the United States of America, 105*(3), 1044–9.

Taylor, A. H., Ussher, M. H., & Faulkner, G. (2007). The acute effects of exercise on cigarette cravings, withdrawal symptoms, affect and smoking behaviour: A systematic review. *Addiction, 102*(4), 534–43.

Taylor, M. J., Wilder, H., Bhagwagar, Z., & Geddes, J. (2004). Inositol for depressive disorders. *Cochrane Database of Systematic Reviews, 2*, CD004049.

Teicher, M. H., Glod, C. A., Surrey, J., & Swett, C., Jr. (1993). Early childhood abuse and limbic system ratings in adult psychiatric outpatients *Journal of Neuropsychiatry and Clinical Neurosciences, 5*(3), 301–6.

Teschke, R., Sarris, J., & Lebot, V. (2012). Contaminant hepatotoxins as culprits for kava hepatotoxicity—fact or fiction? *Phytotherapy Research*. doi: 10.1002/ptr.4729 [Epub ahead of print.]

Thibodeau, R., Jorgensen, R. S., & Kim, S. (2006). Depression, anxiety, and resting frontal EEG asymmetry: A meta-analytic review. *Journal of Abnormal Psychology, 115*, 715–29.

Tillman, R., Geller, B., Bolhofner, K., Craney, J. L., Williams, M., & Zimerman, B. (2003). Life events in a prepubertal and early adolescent bipolar disorder phenotype compared to attention-deficit hyperactive and normal controls. *Journal of the American Academy of Child and Adolescent Psychiatry, 13*(3), 1486–93.

Tomkinson, G. R., & Olds, T. S. (2007). Secular changes in aerobic fitness test performance of Australasian children and adolescents. *Medicine and Sports Science, 50,* 168–82.

Torrey, E. F. (1992). Are we overestimating the genetic contribution to schizophrenia? *Schizophrenia Bulletin, 18*(2), 159–70.

Tough, P. (2001, Sept. 14). What if the secret to success is failure? *New York Times Magazine.*

Travis, J. (2000). Human genome work reaches milestone. *Science News, 158*(1), 4.

Tsang, H. W., Chan, E. P., & Cheung, W. M. (2008). Effects of mindful and non-mindful exercises on people with depression: A systematic review. *British Journal of Clinical Psychology, 47*(Pt 3), 303–22.

Tsapakis, E. M., Soldani, F., Tondo, L., & Baldessarini, R. J. (2008). Efficacy of antidepressants in juvenile depression: Meta-analysis. *British Journal of Psychiatry, 193*(1), 10–17.

Tseng, W. S., & McDermott, J. F. (1975). Psychotherapy, historical roots, universal elements, and cultural variations. *American Journal of Psychiatry, 132*(4), 378–84.

Turner, E. H., Matthews, A. M., Linardatos, E., Tell, R. A., & Rosenthal, R. (2008). Selective publication of antidepressant trials and its influence on apparent efficacy. *New England Journal of Medicine, 358*(3), 252–60.

Twenge, J. M., Zhang, L., & Im, C. (2004). It's beyond my control: A cross-temporal meta-analysis of increasing externality in locus of control, 1960–2002. *Personality and Social Psychology Review, 8*(3), 308–19.

Vaknin, A., Eliakim, R., Ackerman, Z., & Steiner, I. (2004). Neurological abnormalities associated with celiac disease. *Journal of Neurology, 251*(11), 1393–97.

Van der Oord, S., Prins, P. J., Oosterlaan, J., & Emmelkamp, P. M. (2008). Efficacy of methylphenidate, psychosocial treatments and their combination in school-aged children with ADHD: A meta-analysis. *Clinical Psychology Review, 28*(5), 783–800.

Van der Watt, G., Laugharne, J., & Janca, A. (2008). Complementary and alternative medicine in the treatment of anxiety and depression. *Current Opinion in Psychiatry, 21*(1), 37–42.

Van Ljzendoorn, M. (1995). Adult attachment representations. *Psychological Bulletin, 117*(3), 387–403.

Van Praag, H. M. (2004). Can stress cause depression? *Progress in Neuro-Psychopharmacology and Biological Psychiatry, 28*(5), 891–907.

Vasilev, C. A., Crowell, S. E., Beauchaine, T. P., Mead, H. K., & Gatzke-Kopp, L. M. (2009). Correspondence between physiological and self-report measures of emotion dysregulation: A longitudinal investigation of youth with and without psychopathology. *Journal of Child Psychology and Psychiatry, 50*, 1357–64.

Versino, M., Franciotta, D., Colnaghi, S., Biagi, F., Zardini, E., Corazza, G. R., . . . Cosi, V. (2009). Cerebellar signs in celiac disease. *Neurology, 72*(23), 2046–48.

Vidair, H. B., Reyes, J. A., Shen, S., Parrilla-Escobar, M. A., Heleniak, C. M., Hollin, I. L., . . . Rynn, M. A. (2011). Screening parents during child evaluations: Exploring parent and child psychopathology in the same clinic. *Journal of the American Academy of Child and Adolescent Psychiatry, 50*(5), 441–50.

Vilensky, J. A., Damasio, A. R., & Maurer, R. G. (1981). Gait disturbances in patients with autistic behavior: A preliminary study. *Archives of Neurology, 38*(10), 646–49.

Vitiello, B., Silva, S. G., Rohde, P., Kratochvil, C. J., Kennard, B. D., Reinecke, M. A. . . March, J. S. (2009). Suicidal events in the treatment for adolescents with depression study (TADS). *Journal of Clinical Psychiatry, 70*(5), 741–7.

von Bonsdorff, M. B., & Rantanen, T. (2011). Benefits of formal voluntary work among older people: A review. *Aging Clinical and Experimental Research, 23*(3), 162–69.

Wagstaff, A. J., Ormrod, D., & Spencer, C. M. (2001). Tianeptine: A review of its use in depressive disorders. *CNS Drugs, 15*(3), 231–59.

Waldron, H. B., & Turner, C. W. (2008). Evidence-based psychosocial treatments for adolescent substance abuse. *Journal of Clinical Child and Adolescent Psychology, 37*(1), 238–61.

Walsh, B. T., Seidman, S. N., Sysko, R., & Gould, M. (2002). Placebo response in studies of major depression: Variable, substantial, and growing. *Journal of the American Medical Association, 287*(14), 1840–47.

Waschbusch, D. A., Pelham, W. E., Jr., Waxmonsky, J., & Johnston, C. (2009). Are there placebo effects in the medication treatment of children with attention-deficit hyperactivity disorder? *Journal of Developmental and Behavioral Pediatrics, 30*(2), 158–68.

Wasilewska, J., Jarocka-Cyrta, E., & Kaczmarski, M. (2009). Gastrointestinal abnormalities in children with autism. *Polski Merkuriusz Lekarski: Organ Polskiego Towarzystwa Lekarskiego, 27*(157), 40–43.

Waterland, R. A., & Jirtle, R. L. (2003). Transposable elements: Targets for early nutritional effects on epigenetic gene regulation. *Molecular and Cellular Biology, 23*(15), 5293–300.

Waters, A. M., Schilpzand, E., Bell, C., Walker, L. S., & Baber, K. (2012). Functional gastrointestinal symptoms in children with anxiety disorders. *Journal of Abnormal Child Psychology, 41*(1),151–163. [Epub ahead of print].

Waters, E., Merrick, S., Treboux, D., Crowell, J., & Albersheim, L. (2000). Attachment security in infancy and early adulthood: A twenty-year longitudinal study. *Child Development, 71*(3), 684–89.

Weber, M., & Baumann, J. U. (1988). Muscle contractures of football players—relationship with knee complaints and the effect of stretching exercises. *Schweizerische Zeitschrift für Sportmedizin, 36*(4), 175–78.

Weil, A. (1983). *Health and healing*. Boston: Houghton Mifflin.

Weil, A. (1995). *Spontaneous healing*. New York: Alfred Knopf.

Weil, A. (2004). *Health and healing: The philosophy of integrative medicine and optimal health*. New York: Mariner.

Weinstock, J., Barry, D., & Petry, N. M. (2008). Exercise-related activities are associated with positive outcome in contingency management treatment for substance use disorders. *Addictive Behaviors, 33*(8), 1072–5.

Weissman, M. M., John, K., & Merikangas, K. R. (1986). Depressed parents and their children: General health, social, and psychiatric problems. *American Journal of Diseases of Children, 140*(8), 801–5.

Weissman, M. M., Pilowsky, D. J., Wickramaratne, P. J., Talati, A., Wisniewski, S. R., Fava, M., . . . Rush, A. J. (2006). Remissions in maternal depression and child psychopathology: A STAR*D-child report. *Journal of the American Medical Association, 295*(12), 1389–98.

Welch, L. (2012, May). The ADHD CEO: Karmaloop's Greg Selkoe. *Inc. Magazine*, 122.

Werner, E. E. (1992). The children of Kauai: Resiliency and recovery in adolescence and adulthood. *Journal of Adolescent Health, 13*(4), 262–68.

West, A. E., Henry, D. B., & Pavuluri, M. N. (2007). Maintenance model of integrated psychosocial treatment in pediatric bipolar disorder: A pilot feasibility study. *Journal of the American Academy of Child and Adolescent Psychiatry, 46*(2), 205–12.

West, S. A., McElroy, S. L., Strakowski, S. M., Keck, P. E., Jr., & McConville, B. J. (1995). Attention deficit hyperactivity disorder in adolescent mania. *American Journal of Psychiatry, 152*(2), 271–73.

Whitaker, R. (2002). *Mad in America: Bad science, bad medicine, and the enduring mistreatment of the mentally ill.* New York: Perseus.

Whiteley, P., Haracopos, D., Knivsberg, A. M., Reichelt, K. L., Parlar, S., Jacobsen, J., . . . Shattock, P. (2010). The ScanBrit randomised, controlled, single-blind study of a gluten- and casein-free dietary intervention for children with autism spectrum disorders. *Nutritional Neuroscience, 13*(2), 87–100.

Wilens, T. E., Biederman, J., Brown, S., Tanguay, S., Monuteaux, M. C., Blake, C., & Spencer, T. J. (2002). Psychiatric comorbidity and functioning in clinically referred preschool children and school-age youths with ADHD. *Journal of Child and Adolescent Psychiatry, 41*(3), 262–68.

Wilkinson, P. O., & Goodyer, I. M. (2011). Childhood adversity and allostatic overload of the hypothalamic-pituitary-adrenal axis: A vulnerability model for depressive disorders. *Developmental Psychopathology, 23*(4), 1017–37.

Willcutt, E. G. (2012). The prevalence of DSM-IV attention-deficit/hyperactivity disorder: A meta-analytic review. *Neurotherapeutics, 9*(3), 490–99.

Willcutt, E. G., & Pennington, B. F. (2000). Comorbidity of reading disability and attention-deficit/hyperactivity disorder: Differences by gender and subtype. *Journal of Learning Disabilities, 33*(2), 179–91.

Williams, J. K., Smith, D. C., An, H., & Hall, J. A. (2008). Clinical outcomes of traumatized youth in adolescent substance abuse treatment: A longitudinal multisite study. *Journal of Psychoactive Drugs, 40*(1), 77–84.

Williams, J. M., Barnhofer, T., Crane, C., Duggan, D. S., Shah, D., Brennan, K., . . . Russell, I. T. (2012). Pre-adult onset and patterns of suicidality in patients with a history of recurrent depression. *Journal of Affective Disorders, 138*(1–2), 173–79.

Williamson, D. E., Birmaher, B., Frank, E., Anderson, B. P., Matty, M. K., & Kupfer, D. J. (1998). Nature of life events and difficulties in depressed adolescents. *Journal of the American Academy of Child and Adolescent Psychiatry, 37*(10), 1049–57.

Williamson, D. E., Birmaher, B., Ryan, N. D., Shiffrin, T. P., Lusky, J. A., Protopapa, J., . . . Brent, D. A. (2003). The stressful life events schedule for children and adolescents: Development and validation. *Psychiatric Research, 119*(3), 225–41.

Wilson, A. C., Lengua, L. J., Meltzoff, A. N., & Smith, K. A. (2010). Parenting and temperament prior to September 11, 2001, and parenting specific to 9/11 as predictors of children's posttraumatic stress symptoms following 9/11. *Journal of Clinical Child and Adolescent Psychology, 39*(4), 445–59.

Wilson, C. R., Sherritt, L., Gates, E., & Knight, J. R. (2004). Are clinical impressions of adolescent substance use accurate? *Pediatrics, 114*(5), e536–40.

Winnicott, D. W. (1965). *Maturational processes and the facilitating environment: Studies in the theory of emotional development.* New York: International Press.

Wirz-Justice, A., Graw, P., Roosli, H., Glauser, G., & Fleischhauer, J. (1999). An open trial of light therapy in hospitalised major depression. *Journal of Affective Disorders, 52*(1–3), 291–92.

Wong, H. H., & Smith, R. G. (2006). Patterns of complementary and alternative medical therapy use in children diagnosed with autism spectrum disorders. *Journal of Autism and Developmental Disorders, 36*(7), 901–9.

Wozniak, J., Biederman, J., Kiely, K., Ablon, J. S., Faraone, S. V., Mundy, E., & Mennin, D. (1995). Mania-like symptoms suggestive of childhood-onset bipolar disorder in clinically referred children. *Journal of the American Academy of Child and Adolescent Psychiatry, 34*(7), 867–76.

Wozniak, J., Biederman, J., Mick, E., Waxmonsky, J., Hantsoo, L., Best, C. . . . Laposata, M. (2007). Omega-3 fatty acid monotherapy for pediatric bipolar disorder: A prospective open-label trial. *European Neuropsychophamacology, 17*(6–7), 440–47.

Wray, N. R., Pergadia, M. L., Blackwood, D. H., Penninx, B. W., Gordon, S. D., Nyholt, D. R., . . . Sullivan, P. F. (2012). Genome-wide association study of major depressive disorder: New results, meta-analysis, and lessons learned. Molecular *Psychiatry, 17*(1), 36–48.

Wu, J., Yeung, A. S., Schnyer, R., Wang, Y., & Mischoulon, D. (2012). Acupuncture for depression: A review of clinical applications. *Canadian Journal of Psychiatry, 57*(7), 397–405.

Wu, L. T., Woody, G. E., Yang, C., Pan, J. J., & Blazer, D. G. (2011). Racial/Ethnic variations in substance-related disorders among adolescents in the United States. *Archives of General Psychiatry, 68*(11), 1176–85.

Zelnik, N., Pacht, A., Obeid, R., & Lerner, A. (2004). Range of neurologic disorders in patients with celiac disease. *Pediatrics, 113*(6), 1672–76.

Zeman, J., Cassano, M., Perry-Parrish, C., & Stegall, S. (2006). Emotion regulation in children and adolescents. *Journal of Developmental and Behavioral Pediatrics, 27*, 155–68.

Zimmerman, M., Mattia, J. I., & Posternak, M. A. (2002). Are subjects in pharmacological treatment trials of depression representative of patients in routine clinical practice? *American Journal of Psychiatry, 159*(3), 469–73.

Zoladz, J. A., & Pilc, A. (2010). The effect of physical activity on the brain derived neurotrophic factor: From animal to human studies. *Journal of Physiology and Pharmacology, 61*(5), 533–41.

Zuvekas, S. H., & Vitiello, B. (2012). Stimulant medication use in children: A 12-year perspective. *American Journal of Psychiatry, 169*(2), 160–66.

Zwi, M., Jones, H., Thorgaard, C., York, A., & Dennis, J. A. (2011). Parent training interventions for attention deficit hyperactivity disorder (ADHD) in children aged 5 to 18 years. *Cochrane Database of Systematic Reviews, 12*, CD003018.

INDEX